Nutrition and the Developing Brain

Nutrition and the Developing Brain

Edited by

Victoria Hall Moran
Nicola M. Lowe

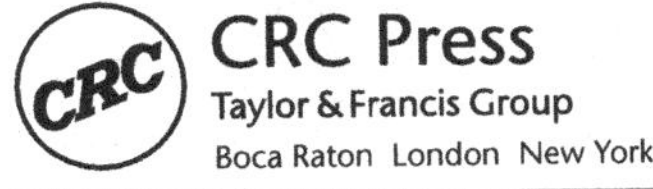
CRC Press
Taylor & Francis Group
Boca Raton London New York

CRC Press is an imprint of the
Taylor & Francis Group, an **informa** business

CRC Press
Taylor & Francis Group
6000 Broken Sound Parkway NW, Suite 300
Boca Raton, FL 33487-2742

First issued in hardback 2019

ISBN 13: 978-1-03-209775-6 (pbk)
ISBN 13: 978-1-4822-5473-0 (hbk)

Publisher's Note
The publisher has gone to great lengths to ensure the quality of this reprint but points out that some imperfections in the original copies may be apparent.

Library of Congress Cataloging-in-Publication Data

Names: Moran, Victoria Hall, editor. | Lowe, Nicola, editor.
Title: Nutrition and the developing brain / editors, Victoria Hall Moran and Nicola M. Lowe.
Other titles: Nutrition and the developing brain (Moran)
Description: Boca Raton : Taylor & Francis, 2017. | Includes bibliographical references and index.
Identifiers: LCCN 2016006498 | ISBN 9781482254730 (alk. paper)
Subjects: | MESH: Brain--growth & development | Micronutrients--metabolism | Nutrition Disorders--complications | Nutrition Disorders--prevention & control | Infant Nutritional Physiological Phenomena
Classification: LCC QP376 | NLM WL 300 | DDC 612.8/2--dc23
LC record available at http://lccn.loc.gov/2016006498

Visit the Taylor & Francis Web site at
http://www.taylorandfrancis.com

and the CRC Press Web site at
http://www.crcpress.com

Contents

Preface

Adequate nutrition for pregnant women and infants is necessary for normal brain development. Pregnancy and infancy are critical periods for the formation of the brain, laying the foundation for the development of cognitive, motor, and socio-emotional skills throughout childhood and adulthood. Evidence for the critical role of several nutrients on brain growth and development, for example, the relationship between iron and iodine deficiencies in early life and compromised cognitive and motor functions in young children, is now well established. However, more recent research has indicated that many other micronutrients, such as zinc and docosahexaenoic acid (DHA), may also play a role in early brain development. Many of these nutrients are found in high levels in the brain, particularly the hippocampus, the area of the brain involved in learning and memory.

The impact of a lack of both macro- and micronutrients during pregnancy, infancy, and childhood must be understood in the context of multiple biological and environmental influences as well as the interactions between them. For example, low-birthweight infants born into families with high socio-economic status are at a lower risk for poor developmental outcomes than those born into disadvantaged environments. Thus, protective environmental factors can, in some cases, buffer the potential negative effects of undernutrition. Conversely, undernourished children from disadvantaged homes where protective factors are lacking may show more response to nutrition (and other forms of) intervention.

This book takes a unique, integrative approach to the nutritional, environmental, and genetic influences on brain development, including evidence from both animal and human research. Issues surrounding single versus multiple limiting nutrients, critical periods of deficiency, and the impact of a child's early 'environment of relationships' on the developing brain architecture are considered.

In Chapter 1, Professor Bryan Kolb and colleagues introduce key concepts in brain development and how this process is influenced by a wide range of experiences, exhibiting a remarkable capacity for a change in plasticity. They explain that although the impact of nutrition on brain development is well established, little is known about how nutritional changes interact with the many other factors that influence brain development. In particular, we still know little about how nutrition might alter the effects of other negative early experiences such as stress, abnormal parent and peer relationships, and intestinal flora and which mechanism(s) might mediate these effects.

Jenalee Doom and Professor Michael Georgieff outline the neurodevelopmental effects of pre- and postnatal macronutrient deprivation and biological mechanisms of action in Chapter 2. The beneficial impact of macronutrient supplementation, even in the absence of specific micronutrient supplementation, is described. The authors advocate that for populations that are experiencing or are at risk for prenatal or postnatal malnutrition, macronutrient supplementation should be considered, as macronutrient deficiencies are an independent risk factor for poorer developmental outcomes. With appropriate intervention during optimal developmental periods, it has been claimed that millions of individuals who are currently experiencing macronutrient deficiencies may become closer to fulfilling their developmental potential.

Professor Lotte Lauritzen and colleagues summarize the accumulating evidence for the role of certain long-chain polyunsaturated fatty acids (LCPUFAs) in early brain development in Chapter 3. Available evidence, specifically from more recently conducted studies, suggests that docosahexaenoic acid could play a role in brain development in a sex-specific way, although presently, it is not easy to interpret whether an early DHA supply results in improved brain function or merely a change in development. It is possible that DHA may not only affect intellectual abilities as such, but rather certain basic aspects of brain function related to the way in which we interact with the world, for example, personality traits, monoaminergic-controlled emotions, or stress vulnerability, which may be linked to potential effects on attention-deficit hyperactivity disorder (ADHD)-like outcomes. More follow-up studies investigating the effect of early supplementation in later childhood and in different age groups are called for to help determine whether the effects are transient or, in fact, result in real programming effects on brain function later in life.

In Chapter 4, Dr. Stephanie Dillon and Heather Ohly describe the role of vitamins A, C, and E on the developing brain. The antioxidant effects of these vitamins become particularly important during the periods of intense growth and development where there is an increased production of reactive oxygen/nitrogen species. Studies in animals show clear, cognitive implications from deficiencies of vitamins A and C, in particular, but limited human studies restrict the ability to form firm conclusions at this point in time.

Chapter 5 describes the role of B vitamins and choline, all are essential nutrients in cell proliferation, myelination, neurotransmitter synthesis and functioning, and brain energy metabolism. There is increasing evidence that folate, thiamin, and vitamin B_{12}, in particular, influence cognitive development through two related neurochemical mechanisms involving hypomethylation and homocysteine metabolism. While most vitamin B deficiencies have become rare in high-income countries where food has been enriched with several B vitamins, recent evidence suggests that the prevalence of deficiencies in B vitamins such as thiamin and vitamin B_{12} may be common in some low-income countries. Fortification of foodstuffs with B vitamins, in addition to other key nutrients, has shown promising results for preventing deficiencies and subsequent developmental delays, but further robust research in low- and middle-income countries that evaluate the long-term impacts is needed.

In Chapter 6, Professor Harry McArdle, Professor Michael Georgieff, and Dr. William Rees examine the role that iron plays in brain development; iron metabolism is crucial for the functioning of the central nervous system (CNS). In doing so, the authors clarify how important it is for a woman to enter pregnancy with an adequate reserve of iron and they illustrate how, if this is insufficient, her developing baby is at risk for not achieving its genetic potential for brain development and function.

The impact of zinc on brain development is discussed by Dr. Andreas Grabrucker in Chapter 7. The chapter describes how embryonic brain development is particularly susceptible to changes in maternal zinc levels and that only a few days of zinc deficiency might severely affect brain development. Although animal models have shown that pre- and perinatal zinc deficiency cause deficits in activity, social behaviour, attention, learning, and memory, data on the benefits of zinc supplementation during pregnancy or infancy on child cognitive development in humans show mixed results. Problems with detection and quantification of zinc deficiency may contribute to the lack of clarity. Nevertheless, it is argued that there are sufficient data to support the clinical relevance and public health importance of zinc deficiency. The observation that mild zinc deficiency may be widespread in human populations, even among adequately nourished groups, raises questions as to how the complexities of zinc metabolism can be better understood, how biomarkers of zinc status are identified to assess populations or individuals at special risk, and how strategies such as zinc supplementation or fortification for the management and prevention of zinc deficiency can be implemented.

In Chapter 8, Professor Sheila Skeaff and Dr. Shao Zhou discuss the current knowledge describing the influence of iodine on the developing brain. The role of iodine in brain development originates from the nutrient's essentiality in thyroid hormone syntheses, which are involved in almost all aspects of brain development. The chapter describes the well-established implications of severe iodine deficiency, as well as growing evidence of the detrimental effects of less severe iodine deficiency in pregnancy on the growing brain. The authors emphasize that a lack of iodine in the diet results in a lowered cognitive capacity and therefore limits a child's future and eventually the capacity of the country. The elimination of iodine deficiency has been ranked as the world's third best economic investment highlighting the importance of nutritional strategies to strengthen human capital.

Professor Nicola Lowe describes the essential roles of copper and selenium that operate primarily as cofactors for enzymes involved in brain tissue function in Chapter 9. The prevalence of copper deficiency, in the absence of generalized malnutrition, is low, however, and potential issues relating to copper deficiency are not easily defined due to a lack of specific and sensitive indicators of copper status. In contrast, suboptimal dietary selenium intake is prevalent in some parts of the world, and the correlation between maternal selenium status, transfer to the fetus, and breast milk concentration is therefore a concern. However, it should be noted that when considering selenium supplementation, there is a relatively narrow range between deficiency, essentiality, and toxicity doses, which when coupled with the U-shaped relationship between cord selenium concentration and neonatal neurological development indicates that a cautious approach to optimizing dietary intakes is warranted.

Professor Parul Christian and Dr. Laura Murray-Kolb describe nutrient interactions and multiple micronutrient supplementation to improve brain development and functioning in Chapter 10. The chapter discusses how micronutrient deficiencies often coexist and are highly prevalent, most commonly occurring in pregnant women and young children in under-resourced settings. The effects on cognitive function by increasing supplementation with multiple micronutrients both during prenatal and postnatal periods have been examined; with some studies following children at later ages to investigate the long-term consequences of early life exposure. Although observational data linking micronutrient status in pregnancy with developmental outcomes exist, data from randomized controlled trials remain limited. The heterogeneity of interventions and assessed outcomes also make it difficult to draw clear conclusions on the benefits of micronutrient interventions at different life stages on childhood developmental outcomes. Further research is needed to elucidate which combinations of micronutrients and at what critical periods in early and later life are likely to result in beneficial outcomes of child development.

Professor Maureen Black and Jennifer Reid complete this collection with their chapter which investigates the relationship between integrated nutrition, child development, and environmental factors. The chapter explains how early brain development, when plasticity is high, form the foundations of adult health and well-being. Nutrition plays an important role throughout early brain development, and when faced with undernutrition, children may experience lasting deficits to their growth and development. The process is influenced by poverty and by opportunities for early learning and responsive caregiving. Through associations with adversity, poverty undermines brain development, potentially interfering with regulatory processes and higher-order functioning. However, the nurturance associated with breastfeeding and responsive caregiving can mitigate some of the neuropsychological effects of adversity, emphasizing the importance of interventions to children's health and well-being. In spite of the positive evaluations of the impact of early learning and responsive caregiving interventions, there are far fewer intervention options available for children and families. Future recommendations include strategies to integrate, monitor, and sustain effective interventions for infants and preschool children.

The effect of undernutrition on the developing brain of infants and young children can be devastating and enduring. It can impede behavioural and cognitive development and educability, thereby undermining future work productivity. An estimated 200 million children under 5 years old in low- and middle-income countries are at risk of failing to reach their developmental potential in cognitive, motor, and socio-emotional abilities, partly due to undernutrition. The effects of undernutrition must be understood in the context of multiple biological and environmental influences as well as the interactions between them. The chapters in this book address this issue by providing the latest knowledge from leading experts in this field, who have generously given their time and expertize to contribute to this book. We hope that readers find this collection useful and that it stimulates further discussion and research in this important, interdisciplinary field.

Victoria Hall Moran
Nicola M. Lowe
University of Central Lancashire
Preston, United Kingdom

Editors

Victoria Hall Moran, PhD, is an associate professor within the Maternal and Infant Nutrition and Nurture Unit (MAINN) at the University of Central Lancashire (UCLan). Her research has focused on the nutritional needs of pregnant and lactating women, and women's experiences with infant feeding and related support services. Recently, she became a partner in the European Commission–funded EURRECA project, a Network of Excellence established to address the variance in micronutrient recommendations across Europe. Dr. Moran's current research includes a realist evaluation of Best Beginnings resources to support breastfeeding and the RESPITE postnatal study, exploring whether different forms of pain relief in labour can influence breastfeeding and maternal and infant behaviours. Together with Professor Rafael Pérez-Escamilla of the Yale School of Public Health, she edits the international, interdisciplinary journal *Maternal and Child Nutrition* (Wiley-Blackwell).

Nicola M. Lowe, PhD, is professor of nutritional sciences at the University of Central Lancashire and co-director of the International Institute of Nutritional Sciences and Food Safety Studies. After graduating from the University of Liverpool with a PhD in trace mineral metabolism, Dr. Lowe spent 4 years as a postdoctoral research fellow at the University of California, Berkeley, where she conducted research examining the homeostatic response to dietary zinc depletion. She joined UCLan as a senior lecturer in 2000. Her primary area of research is micronutrient metabolism with a particular focus on zinc. She is currently involved in projects in Europe, the United States, and Pakistan and is chair of the Network for the Biology of Zinc (http://www.cost.eu/COST_Actions/fa/Actions/TD1304 [Zinc-Net]), a COST Action network supported by the European Commission. Dr. Lowe is the author of more than 50 peer-reviewed publications. She is a Fellow of the Association for Nutrition and a Fellow of the Higher Education Academy. She is also the research director and trustee for the Abaseen Foundation UK. This Lancashire-based charity is working alongside community members in rural villages in North West Pakistan to improve education, nutritional status, and health care provision.

Contributors

Maureen M. Black
Department of Pediatrics
University of Maryland School of Medicine
Baltimore, Maryland

and

RTI International
Research Triangle Park, North Carolina

Parul Christian
Global Development
Bill & Melinda Gates Foundation
Seattle, Washington

Camilla T. Damsgaard
Department of Nutrition, Exercise and Sports
University of Copenhagen
Copenhagen, Denmark

Stephanie A. Dillon
Division of Sport, Exercise and Nutritional Sciences
University of Central Lancashire
Preston, United Kingdom

Jenalee R. Doom
Institute of Child Development
University of Minnesota
Minneapolis, Minnesota

and

Center for Human Growth and Development
University of Michigan
Ann Arbor, Michigan

Michael K. Georgieff
School of Medicine
University of Minnesota
Minneapolis, Minnesota

Robbin Gibb
Department of Neuroscience
University of Lethbridge
Lethbridge, Alberta, Canada

Andreas M. Grabrucker
Department of Neurology
Ulm University
Ulm, Germany

Celeste Halliwell
Department of Neuroscience
University of Lethbridge
Lethbridge, Alberta, Canada

Laurine B.S. Harsløf
Department of Nutrition, Exercise and Sports
University of Copenhagen
Copenhagen, Denmark

Bryan Kolb
Department Neuroscience
University of Lethbridge
Lethbridge, Alberta, Canada

Lotte Lauritzen
Department of Nutrition, Exercise and Sports
University of Copenhagen
Copenhagen, Denmark

Harry J. McArdle
Rowett Institute of Nutrition and Health
University of Aberdeen
Aberdeen, United Kingdom

Laura E. Murray-Kolb
Department of Nutritional Sciences
The Pennsylvania State University
University Park, Pennsylvania

Heather Ohly
Maternal and Infant Nutrition
and Nurture Unit
University of Central Lancashire
Preston, United Kingdom

William D. Rees
Rowett Research Institute of Nutrition
and Health
University of Aberdeen
Aberdeen, United Kingdom

Jennifer M. Reid
University of Maryland School
of Medicine
Baltimore, Maryland

Sheila A. Skeaff
Department of Human Nutrition
University of Otago
Dunedin, New Zealand

Louise B. Sørensen
Department of Nutrition, Exercise
and Sports
University of Copenhagen
Copenhagen, Denmark

Shao J. Zhou
School of Agriculture, Food and Wine
University of Adelaide
Adelaide, Australia

1 Nutritional and Environmental Influences on Brain Development

Critical Periods of Brain Development, Pathways, and Mechanisms of Effect

Bryan Kolb, Celeste Halliwell, and Robbin Gibb

CONTENTS

1.1 INTRODUCTION

Brain and behavioural development is influenced by a wide range of factors, including nutrients. Although there is a considerable literature on the effects of early life nutrition on normal and abnormal behavioural development (e.g. Georgieff 2007; Georgieff & Rao 2001; Leung et al. 2011; Rucklidge & Kaplan 2013), far less is known about how early nutrition affects either brain plasticity or the effects of perinatal brain injury. The goal of this chapter is to introduce the reader to these issues. We begin with a brief review of brain development and plasticity, consider a model of early brain injury in rats, and then consider the role of nutrition in stimulating recovery and brain plasticity.

1.2 BRAIN DEVELOPMENT IN HUMANS AND RODENTS

Brain development is a long and complex process that can broadly be divided into two phases in mammals. The first phase is in utero and reflects a genetically determined sequence of events that are modulated by the internal maternal environment and external factors that influence this environment. The second phase of the development is largely postnatal in species such as the rat but occurs in both pre- and postnatal periods in species such as humans. This phase represents a period where the developing connectivity and organization of the brain is very sensitive to internal and external environmental stimuli.

Table 1.1 summarizes seven general stages of brain development characteristic of all mammals (for extensive reviews, see Molnar & Clowry 2012; Semple et al. 2013). The generation of neurons begins around 6 weeks after conception in humans and on embryonic (E) day 10.5–11 in rats. Neurogenesis in the cerebral cortex is largely complete in humans around 30 weeks and in rats by birth (E21–22). Neuronal migration begins after neuron generation, and in humans, it continues for about 6 weeks and in rats until about postnatal (P) day 5. Cell differentiation is essentially complete at birth in humans, although neuron maturation, which includes the growth of dendrites, axons, and synapses, goes on for years. Synapse formation in the human cerebral cortex is a daunting challenge for the brain, with a total of more than 100,000 trillion (10^{14}). This enormous number could not possibly reflect a predetermined genetic programme but rather reflects an unusual process of overproduction of both

TABLE 1.1
Stages of Brain Development

1. Cell birth (neurogenesis, gliogenesis)
2. Cell migration
3. Cell differentiation
4. Cell maturation (dendrite and axon growth)
5. Synaptogenesis (formation of synapses)
6. Cell death and synaptic pruning
7. Myelogenesis (formation of myelin)

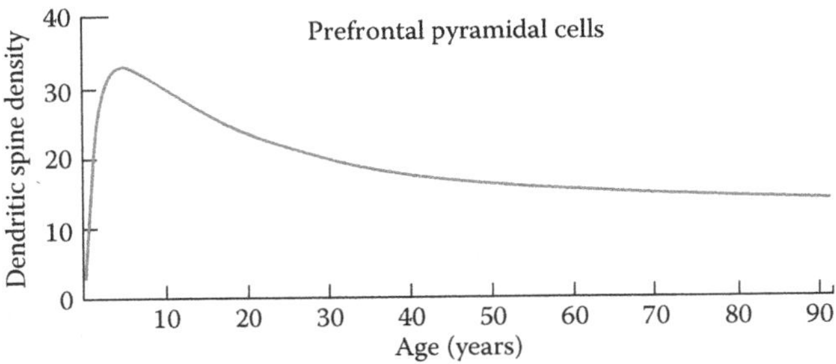

FIGURE 1.1 Spine pruning in the dorsolateral prefrontal cortex of humans. Spine density in layer III pyramidal cells reaches a peak around age 5, and then declines into the 30s, before stabilizing at adult levels. (Data from Petanjek, Z. et al., *Proc. Natl. Acad. Sci. USA*, 108, 13283, 2011, Figure 1.2b.)

neurons and synapses that are pruned back by a variety of environmental cues and signals (see Figure 1.1).

The pruning of synapses follows, beginning in the visual cortex after 1 year but not until a couple of years later in some parts of the brain such as the prefrontal cortex (e.g. Huttenlocher 1984; Petanjek et al. 2011). Cell differentiation peaks around P7–10 in rats, followed by a rapid increase in synapse production from about P10 to P30, depending upon the brain region. Synaptic pruning is not well studied in the rat, but Van Eden et al. (1990) showed a decline in cortical thickness in the prefrontal cortex from P60 to P90, and Vinish et al. (2013) showed a decrease in spine density over a similar time period in the medial prefrontal cortex (mPFC).

One surprising effect of pruning, as well as other factors, is that the cortex actually becomes measurably thinner in a caudal–rostral gradient in humans, beginning around age 2 and continuing until at least 20 years of age (e.g. O'Hare & Sowell 2008). Using structural MRI scans, Houston et al. (2014) examined the relationship between reading skill and cortical grey matter volume change in boys aged 5–15 years who received two scans about 2 years apart. The authors found an inverse correlation between improved scores on various reading-related cognitive tests and reduced volume of grey matter in the left inferior parietal cortex and left inferior frontal cortex. It appeared that children who were better readers had a different trajectory of cortical maturation than those who read less well.

One important additional aspect for understanding brain development is the effect of epigenetics, which is the heritable change in gene expression that does not result from changes in the sequence of DNA. Epigenetic mechanisms create variation in phenotypes, without altering the base-pair nucleotide sequence of the genes. Thus, the environment can allow a gene to be expressed or to be prevented from its expression. Although epigenetic mechanisms are at work throughout the lifetime, they are especially important during brain development: our early experiences induce changes in our brains that make us unique. For example, developing brains exposed to different environmental events such as sensory stimuli, stress, injury, diet, drugs, gut bacteria, peer play, and social relationships can show dramatically different phenotypes later in life. Furthermore, there is growing evidence

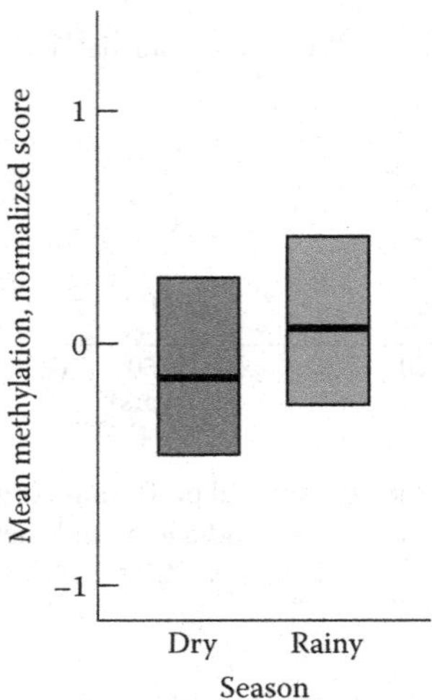

FIGURE 1.2 Diet and gene expression. The diets of women in rural Gambia vary with the season. Babies conceived in the rainy season show significantly higher gene methylation (fewer genes expressed) compared with babies conceived in the dry season. The dark horizontal bar represents the median and the box is the range. (Data from Dominguez-Salas et al. 2014, Figure 1.3b.)

that epigenetic changes can cross generations. One especially powerful influence is gestational stress, which affects not only epigenetics and behaviour in the offspring but also their offspring (see the review by Babenko et al. 2015).

A maternal diet during gestation has long been known to alter the offspring's brain development and later behaviour, but the mechanisms are only beginning to be examined. For example, Dominguez-Salas et al. (2014) showed that maternal diet at conception significantly altered gene methylation in newborns (i.e. gene methylation is a measure of epigenetic change). The researchers studied infants in rural Gambia who had been conceived in either the dry season or the rainy season. Gambians' diets are dramatically different during these two seasons and so was gene methylation in the infants' blood (see Figure 1.2). The level of gene methylation reflects the number of genes expressed. Increased gene methylation, for instance, means that fewer genes are expressed, and thus, the body and brain will develop differently.

1.3 SPECIAL FEATURES OF BRAIN DEVELOPMENT

Two features of brain development are especially important in understanding how experiences can modify cerebral organization: stem cells and plasticity.

1.3.1 Stem Cells

The cells residing in the subgranular zone (SGZ) in the hippocampus are stem cells that remain active throughout life, producing neurons and astrocytes at a fairly stable rate, although there is a decline with senescence. The cells lining the subventricular zone (SVZ) lying below the neocortex can produce neural or glial progenitor cells that are capable of migrating into the white or grey matter throughout life. These cells remain quiescent for extended periods of time, however, and their role remains poorly understood, but their generation is influenced by many factors including experience, drugs, hormones, and injury.

1.3.2 Plasticity

Brain plasticity refers to the capacity of the brain to change its structure and ultimately its function (e.g. Kolb 1995). Changes in the brain can be shown at many levels of analysis ranging from molecules to behaviour. One advantage of using laboratory animals is that it is possible to measure anatomical and molecular changes in post-mortem tissue of animals with different experiences and to correlate these changes with behaviour.

Three types of plasticity can be distinguished in the normal developing brain: experience-independent, experience-expectant, and experience-dependent plasticity (Greenough et al. 1987; Shatz 1992). *Experience-independent* plasticity is largely a prenatal developmental process. It is impractical for the genome to specify the connectivity of every connection in neuron development. Instead, the brain produces a rough structure in which there is an overproduction of neurons and, later, connections, which are sculpted in response to internal and external events. A good example is the development of the eye-specific layers of the lateral geniculate nucleus (LGN) of the cat (Campbell & Shatz 1992). The mature LGN has several layers that receive specific connections from each eye. To segregate the layers correctly, the retinal ganglion cells spontaneously fire so as to correlate their firing with nearby cells in the same eye but independent of those in the other eye. Cells which are active together increase their connections, whereas those out of synch weaken their connections and eventually die out. Experience-independent plasticity allows the nervous system more precision in connectivity without requiring overwhelmingly complex genetic instructions.

Experience-expectant plasticity largely occurs during development, often during sensitive periods. For example, the human brain expects to hear speech sounds, but it typically hears only those of one or two languages. Because different languages are composed of language-specific sounds, the early exposure to these sounds activates certain groups of neurons, which are sustained by the activity, whereas other sounds are not encountered, and the ability to distinguish them is reduced. Later in life, it becomes difficult to learn to distinguish certain sounds in other languages, even though all babies can do so, leading sometimes to strong accents in adults learning new languages.

Finally, *experience-dependent* plasticity refers to a process of changing neuronal ensembles that are growing or already present. This can be seen in situations such as when animals learn problems (e.g. Comeau et al. 2010; Greenough & Chang 1989), when animals receive intense environmental manipulations (e.g. Greenough & Chang 1989), have brain injury (e.g. Kolb et al. 2013), or response to psychoactive drugs (e.g. Robinson & Kolb 2004). These types of experiences can both increase and decrease synapse numbers concurrently but in different regions in the same animals.

Although experience-dependent plasticity occurs throughout the lifespan, it occurs extensively during development and will influence both how a brain responds to injury and post-injury interventions.

Two features of brain plasticity are especially important in the current context. First, plastic changes are age-dependent. It is generally expected that the developing brain will be more responsive to experiences than the adult or senescent brain, and this is true. One unexpected age-related effect, however, is that there are qualitatively different plastic changes in the brain at different ages. One of the most powerful ways to change the brain of the laboratory rat is to place it in a complex environment which provides extensive social interaction and activity. Rats placed in such environments as adults show a widespread *increase* in spine density, reflecting an increase in excitatory synapses. In contrast, rats placed in the same environments as juveniles show a *decrease* in spine density, although the cells remain the same size (Kolb et al. 2003). Importantly, both groups of stimulated animals show similar enhanced cognitive and motor capacities. A parallel example comes from the effects of nicotine. When administered in adulthood, nicotine increased spine density in the medial frontal cortex, but when administered prenatally, it decreased spine density (Brown & Kolb 2001; Mychasiuk et al. 2013a). A final example can be seen in the effects of early cortical injury. In rats, injury in the first few days of life drastically reduced neuronal complexity and spine density in the cortex, whereas a similar injury in the second week of life produced the opposite effect (e.g. Kolb & Gibb 2007 review). In this case, the changes in spine density are correlated with a dismal behavioural outcome in adulthood following the early injury but a much better recovery and increased spine density after the later one.

Second, experience-dependent effects interact with one another. As we travel through life, we have hundreds of thousands of experiences, and these experiences interact to influence later plastic changes. For example, play behaviour in juvenile rats acts to increase the pruning of neurons in the medial prefrontal cortex (Bell et al. 2010). This pruning acts to alter the effect of nicotine given later in adolescence (Himmler et al. 2013). Similarly, if rats are exposed to nicotine prenatally, there is a change in the pattern of experience-dependent changes related to complex housing (Mychasiuk et al. 2014b). Thus, as we consider the effects of nutrients on brain plasticity, we need to be wary not only of the possibility of age-dependent effects but also of the interaction between early experiences, including nutrition. One possible example might be the effect of gestational stress on the effect of specific diets later in the development.

1.4 FACTORS INFLUENCING BRAIN DEVELOPMENT IN THE NORMAL BRAIN

Brain development is sculpted not only by the emergence of brain structures but also by each individual's environments and experiences. Each type of experience has a unique way of influencing brain organization and behaviour. We consider here a range of factors that both change brain development on their own and in combination with one another (see Table 1.2).

TABLE 1.2
Factors Affecting Brain Development

1. Sensory and motor experiences (complex housing, tactile stimulation)
2. Psychoactive drugs
3. Gonadal hormones
4. Parent–child relationships
5. Peer relationships
6. Early stress
7. Intestinal flora
8. Diet

1.4.1 Sensory and Motor Experiences

Research on experience-dependent effects in brain development began with researchers placing animals in severely impoverished conditions, such as being raised in the dark (e.g. Reisen 1961). Such extreme experiences certainly disrupted development but were not 'normal' in any real sense of the word. By the 1970s, it had become clear that a wide range of less drastic, and sometimes seemingly innocuous, experiences could also produce large changes in the brain.

As noted earlier, placing animals in complex environments with many social and sensorimotor experiences changes not only spine density, but it also changes brain size, cortical thickness, neuron size, dendritic branching and length, glial numbers and complexity, the expression of neurotransmitters and growth factors, and vascular arborization (e.g. Greenough & Chang 1989; Sirevaag & Greenough 1988). More recently, there is evidence that the effects of complex housing can cross generations. For example, Gibb et al. (2014) showed that if pregnant rats are housed in complex environments until their pups are born, there is an increase in dendritic spines in the cortex of adult offspring. In a parallel study, Mychasiuk et al. (2012) showed that the weanling offspring also show a significant (4%) drop in global methylation from maternal (gestational) complex housing. Although this does not sound like a large change, it would mean that over 800 genes were being expressed in the cortex of the animals that experienced 'gestational complex housing'. The same authors also placed male rats in complex environments for 28 days before mating with control females and once again found an effect on the offspring's brains – the epigenetic effect being nearly identical to that observed in the maternal housing study.

One especially powerful sensory experience in the development is touch. Schanberg & Field (1987) showed that tactile stimulation of preterm infants accelerated growth, leading to an earlier release from the hospital. Further studies have shown serum changes in neurotrophic factors and accelerated neurophysiological maturation under the same conditions (Field et al. 2008; Guzzetta et al. 2009). Parallel studies in rats have also shown persisting changes in the brain and behaviour of adult animals receiving tactile stimulation for 15 min three times per day from birth until weaning (e.g. Richards et al. 2012).

The actual mechanism of the effect of tactile stimulation is not known, although it has been shown that tactile stimulation increases the production of a neurotrophic factor (fibroblast growth factor-2 or FGF-2) in the skin and FGF-2 has receptors in the brain (Gibb et al. 2016). We have previously found that FGF-2 influences brain development, and experiences such as complex housing increased the expression of FGF-2 in the brain, suggesting that FGF-2 is an important component of experience-dependent neural plasticity (Kolb et al. 1998a).

1.4.2 Psychoactive Drugs

It is likely that all psychoactive drugs, including prescription drugs, change the structure of the brain. For example, the exposure of adults to psychomotor stimulants, opioids, marijuana, or phencyclidine all chronically changes the synaptic organization of the prefrontal cortex and nucleus accumbens (e.g. Robinson & Kolb 2004), and these changes are correlated with changes in gene expression in the prefrontal cortex and hippocampus (Mychasiuk et al. 2013b). There is now evidence that prenatal exposure to psychoactive drugs, including amphetamine, nicotine, diazepam, valproic acid, fluoxetine, morphine, and of course alcohol, produce parallel changes (e.g. Muhammad et al. 2013; Mychasiuk et al. 2013a). Similarly, administration of amphetamine, methylphenidate, haloperidol, and olanzapine in the juvenile period also leads to impaired behaviour and dendritic changes in adulthood (e.g. Diaz Heijtz et al. 2003; Frost et al. 2010).

One important aspect of perinatal drug exposure is that the brain's response to other experiences is altered. For example, if rats receive nicotine prenatally, the response to complex housing in adulthood is altered (Mychasiuk et al. 2014b), and this is reflected in the effect of later training on cognitive tasks (Muhammad et al. 2013). It would be interesting to see how early nutrition might modulate these drug effects.

1.4.3 Stress

Stress has significant effects on the brain throughout the life course (e.g. McEwen & Morrison 2013). Until recently, most of the research focused on stress in adulthood, but there is a rapidly growing literature on the effects of gestational and early life stress. For example, prenatal stress is now known to be a risk factor in the development of disorders such as schizophrenia, depression, drug addiction, and attention-deficit hyperactivity disorder (ADHD) (e.g. Anda et al. 2006; van den Bergh & Marcoen 2004). Studies with laboratory animals have shown that perinatal stress produces a wide range of behavioural changes when measured in adulthood, including impaired learning and memory, high anxiety, altered social behaviour, and a preference for alcohol (e.g. review by Weinstock 2008). These behavioural changes are correlated with synaptic changes in many cerebral structures including the prefrontal cortex, hippocampus, and amygdala (e.g. Muhammad & Kolb 2011a, 2011b; Murmu et al. 2006).

The effects of gestational stress can also be indirect. Mychasiuk et al. (2011, 2012) and housed pregnant females together for the duration of their pregnancies. One rat was removed daily for 20 min for exposure to a moderate stressor during embryonic days 12–16. The other dam (the bystander) was left alone. Both sets of offspring showed significant changes in gene expression and dendritic organization, compared to the offspring of unstressed mothers, although the effects were different in the directly stressed and bystander-stressed offspring. We are currently examining the effects of bystander stress when the father is removed daily and exposed to the same stress paradigm, which would be somewhat more likely to be an ecological scenario in humans.

1.4.4 Peer Relationships

Play behaviour has a powerful influence on brain development (e.g. Pellis & Pellis 2010). The prefrontal cortex is critical for the control of play behaviour, and prefrontal development is strongly influenced by play. One example is that play behaviour promotes the pruning of the medial prefrontal cortex of rats (Bell et al. 2010), and this pruning appears to alter the response of this region to nicotine in adolescence (Himmler et al. 2013). Furthermore, perinatal experiences including prenatal stress and tactile stimulation have been found to alter play behaviour and prefrontal organization (e.g. Muhammad et al. 2011b). These experiences also include feeding young animals a vitamin/mineral-supplemented diet (Halliwell 2011). We return to this finding later.

1.4.5 Parent–Child Relationships

Mammals are born in various states of helplessness, but all are immature and require parental care, sometimes for extended periods. There is little doubt that parent–child relationships have a profound effect on the development of both brain and behaviour (e.g. Myers et al. 1989). There have been extensive studies of mother–infant interactions in rodents where aspects of mothering, such as contact time, correlate with a range of behavioural and somatic outcomes. Meany and his colleagues have done extensive studies showing that maternal–infant interactions modulate changes in the hypothalamic–pituitary–adrenal (HPA) stress response, gene expression in the hippocampus, and changes in emotional and cognitive behaviours (e.g. Cameron et al. 2005; Weaver et al. 2006). Other studies which have followed a similar experimental paradigm have also shown changes in the hypothalamus, amygdala (Fenoglio et al. 2006), and the prefrontal cortex (Muhammad & Kolb 2011a,b).

1.4.6 Intestinal Flora

We have emphasized factors that affect the central nervous system directly, but there is a less direct route via the enteric nervous system (ENS), which is a mesh of neurons embedded in the lining of the gut. The ENS is sometimes considered a part of the autonomic nervous system, but it largely functions independently. Digestion is complicated, and evolution has provided a dedicated nervous system to control it. The ENS is estimated to have 200–500 million neurons (about the same as the spinal cord) and is sometimes referred to as the 'second brain' because of the diversity of neuron types, large number of glial cells, and complex integrated circuits it contains. The ENS functions to control bowel motility, secretion, and blood flow to permit fluid and nutrient absorption and support waste elimination (see Avetisyan et al. 2015). The ENS sends information to the brain that affects our mental state and the brain can act to modify the gut function.

An important component of the ENS is that it interacts with the bacteria in the gut, known collectively as the microbiome. About 10^{14} microbiota populate the adult gut, which means that microbiota outnumber the host cells by a factor of 10 (Farmer et al. 2014). The microbiota influence the absorption of nutrients and are a source of neurochemicals that regulate an array of physiological and psychological processes. This influence can be innervation of the vagus nerve or through the bloodstream independent of the vagus nerve. The ENS and microbiome are clearly important in our understanding of how nutrients are extracted from food and how they can influence brain and behavioural functions.

Although the gut has no microbiota before birth, it is populated from the mother from both vaginal and anal fluids as well as the skin (especially breast) after birth. It has been suggested that many neurodevelopmental disorders, including autism, may be related to microbial infections early in life (e.g. Finegold et al. 2002; Kohane et al. 2012). Hsiao et al. (2013) studied a mouse model which is known to display features of autism spectral disorder. These mice have a very low production of social auditory vocalizations which measure about 1/3 of the normal levels. Manipulation of the gut bacteria towards strain typical levels restored the vocalizations to normal, thus demonstrating that gut bacteria can alter behaviour.

1.4.7 Early Brain Injury

The most common cause of early brain injury in humans is hypoxic–ischemic encephalopathy (HIE), which is a condition that results from brain not receiving enough oxygen during birthing. Because birth is a traumatic event for the brain, it is quite possible for the brain to be injured or deprived of oxygen. The brain damage in HIE tends to be diffuse, often affecting the white matter more severely than the grey matter, and it is estimated that HIE accounts for 25% of developmental disabilities in children. Another common form of early brain injury in children is traumatic brain injury (TBI), which is estimated to affect about 0.5 million children from 0 to 14 years per year in the United States alone. Children also receive neurosurgery for various reasons, especially as a treatment for uncontrolled epilepsy, which usually requires the removal of the abnormal brain tissue. Although it was once believed that infants and children could recover better than adults with similar injuries (the so-called Kennard principle), it is now clear that the developing brain responds differently to injury than the adult brain. It is also clear that there are especially sensitive periods during the development when functional outcome from an injury incurred during the early years may be worse or better than from a similar injury incurred in adulthood (e.g. Crowe et al. 2015; Kolb et al. 2013).

Rodent models of early brain injury are often used to investigate the processes which regulate functional outcomes and to identify the underlying plastic mechanisms which may provide insight into therapies. HIE models typically study animals with ischemia at about 7 days of age, which is usually taken as developmentally equivalent to birth in humans (e.g. Yager & Ashwal 2009). It is possible to inflict HIE as early as postnatal day 3 (P3), which would mimic HIE in premature humans, although there are few such studies (but see Williams 2009). TBI is difficult to mimic in young animals, although recent studies have been promising (e.g. Mychasiuk et al. 2014a). Over the past 40 years, we have developed a focal model of early brain injury that has advantages over animal models of HIE (e.g. Kolb & Gibb 2007; Kolb & Whishaw 1989). For example, it is possible to make more precise localized injuries than those seen in HIE or TBI. This makes comparison across different ages easier because the location and extent of the injuries are more consistent. In addition, there can be more white matter inclusion than in other models. And it is possible to make prenatal injuries in rodents, thus mimicking earlier injury seen in very premature infants (e.g. Kolb et al. 1998b). We have demonstrated that in both rats and mice, damage on postnatal days 1–5 can have devastating consequences on behaviour, depending upon the extent of injury and regardless of which cerebral region is injured. In contrast, similar damage on days 7–12 permits a much better functional outcome, and depending upon the behavioural measure, there can be surprisingly normal behavioural outcomes, despite the fact that the brain is significantly smaller than in normal control animals. The better functional outcomes at P7–12 are correlated with dendritic sprouting, increased astrocyte formation, and, in special circumstances, neurogenesis that fills in the injured regions (e.g. Kolb et al. 1998c). Furthermore, we have been able to show that a wide range of pre- and post-injury experiences can influence both the behavioural outcomes and corresponding compensatory neural changes, including pre- and postnatal tactile stimulation, pre- and postnatal complex housing, gestational stress, administration of growth factors such as FGF-2, depletion of noradrenalin, gonadal hormones, and diets (for a review, see Kolb et al. 2013).

There are also some disadvantages to our focal model too. In particular, it does not mimic the more common HIE injuries found in human infants. We do not see this as a particular problem, however, because our model provides suggestions of possible rehabilitation treatments that can be applied to infants (or rodents) with HIE injuries. We have shown that treatments such as nicotine and FGF-2 stimulate recovery from P3 to P5 suction lesions (see the review by Kolb et al. 2013), and both of these treatments are also effective after P7 HIE (Williams 2009).

1.4.8 Nutrition and Brain Development

There is a large amount of literature showing that nutrients influence brain development when administered beginning in the first day of the postnatal period and continuing into adulthood, so we will not try to summarize it here. The role of nutrients has largely been studied by examining the effects of nutrient deficiencies (see the review by Georgieff 2007), particularly related to protein energy, iron, zinc, copper, and choline. Such nutritional deficiencies can have global effects on the developing brain or brain circuit–specific effects, depending upon the precise timing of the nutrient deficit. It is reasonable to suspect that brain development might be enhanced by vitamin and/or mineral supplements, although this is somewhat harder to demonstrate than the effects of deficiencies, owing to ceiling effects in many behavioural tasks. Dietary choline supplementation during the perinatal period leads to enhanced spatial memory in various spatial navigation tasks (e.g. Meck & Williams 2003; Tees & Mohammadi 1999), which correlated with increased levels of nerve growth factor in the hippocampus and neocortex (e.g. Sandstrom et al. 2002). Although these studies did not have a direct measure of neuroplastic changes underlying the effects of choline, we can infer that there would have been neuroplastic changes that mediated the behavioural changes. Indeed, to date, there has been little research on the effects of nutrient-supplemented diets on synaptic organization of otherwise healthy infants.

Although the study of deficiencies in, or supplements of, single nutrients is important, there is growing interest in the idea that a combination of nutrients should work synergistically for an optimal metabolic activity (e.g. Leung et al. 2011; Rucklidge et al. 2013). It should also be noted that the metabolism and biochemistry of macronutrients (protein, carbohydrates, and fats) and micronutrients (vitamins and minerals) are generally engaged within various biochemical pathways with the aid of enzymes and cofactors. Because the body requires all nutrients, supplementation of only one large dose could skew affiliated biochemical cascades. Conversely, supplementation of a spectrum of nutrients that are required in a number of biochemical pathways will propagate a cascade of reactions and promote more activity in biochemical systems that support physiological systems. In the brain, the increases in physiology and metabolic activity would engage the neural activity which in turn increases trophic factor production which is necessary for neuroplasticity and could contribute to neurogenesis.

With this in mind, we have administered a broad mixture of vitamins and minerals by enriching the usual diet of rats with a product called EmpowerPlus™. This product is a blend of 36 vitamins, minerals, and antioxidants and includes a proprietary blend of herbal supplements such as gingko biloba and amino acid precursors for neurotransmitters; choline, phenylalanine, glutamine, and methionine. The minerals in this formula are also chelated to increase absorption and utilization for efficacy. It should also be noted that glutamine contributes to repair function in the gastrointestinal tract, thereby enabling greater nutrient absorption (Gropper & Smith 2012).

EmpowerPlus has been studied extensively for its effects on a wide range of behavioural problems (e.g. Simpson et al. 2011). Rats fed this diet either in adulthood or during the development showed significant increases in dendritic length in pyramidal neurons in the parietal cortex, as illustrated in Figure 1.3 (Halliwell 2011; Silasi 2005). Unfortunately, animals which had stroke showed no advantage on cognitive and motor tests. The likely problem is that the tests used were likely not sensitive enough as they were designed to show deficits, not improvements, in performance. It is also possible that rats were not fed the supplemented diet long enough. This led us to take a different approach, which was to examine whether nutrients might enhance brain development after perinatal injury (see the following text).

1.5 NUTRITION AND EARLY BRAIN INJURY

It is generally presumed that the body heals better when it is given good nutrition, so it is reasonable to predict that recovery from early brain perturbations might be facilitated by nutritional supplements. For example, there is growing interest in using nutrition as a treatment after preterm birth, with a special emphasis on nutritional components that might positively influence the gut microbiome (e.g.

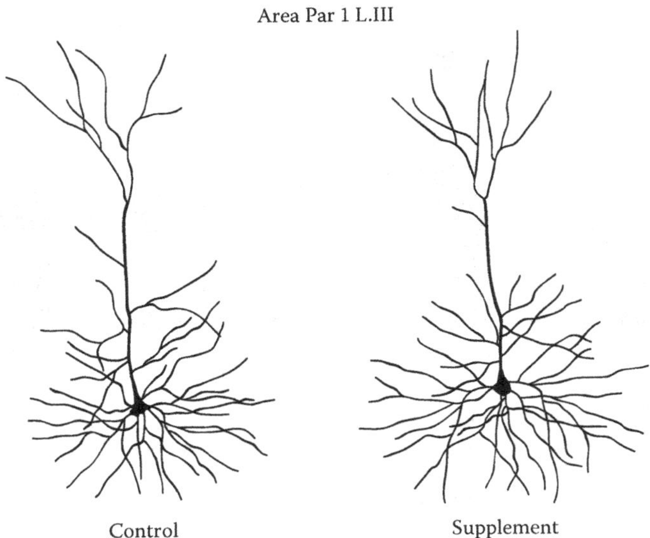

FIGURE 1.3 Examples of layer III pyramidal neurons from the parietal cortex of a rat. The cell on the right is from an adult animal given a vitamin/mineral supplement from conception until weaning. There is about a 15% increase in the dendritic length in the neuron from the supplement-treated animal.

Keunen et al. 2015). The possibility that diet might be important for stimulating recovery after early cortical injury is further supported in a study by Dabydeen et al. (2008). Human neonates with perinatal brain damage were randomly allocated to receive either a high (120% recommended average intake) or average (100% recommended average intake) energy and protein diet. The effect on recovery was dramatic. Infants fed the enhanced diet showed significantly larger head circumference (>1 SD difference) and heavier body weight at 1 year relative to untreated infants. In addition, non-invasive imaging showed that axonal diameters in the corticospinal tract, length, and weight were also significantly increased. Finally, there have been suggestions that nutrition may be a useful treatment for traumatic brain injury in both adults and children (e.g. Costello et al. 2014; Redmond & Lipp 2006).

We are only aware of two preclinical studies using nutrition as a treatment for rats with perinatal brain injury, one using choline and the other a concoction of vitamins and minerals. Both studies examined the behaviour and brain of rats receiving mPFC lesions at 3–5 days of age. In the choline study, supplementation began prenatally via drinking water given to pregnant dams and is continued until weaning (Halliwell et al. 2016). When tested as adults, the rats with mPFC lesions showed marked recovery of both cognitive (spatial learning) and motor (skilled reaching). This was correlated with increased brain weight, increased cortical thickness, and increased dendritic length in the perilesional sensorimotor cortex (see Figure 1.4) of the choline-treated lesion rats relative to untreated lesion of animals.

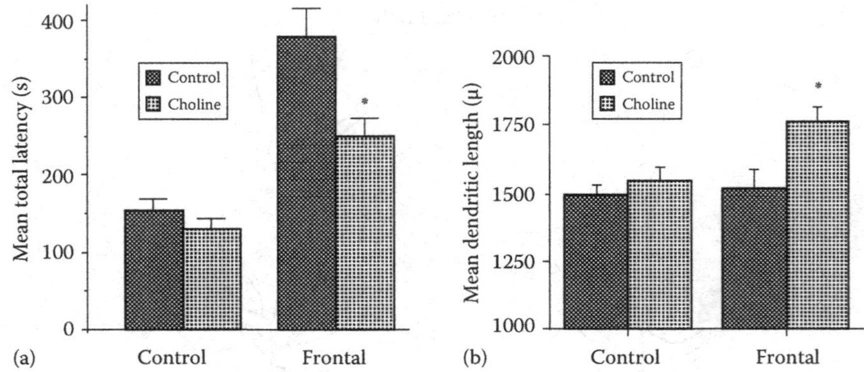

FIGURE 1.4 Effects of a choline-enriched diet on spatial learning (Morris water task) and dendritic length of layer III pyramidal cells in the sensorimotor cortex. "*" indicates a significant difference from the untreated frontal lesion group ($p < 0.05$ or better). (a) Morris water task performance; (b) Parietal dendritic length.

The second study supplemented the diet of pregnant dams with EmpowerPlus as noted earlier (Halliwell 2004, 2011). The results were similar with complete recovery of cognitive and motor tasks as well as increased brain weight and cortical thickness. There was one additional, unexpected finding as well. The lesion cavities in many, although not all, of the diet-supplemented animals appeared to have regrown much of the lost tissue. There is a precedent for this in previous studies where we have shown that regrowth appears spontaneously after mPFC lesions around postnatal days 7–12, but not with lesions before or after this age (Kolb et al. 1998a), and regrowth can be stimulated with subcutaneous injections of FGF-2 following day 10 motor cortex lesions (e.g. Monfils et al. 2006).

One challenge for the vitamin/mineral supplement neuroanatomical results is the question of what mechanism might stimulate cortical regrowth. One possibility is that the diet increased the production of neurotrophic factors such as FGF-2 or epidermal growth factor (EGF), both of which stimulate the production of neural progenitor cells both *in vitro* and *in vivo* (e.g. Morshead et al. 1994; Reynolds & Weiss 1992) and can stimulate functional recovery from cortical injury (Kolb et al. 2007; Monfils et al. 2008). Another explanation might be that the vitamin/mineral supplement induced epigenetic changes, which in turn led to the neural generation. It is known that diet supplements can produce large changes in gene expression that produce differences in body structure and behaviour of mice that are essentially clones (Gilbert & Epel 2009). Recall, too, the effects of diet on the epigenetic pattern in infants in Gambia illustrated in Figure 1.2.

1.6 CONCLUSION

We have shown that the developing brain is influenced by a wide range of experiences and shows a remarkable capacity for plastic change, for better or worse. Although nutrition has been known to influence brain development for some time, little is known about how nutritional changes interact with many other factors that influence brain development. In view of the effect of nutritional supplements on recovery from perinatal injury, it would be especially interesting to determine how nutrition might alter the effects of other negative early experiences including stress, psychoactive drugs, abnormal parent and peer relationships, and intestinal flora. A remaining question too will be what the mechanism(s) might be that would mediate these effects.

ACKNOWLEDGEMENT

The research by the authors discussed in this chapter was supported by NSERC of Canada grants to B.K. and R.G.

REFERENCES

Anda, R.F., Felitti, V.J., Bremner, J.D., Walker, J.D., Whitfield, C., Perry, B.D., & Giles, W.H. (2006). The enduring effects of abuse and related adverse experiences in childhood. A convergence of evidence from neurobiology and epidemiology. *European Archives of Psychiatry and Clinical Neuroscience,* 256, 174–186.

Avetisyan, M., Schill, E.M., & Heuchkeroth, R.O. (2015). Building a second brain in the bowel. *Journal of Clinical Investigation*, 125, 899–907.

Babenko, O., Kovalchuk, I., & Metz, G.A. (2015). Stress-induced perintal and transgeneration epigenetic programming of brain development and mental health. *Neuroscience and Biobehavioral Reviews*, 48, 70–91.

Bell, H.C., Pellis, S.M., & Kolb, B. (2010). Juvenile peer play experience and the development of the orbitofrontal and medial prefrontal cortex. *Behavioural Brain Research*, 207, 7–13.

Brown, R.W. & Kolb, B. (2001). Nicotine sensitization increases dendritic length and spine density in the nucleus accumbens and cingulate cortex. *Brain Research*, 899, 94–100.

Cameron, N.M., Champagne, F.A., Carine, P., Fish, E.W., Ozaki-Kuroda, K., & Meaney, M. (2005). The programming of individual differences in defensive responses and reproductive strategies in a rat through variations in maternal care. *Neuroscience and Biobehavioral Reviews*, 29, 843–865.

Campbell, G. & Shatz, C.J. (1992). Synapses formed by identified retinogeniculate axons during the segregation of eye input. *Journal of Neuroscience*, 12, 1847–1858.

Comeau, W., McDonald, R., & Kolb, B. (2010). Learning-induced structural changes in the prefrontal cortex. *Behavioural Brain Research*, 214, 91–101.

Costello, L.A., Lithander, F.E., Gruen, R.L., & Williams, L.T. (2014). Nutrition therapy in the optimisation of health outcomes in adult patients with moderate to severe traumatic brain injury: Findings from a scoping review. *Injury*, 45, 1834–1841.

Crowe, L.M., Catroppa, C., & Anderson, V. (2015). Sequelae in children: Developmental consequences. *Handbook of Clinical Neurology*, 128, 661–677.

Dabydeen, L., Thomas, J.E., Aston, T.J., Hartley, H., Sinha, S.K., & Eyre, J.A. (2008). High-energy and -protein diet increases brain and corticospinal tract growth in term and preterm infants after perinatal brain injury. *Pediatrics*, 12, 181–182.

Diaz Heijtz, R., Wang, S., Anuar, F., Qian, Y., Björkholm, B., Samuelsson, A., & Pettersson, S. (2003). Normal gut microbiota modulates brain development and behavior. *Proceedings of the National Academy of Science of the United States of America*, 108, 3047–3052.

Dominguez-Salas, P., Moore, S.E., Baker, M.S., Bergen, A.W., Cox, S.E., Dyer, R.A., Fulford, A.J., Guan, Y., Laritsky, E., Silver, M.J., Swan, G.E., Zeisel, S.H., Innis, S.M., Waterland, R.A., Prentice, A.M., & Hennig, B.J. (2014). Maternal nutrition at conception modulates DNA methylation of human metastable epialleles. *Nature Communications*, 5, 3746. doi: 10.1038/ncomms4746.

Farmer, A.D., Randall, H.A., & Aziz, Q. (2014). It's a gut feeling: How the gut microbiota affects the state of mind. *Journal of Physiology*, 592, 2981–2988.

Fenoglio, K.A., Chen, Y., & Baram, T.Z. (2006). Neuroplasticity of the hypothalamic-pituitary-adrenal axis early in life requires recurrent recruitment of stress-regulating brain regions. *Journal of Neuroscience*, 26, 2434–2442.

Field, T., Diego, M., Hernandez-Reif, M., Dieter, J., Kumar, A., Schanberg, S., & Kuhn, C. (2008). Insulin and insulin-like growth factor-1 increased in preterm neonates following massage therapy. *Journal of Developmental and Behavioral Pediatrics*, 29, 463–466.

Finegold, S.M., Molitoris, D., Song, Y., Liu, C., Vaisanen, M.L., Bolte, E., McTeague, M., Sandler, R., Wexler, H., Marlowe, E.M. et al. (2002). Gastrointestinal microflora studies in late-onset autism. *Clinical Infective Diseases*, 35, S6–S16.

Frost, D.O., Gibb, R., & Kolb, B. (2010). Trick or treat? Neurodevelopmental consequences of pharmacotherapy for affective disorders. *Neuropsychopharmacology Reviews*, 35, 344–345.

Georgieff, M.K. (2007). Nutrition and the developing brain: Nutrient priorities and measurement. *The American Journal of Clinical Nutrition*, 85S, 614–620.

Georgieff, M.K. & Rao, R. (2001). The role of nutrition in cognitive development. In: Nelson, C.A. & Luciana, M. (eds), *Handbook in Developmental Cognitive Neuroscience*. Cambridge, MA: MIT Press, pp. 491–504.

Gibb, R., Gonzalez, C., & Kolb, B. (2014). Prenatal enrichment and recovery from perinatal cortical damage: Effects of maternal complex housing. *Frontiers in Behavioral Neuroscience*, 8, 223.

Gibb, R., Kovalchuk, A., & Kolb, B. (2016). Tactile stimulation of functional recovery after perinatal cortical injury is mediated by FGF-2. Manuscript in submission.

Gilbert, S.F. & Epel, D. (2009). *Ecological Developmental Biology: Integrating Epigenetics, Medicine, and Evolution*. New York: Sinauer.

Greenough, W., Black, J., & Wallace, C. (1987). Experience and brain development. *Child Development*, 58, 539–559.

Greenough, W. & Chang, F. (1989). Plasticity of synapse structure and pattern in the cerebral cortex. In: Peters, A. & Jones, E. (eds.), *Cerebral Cortex*. New York: Plenum Press, pp. 391–440.

Gropper, S.S. & Smith, J.L. (2012). *Advanced Nutrition and Human Metabolism*. St. Paul, MN: West Publishing Company.

Guzzetta, G., Manfredi, P., Gasparini, R., Panatto, D., & Edmunds, W.J. (2009). Massage accelerates brain development and the maturation of visual function. *Journal of Neuroscience*, 29, 6042–6051.

Halliwell, C. (2004). Dietary factors and recovery from brain damage. Unpublished MSc thesis, University of Lethbridge, Lethbridge, Alberta, Canada.

Halliwell, C. (2011). Treatment interventions following prenatal stress and neonatal cortical injury. Unpublished PhD thesis, University of Lethbridge, Lethbridge, Alberta, Canada.

Halliwell, C., Tees, R.C., & Kolb, B. (2016). Neonatal dietary choline supplementation facilitates functional recovery and morphological change after neonatal frontal or parietal lesions in rats. Manuscript in submission.

Himmler, B.T., Pellis, S.M., & Kolb, B. (2013). Juvenile play experience primes neurons in the medial prefrontal cortex to be more responsive to later experiences. *Neuroscience Letters*, 556, 42–45.

Houston, S.M., Katzir, L.C., Manis, F.R., Kan, E., Rodriguez, G.G., & Sowell, E.R. (2014). Reading skill and structural brain development. *Neuroreport*, 25, 347–352.

Hsiao, E.Y., McBride, S.W., Hsien, S., Sharon, G., Hyde, E.R., McCue, T., Codelli, J.A., Chow, J., Reisman, S.E., Petrosino, J.F. et al. (2013). Microbioata modulate behavioral and physiological abnormalities associated with neurodevelopmental disorders. *Cell*, 155, 1451–1463.

Huttenlocher, P.R. (1984). Synapse elimination and plasticity in developing human cerebral cortex. *American Journal of Mental Deficiency*, 88, 488–496.

Keunen, K., van Elburg, R.M., van Bel, F., & Benders, M.J. (2015). Impact of nutrition on brain development and its neuroprotective implications following preterm birth. *Pediatric Research*, 77, 148–155.

Kohane, I.S., McMurry, A., Weber, G., MacFadden, D., Rappaport, L., Kunkel, L., Bicke, J., Wattanasin, N., Spence, S., Murphy, S. et al. (2012). The co-morbidity burden of children and young adults with autism spectrum disorders. *PLoS One*, 7, e33224.

Kolb, B. (1995). *Brain Plasticity and Behavior*. Hillsdale, NJ: Lawrence Erlbaum.

Kolb, B., Cioe, J., & Muirhead, D. (1998a). Cerebral morphology and functional sparing after prenatal frontal cortex lesions in rats. *Behavioural Brain Research*, 91, 143–155.

Kolb, B., Forgie, M., Gibb, R., Gorny, G., & Rowntree, S. (1998b). Age, experience, and the changing brain. *Neuroscience and Biobehavioral Reviews*, 22, 143–159.

Kolb, B. & Gibb, R. (2007). Brain plasticity and recovery from early cortical injury. *Developmental Psychobiology*, 49, 107–118.

Kolb, B., Gibb, R., & Gorny, G. (2003). Experience-dependent changes in dendritic arbor and spine density in neocortex vary with age and sex. *Neurobiology of Learning and Memory*, 79, 1–10.

Kolb, B., Gibb, R., Gorny, G., & Whishaw, I.Q. (1998c). Possible brain regrowth after cortical lesions in rats. *Behavioural Brain Research*, 91, 127–141.

Kolb, B., Morshead, C., Gonzalez, C., Kim, N., Shingo, T., & Weiss, S. (2007). Growth factor-stimulated generation of new cortical tissue and functional recovery after stroke damage to the motor cortex of rats. *Journal of Cerebral Blood Flow and Metabolism*, 27, 983–997.

Kolb, B., Mychasiuk, R., Muhammad, A., & Gibb, R. (2013). Brain plasticity in the developing brain. *Progress in Brain Research*, 207, 35–64.

Kolb, B. & Whishaw, I.Q. (1989). Plasticity in the neocortex: Mechanisms underlying recovery from early brain damage. *Progress in Neurobiology*, 32, 235–276.

Leung, B.M.Y., Wiens, K.P., & Kaplan, B.J. (2011). Does prenatal micronutrient supplementation improve children's mental development? A systematic review. *BMC Pregnancy and Childbirth*, 11, 12. doi: 10.1186/1471-2393-11-12.

McEwen, B.S. & Morrison, J.H. (2013). The brain on stress: vulnerability and plasticity of the prefrontal cortex over the life course. *Neuron*, 79, 16–29.

Meck, W.H. & Williams, C.L. (2003). Metabolic imprinting of choline by its availability during gestation: Implications for memory and attentional processing across the lifespan. *Neuroscience and Biobehavioral Reviews*, 27, 385–399.

Molnár, Z. & Clowry, G. (2012). Cerebral cortical development in rodents and primates. *Progress in Brain Research*, 195, 45–70.

Monfils, M.-H., Driscoll, I., Kamitakahara, H., Wilson, B., Flynn, C., Teskey, G.C., Kleim, J.A., & Kolb, B. (2006). FGF-2-induced cell proliferation stimulates anatomical, neurophysiological, and functional recovery from neonatal motor cortex injury. *European Journal of Neuroscience*, 24, 739–749.

Monfils, M.-H., Driscoll, I., Vavrek, R., Kolb, B., & Fouad, K. (2008). FGF-2 induced functional improvement from neonatal motor cortex injury via corticospinal projections. *Experimental Brain Research*, 185, 453–460.

Moreshead, C.M., Reynolds, B.A., Craig, C.G., McBurney, M.W., Staines, W.A., Morassutti, D., Weiss, S., & van der Kooy, D. (1994). Neural stem cells in the adult mammalian forebrain: a relatively quiescent subpopulation of subependymal cells. *Neuron*, 13, 1071–1082.

Muhammad, A. & Kolb, B. (2011a). Maternal separation altered behavior and neuronal spine density without influencing amphetamine sensitization. *Behavioural Brain Research*, 223, 7–16.

Muhammad, A. & Kolb, B. (2011b). Mild prenatal stress modulated behaviour and neuronal spine density without affecting amphetamine sensitization. *Developmental Neuroscience*, 33, 85–98.

Muhammad, A., Mychasiuk, R., Hosain, R., Nakahashi, A., Carroll, C., Gibb, R., & Kolb, B. (2013). Training on motor and visual spatial learning tasks in early adulthood produces large changes in dendritic organization of prefrontal cortex and nucleus accumbens in rats given nicotine prenatally. *Neuroscience*, 252, 178–189.

Muhammad, A., Mychasiuk, R., Nakahashi, A., Hossain, S., Gibb, R., & Kolb, B. (2012). Prenatal nicotine exposure alters neuroanatomical organization of the developing brain. *Synapse*, 66, 950–954.

Murmu, M., Salomon, S., Biala, Y., Weinstock, M., Braun, K., & Bock J. (2006). Changes in spine density and dendritic complexity in the prefrontal cortex in offspring of mothers exposed to stress during pregnancy. *European Journal of Neuroscience*, 24, 1477–1487.

Mychasiuk, R., Gibb, R., & Kolb, B. (2011). Prenatal bystander stress induces neuroanatomical changes in the prefrontal cortex and hippocampus of developing rat offspring. *Brain Research*, 1412, 55–62.

Mychasiuk, R., Gibb, R., & Kolb, B. (2012). Prenatal stress produces sexually dimorphic and regionally-specific changes in gene expression in hippocampus and frontal cortex of developing rat offspring. *Developmental Neuroscience*, 33, 531–538.

Mychasiuk, R., Hehar, H., Ma, I., Kolb, B., & Esser, M.J. (2014a). The development of lasting impairments: A mild pediatric brain injury alters gene expression, dendritic morphology, and synaptic connectivity in the prefrontal cortex of rats. *Neuroscience*, 288C, 145–155.

Mychasiuk, R., Muhammad, A., Gibb, R., & Kolb, B. (2013a). Long-term alterations to dendritic morphology and synaptic connectivity associated with prenatal exposure to nicotine. *Brain Research*, 1499, 53–60.

Mychasiuk, R., Muhammad, A., Ilnytsky, S., & Kolb, B. (2013b). Persistent gene expression changes in NAc, mPFC, and OFC associated with previous nicotine or amphetamine exposure. *Behavioural Brain Research*, 256, 655–651.

Mychasiuk, R., Muhammad, A., & Kolb, B. (2014b). Environmental enrichment alters structural plasticity of the adolescent brain but does not remediate the effects of prenatal nicotine exposure. *Synapse*, 68, 293–305.

Mychasiuk, R., Zahir, S., Schmold, N., Ilnystskyyu, S., Kovalchuk, O., & Gibb, R. (2012). Parental enrichment and offspring development: Modifications to brain, behavior, and the epigenome. *Behavioural Brain Research*, 228, 294–298.

Myers, M., Brunelli, S., Squire, J., Shindledecker, R., & Hofer, M. (1989). Maternal behaviour of SHR rats in its relationship to offspring blood pressure. *Developmental Psychobiology*, 22, 29–53.

O'Hare, E. & Sowell, E.R. (2008). Imaging developmental changes in gray and white matter in the human brain. In: Nelson, C. & Luciana, M. (eds.), *Handbook of Developmental Cognitive Neuroscience*. Cambridge, MA: MIT Press.

Pellis, S. & Pellis, V. (2010). *The Playful Brain*. New York: Oneworld Publications.

Petanjek, Z., Judas, M., Simic, G., Rain, M., Uylings, H.B., Rakic, P., & Kostovic, I. (2011). Extraordinary neotony of synaptic spines in the human prefrontal cortex. *Proceedings of the National Academy of Sciences of the United States of America*, 108, 13281–13286.

Redmond, C. & Lipp, J. (2006). Traumatic brain injury in the pediatric population. *Nutrition and Clinical Practice*, 21, 450–461.

Reisen, A. (1961). Studying preceptual development using the technique of sensory deprivation. *Journal of Nervous and Mental Disorders*, 132, 21–25.

Reynolds, B.A. & Weiss, S. (1992). Generation of neurons and astrocytes from isolated cells of the adult mammalian central nervous system. *Science*, 255, 1707–1710.

Richards, S., Mychasiuk, R., Kolb, B., & Gibb, R. (2012). Tactile stimulation during development alters behaviour and neuroanatomical organization of normal rats. *Behavioural Brain Research*, 231, 86–91.

Robinson, T.E. & Kolb, B. (2004). Structural plasticity associated with drugs of abuse. *Neuropharmacology*, 47(Suppl 1), 33–46.
Rucklidge, J.J., Johnstone, J., & Kaplan, B.J. (2013). Magic bullet thinking – Why do we continue to perpetuate this fallacy? *British Journal of Psychiatry*, 203, 313.
Rucklidge, J.J. & Kaplan, B.J. (2013). Broad-spectrum micronutrient formulas for the treatment of psychiatric symptoms: A systematic review. *Expert Reviews Neurotherapy*, 13, 49–73.
Sandstrom, N.J., Loy, R., & Williams, C.L. (2002). Prenatal choline supplementation increase NGF levels in the hippocampus and frontal cortex of young and adult rats. *Brain Research*, 947, 9–16.
Schanberg, S.M. & Field, T.M. (1987). Sensory deprivation stress and supplemental stimulation in the rat pup and preterm human neonate. *Child Development*, 58, 1431–1447.
Semple, B.D., Blomgren, K., Gimlin, K., Ferriero, D.M., & Noble-Haeusslein, L.J. (2013). Brain development in rodents and humans: Identifying benchmarks of maturation and vulnerability to injury across species. *Progress in Neurobiology*, 106, 1–16.
Shatz, C. (1992). The developing brain. *Scientific American*, 267, 60–67.
Silasi, G. (2005). Stroke treatments and neocortical plasticity. Unpublished M.Sc. thesis, University of Lethbridge, Lethbridge, Alberta, Canada.
Simpson, J.S., Crawford, S.G., Goldstein, E.T., Field, C., Burgess, E., & Kaplan, B.J. (2011). Systematic review of safety and tolerability of a complex micronutrient formula used in mental health. *BMC Psychiatry*, 11, 62. doi: 10.1186/1471-244X-11-62.
Sirevaag, A. & Greenough, W. (1988). A multivariate statistical summary of synaptic plasticity measures in rats exposed to complex, social, and individual environments. *Brain Research*, 441, 386–392.
Tees, R.C. & Mohammadi, E. (1999). The effects of neonatal choline dietary supplementation on adult spatial and configural learning and memory in rats. *Developmental Psychobiology*, 35, 226–240.
van den Bergh, B.R. & Marcoen, A. (2004). High antenatal maternal anxiety is related to ADHD symptoms, externalizing problems, and anxiety in 8- and 9-year-olds. *Child Development*, 75, 1085–1097.
Van Eden, C.G., Mrzljak, L., Voorn, P., & Uylings, H.B. (1990). The development of the rat prefrontal cortex: Its size and development of connections with thalamus, spinal cord, and other cortical areas. *Progress in Brain Research*, 85, 169–183.
Vinish, M., Elnabawi, A., Milstein, J., Burke, J., Kallevang, J., Turek, K., Merchenthaler, I., Bailey, A., Kolb, B., Cheer, J. et al. (2013). Olanzapine treatment of adolescent rats alters adult reward behaviour and nucleus accumbens function. *International Journal of Neuropsychopharmacology*, 25, 1–11.
Weaver, I.C.G., Meaney, M., & Szyf, M. (2006). Maternal care effects on the maternal transcriptome and anxiety-mediated behaviors in the offspring that are reversible in adulthood. *Proceedings of the National Academy of Science of the United States of America*, 103, 3480–3486.
Weinstock, M. (2008). The long-term behavioural consequences of prenatal stress. *Neuroscience and Biobehavioral Reviews*, 32, 1073–1086.
Williams, P. (2009). Neonatal stroke in rats impairs behaviour, anatomy, and neurophysiology in adulthood. Unpublished PhD thesis, University of Lethbridge, Lethbridge, Alberta, Canada.
Yager, J.Y. & Ashwal, S. (2009). Animal models of perintal hypoxic-ischemic brain damage. *Pediatric Neurology*, 40, 156–167.

2 Macronutrient Deprivation
Biological Mechanisms and Effects on Early Neurodevelopment

Jenalee R. Doom and Michael K. Georgieff

CONTENTS

2.1 INTRODUCTION

Macronutrient deficiency during the prenatal and early postnatal period is related to poorer cognitive and motor development in both animal models and humans, and these effects can last through adolescence and adulthood. Overall, children and adolescents who suffer severe malnutrition in early life demonstrate IQ deficits and poorer school performance compared to individuals who are not malnourished, especially for those experiencing chronic life stress (Grantham-McGregor 1995). Supplementation trials generally indicate improvements in outcomes depending on the timing of the intervention; specifically, prenatal and early postnatal (aged 0–3 years) interventions have the biggest effects (Christian et al. 2010, 2011; Cusick & Georgieff 2012; Gillespie & Allen 2002). The timing of macronutrient deprivation and subsequent outcomes is in line with the literature on brain development such that many of the effects of macronutrient deprivation in early life parallel the brain structures and circuits rapidly developing during this time period. These findings will be reviewed to understand the specific impact of macronutrient deprivation in the context of early brain development.

The focus of this chapter is to outline the neurodevelopmental effects of pre- and postnatal macronutrient deprivation and biological mechanisms of action, utilizing evidence from preclinical models, infants with intrauterine growth restriction (IUGR), and young children experiencing growth stunting. Supplementation trials will be reviewed to understand timing effects and potential reversibility of deficits due to nutrient deprivation. These findings will be compared and contrasted with other at-risk groups to understand macronutrient effects in groups experiencing high levels of stress.

2.2 BIOLOGICAL MECHANISMS OF MACRONUTRIENT DEPRIVATION

The macronutrients include the two major sources of energy, fat and carbohydrates, and protein. They constitute the major nutritional building blocks which provide the foundation for structure and function during brain development. Reduced availability of these substrates results in changes in brain development that range from profound to subtle and from global to highly specific. Much is known about macronutrient requirements for the developing brain through careful experiments across multiple levels of evidence from cell cultures to whole animals. These experiments are typically developmentally sensitive with respect to approximating human brain development in order to provide biologic plausibility to observations made in human studies (discussed in the following).

2.2.1 Protein

Although the brain has a high fat and water content, amino acids are the building blocks for neuronal architecture, neurotransmitters, and growth factors. Ultimately, much of brain performance is related to neuronal complexity (e.g. dendritic fields in hippocampal area CA1) which relies heavily on appropriate amounts of amino acid substrates, neurotransmitter stimulation within developing circuits, and adequate amounts of cellular energy. Several interacting signalling cascades regulate critical aspects of the neuronal cellular development, for example, neurite extension and retraction, and actin polymerization, by sensing the extra- and intracellular availability of critical metabolites including amino acids. Foremost among these is the mammalian target of rapamycin (mTOR) pathway which senses various availabilities of amino acids, growth factors, iron, oxygen, and energy and, through a complex feedback and feedforward system of kinase-driven reactions, regulates actin polymerization, protein translation rates, cell size, and autophagy (Fretham et al. 2011; Wullschleger et al. 2006). Amino acids regulate the pathway through multiple pathways directly affecting Rheb and mTOR complex 1 (mTORC1) expression and indirectly through regulating the synthesis of growth factors such as insulin-like growth factor (IGF-I) that signal through the PI3K subpathway (Jewell et al. 2015; Wullschleger et al. 2006; Zheng et al. 2014). mTOR also plays an important role in regulating amino acid carriers in the placenta, thus ensuring the appropriate substrate for protein synthesis in the fetal brain (Larque et al. 2013). Growth factors are small-molecular-weight proteins which are necessary for converting a nutritional substrate into growth (via pathways such as mTOR). Without growth factors, such as IGF-I, brain-derived neurotrophic factor (BDNF), nerve growth factor (NGF), and glial cell–derived neurotrophic factor (GDNF), neuronal growth is restricted, the dendritic tree is left simplified, and the neuronal performance is compromised. Fetal macronutrient malnutrition reduces IGF-1 expression (Nishijima 1986), which results in a reduction in regional brain volumes (Lee et al. 1999).

The effect of protein restriction has been well studied in multiple animal models including rodents and non-human primates. The findings at the molecular, cellular, and structural level are remarkably consistent and generally reflect the timing, dose, and duration of the deprivation (Dobbing & Sands 1979; Fuglestad et al. 2008; Kretchmer et al. 1996). Effects are evident not only in neurons but also in supporting cells, including oligodendrocytes, microglia, and astrocytes. The brain has a particularly high need for protein during two major phases of its development: from conception through 3 years of postnatal age when the majority of brain neurogenesis and differentiation takes place and then again in the teenage years when a great deal of remodelling and refinement take place. These two epochs in human development are characterized by the highest dietary protein requirements on a per weight basis.

The consequences of protein malnutrition to the brain include reduced DNA, RNA, and protein content and reduced mRNA for neuronal and glial proteins which provide scaffolding for the fatty acids of myelin (Morgane et al. 2002; Schober et al. 2009). The reduction in myelin is in part mediated through oxidative stress–mediated upregulation of brain morphogenetic protein-4 (BMP-4) expression (Reid et al. 2012). IUGR reduces neuronal cell numbers in the hippocampus and cerebellum accompanied by retarded dendritic and axonal growth (Mallard et al. 2000). mRNA expression for growth factors is also reduced, resulting in lower concentrations of IGF-I and BDNF (Dieni & Rees 2005; Lee et al. 1999). At the structural level, IUGR results in a reduction of dendritic elongation, simplification of the dendritic arbor, and altered synaptic spine density in the hippocampus, which likely has negative effects on learning and memory function (Dieni & Rees 2003). The synthesis of neurotransmitters and their receptors (e.g. glutamate, gamma-aminobutyric acid [GABA], monoaminergic, cholinergic) is compromised (Schober et al. 2009; Wiggins et al. 1984). The combined structural and neurochemical abnormalities likely underlie the brain's compromised electrical potential (Pinto et al. 1981). Overall brain weight and volume are reduced, most likely reflecting both reduced cell number and complexity. These molecular, cellular, electrophysiologic, and anatomic changes manifest as abnormal behaviours, the specificity of which depends on which brain circuits were most rapidly developing and had the highest requirements at the time of the insult. For example, protein malnutrition during late gestation and early postnatal life compromises the hippocampus, an area of the brain that subserves recognition and spatial memory. Abnormalities in spatial memory induced by early life protein malnutrition extend into adulthood and support the concept of a 'critical period' for protein with respect to hippocampal development (see Georgieff et al. 2015 for a discussion of critical periods and nutrition).

2.2.2 Energy

Energy can be derived from any of the macronutrients: carbohydrates, fats, or amino acids. The developing human brain has the highest energy metabolism of any mammal at any time of life (Kuzawa 1998). Sixty percent of the human neonate's total body oxygen consumption occurs in the brain. This figure compares to 20% in the adult human, 10% in the neonatal sheep, and 2% in the adult sheep and rodent (Kuzawa 1998). This enormous energy 'sink' reflects the high demands of rapid neuronal and glial growth and development in our species. Thus, the human brain is highly dependent on a constant source of energy, and, while it highly prefers glucose as a substrate, it has adapted to utilize other energy sources including lactate, amino acids, and ketone bodies derived from fat (Erecinska et al. 2004; Prins 2011; Rao et al. 2010). During gestation, carbohydrate delivery is facilitated from maternal plasma to the fetus by the GLUT transporter and facilitative diffusion (for a review, see Hay 1994). Transport from the fetus' or infant's plasma across the blood–brain barrier is achieved by GLUT1 and 3 (Khan et al. 1999).

The peculiarly high energy demand of the human brain makes modelling of the effects of substrate deprivation (e.g. hypoglycaemia) in animal models quite difficult (Hay et al. 2009). Nevertheless, the effects of early life hypoglycaemia on the developing brain are striking. The cingulate and occipital regions of the cortex, the hippocampus, and the striatum are vulnerable during the neonatal period, while more extensive cortical injury is seen with postnatal hypoglycaemia (Burns et al. 2008; Ennis et al. 2008; Yamada et al. 2004). Early life hypoglycaemia in rats increases fear-related behaviour and alters stress reactivity that persists into adulthood (Moore et al. 2010). Early life hypoglycaemia leads to neuronal death and cell injury through glutamate hyperexcitation and activation of A1 adenosine receptors that promote excessive calcium influx (Turner et al. 2004). Cholinergic and GABAergic neurotransmitter systems are also affected by neonatal hypoglycaemia, as evidenced by a reduction in muscarinic receptors and reduced M1, M2, and M3 receptor gene expression and decreased GABA receptor gene expression in the hippocampus of rats following neonatal hypoglycaemia (Anju & Paulose 2015; Sherin et al. 2012). In cell culture, hypoglycaemia reduces oligodendrocyte precursor cell proliferation, maturation, and migration, while in cerebellar slice culture, hypomyelination occurs. These findings are consistent with a hypomyelination effect (Yan & Rivkees 2006). Thus, neurons are not the only brain cells at risk for the loss of this energy substrate. Ultimately, hypoglycaemia leads to apoptosis, cell loss, and abnormal dendritic structure in vulnerable brain regions. The vulnerability of brain regions is largely dictated by their relative metabolic rates at the time of the insult (Ennis et al. 2011).

Energy can also be derived from fat and utilized by the brain through ketone production, but this process is usually reserved for the neonatal brain in extreme energy crises, for example, hypoglycaemia and hypoxaemia (Ennis et al. 2011; Prins 2008).

Under homeostatic conditions, certain fatty acids are transported from the mother to fetus by direct transport mechanisms. In addition, lipids can also be derived from maternal lipoproteins which are metabolized by the placenta and released as fatty acids into the fetal plasma (for a review, see Hay 1994).

The neurodevelopmental consequences of energy restriction are well described in rodent and monkey models (Schober et al. 2009; Xie et al. 2013). It is useful to consider models of broad profile fatty acid deprivation, as would be seen in generalized malnutrition in humans, and of specific essential fatty acids. The literature on neurodevelopmental effects of deficiency of 'fish oils' is well described and covered in Chapter 3.

The brain needs fats to generate myelin and cell membranes, including synaptosomes. Fatty acid composition of the latter affects their ability to merge with the external presynaptic cell membrane to release neurotransmitters (reviewed in Georgieff & Innis 2005; Uauy & Dangour 2006). Thus, fats play a role in synaptic efficacy beyond myelin's effect on increasing the speed of processing. Fatty acid deficiencies reduce the brain's speed of processing, render neurons more susceptible to membrane disruption and cell death, and profoundly affect cognitive behaviours such as learning and memory (Yehuda et al. 1998, 2005).

2.2.3 Neurodevelopmental Consequences of Intrauterine Growth Restriction in Animal Models

As noted in the following section, human populations rarely have pure deficiencies of single macronutrients. Instead, a combination of protein energy malnutrition with accompanying micronutrient deficiencies is often seen, particularly in the context of intrauterine growth restriction. Multiple models of IUGR exist. IUGR can be induced by food deprivation, protein deprivation, energy deprivation, or restriction of maternal–fetal blood flow. The latter can be accomplished in multiple ways, including via surgical ligation of the uterine arteries, administration of vasoconstrictive chemicals, or increasing maternal body temperature. IUGR has been induced in rodents, sheep, and non-human primates. Overall, the anthropometric phenotype of a small-for-gestational-age (SGA) newborn with loss of muscle and fat mass along signals macronutrient malnutrition. The presence of microcephaly (or low brain weight/volume at necropsy) indicates severe brain involvement, although it must be noted that the lack of microcephaly does not necessarily indicate brain sparing at the microstructural level.

Models of IUGR have elucidated fascinating mechanisms of altered brain form and function including epigenetic modifications of synaptic plasticity genes (Caprau et al. 2012; Fung et al. 2012). The latter findings may be important for understanding the long-term brain/behaviour consequences of early life nutrient deficiency in spite of adequate postnatal growth (Pylipow et al. 2009). It is certainly possible that the long-term behavioural abnormalities following IUGR in humans are a function of abnormal construction of the brain during its critical period and that no amount of postnatal rehabilitation will completely reverse the consequences. An alternative, but not mutually exclusive, possibility is that crucial regulatory set points for genes controlling energy metabolism may be epigenetically modified as the nutrient-restricted brain attempts to maintain a thrifty phenotype (Hanson & Gluckman 2014).

The resultant downregulation of energy utilization may promote brain cell survival but result in more simple cells with less capacity (and less demand on the expected limited resources). The developmental origins of adult health and disease (DOHaD) posit that the fetus and young organism 'make the metabolic assumption' that nutrient availability across the lifespan is likely to be similar to their present condition and set their metabolism accordingly (Gluckman & Hanson 2004). One mechanism to accomplish this is to modify the expression of genes that control metabolic rate with the positive and negative consequences noted earlier. Recent studies demonstrating that IUGR in the rodent model alters the chromatin structure of the hippocampal IGF-1 receptor gene and alters hippocampal neuroprogenitors strongly not only support this possibility but also beg the question whether therapies (e.g. methyl diets; HDAC modifiers) which can alter the epigenetic landscape can rescue the adult brain/behaviour phenotype if proper postnatal macronutrient substrates are provided (Caprau et al. 2012; Fung et al. 2012).

2.3 HUMAN STUDIES

2.3.1 Protein–Energy Malnutrition

Fetal protein–energy malnutrition, which is often the result of maternal malnutrition or hypertension, can result in growth retardation of the fetus (Low & Galbraith 1974). In postnatal life, preterm infants may become malnourished if they are fluid restricted, thereby limiting their nutrients. Protein energy is necessary for global brain cell proliferation and differentiation, synaptogenesis in the cortex, and growth factor synthesis in the hippocampus (Georgieff 2007). Protein intake is generally most important during gestation for global brain development and myelination, as well as for the specific development of the hippocampus, striatum, and cerebellum (Georgieff 2007). Another important sensitive period for protein consumption is 4–12 postnatal months, which is especially important for prefrontal cortex development and myelination (Georgieff 2007). Growth restriction during these periods can result in the failure of the head to grow properly, which is linked to poorer developmental outcomes (Strauss & Dietz 1998; Winer & Tejani 1994). Even when head growth is not severely stunted, around 15% of infants with IUGR have mild cognitive abnormalities (Spinello et al. 1993), and memory systems, especially explicit recognition and working memory, appear especially vulnerable to the effects of macronutrient deprivation during fetal development (Georgieff 2007; Gottlieb et al. 1998; Pollitt and Gorman 1994). Protein–energy malnutrition also has significant effects on motor development which can be detected in infancy (Georgieff 2007).

2.3.2 Intrauterine Growth Restriction

IUGR involves limitations on fetal nutrition often due to poor placental nutrient transfer, poor maternal nutrition, or both at a time when the brain is developing rapidly. The physical manifestations (e.g. low weight for age, low length for age, loss of somatic muscle and fat stores) are due to protein and energy malnutrition. Nevertheless, the syndrome represents a general restriction of nutrients when there is poor placental transport, and thus, micronutrient malnutrition also exists. For example, 50% of infants with IUGR are iron deficient (Chockalingam et al. 1987). Micronutrient malnutrition early in life also negatively affects brain development (see other chapters in this volume). IUGR has frequently been studied in developing countries where maternal undernutrition is more common, with approximately 16% of births being low birthweight (most are IUGR) and up to 27% in South Asia (Walker et al. 2011). Studies of IUGR infants demonstrate that the effects of this early nutritional deprivation can be observed from infancy to adulthood (Strauss 2000). As early as 12 months, IUGR infants in Brazil demonstrate lower developmental quotients than infants of normal birthweight (Grantham-McGregor et al. 1998), and this same result is observed at age 2 and 3 years for IUGR infants in Guatemala (Gorman & Pollitt 1992). Further, Jamaican infants with IUGR showed delays in problem-solving at 7 months (Gardner et al. 2003) and lower developmental quotients at both 15 and 24 months compared to normal birthweight infants (Walker et al. 2004). One study of very-low-birth-weight (VLBW) infants reported that being SGA alone was not associated with lower developmental scores compared with appropriate-for-gestational-age (AGA) infants (Latal-Hajnal et al. 2003). Instead, growth by age 2 years was predictive of motor and physical development. SGA children who remained below <10th percentile in weight showed poorer psychomotor development than SGA children who showed greater catch-up growth (Latal-Hajnal et al. 2003). In contrast, AGA children who fell below the 10th percentile at age 2 showed lower mental development scores than AGA children who remained above the 10th percentile (Latal-Hajnal et al. 2003). As a result, it appears that catch-up growth may be more important for determining neurodevelopment than gestational size for age (discussed further in Section 2.3.4. However, Pongcharoen and colleagues (2012) reported that linear growth at birth and in the first year has stronger associations with IQ than weight and growth between ages 1 and 9 had no effect on IQ.

IUGR appears to be associated with persistent deficits in weight and height catch-up growth in childhood, with approximately 0.5 standard deviation (SD) lower weight-for-age and height-for-age z-scores than children born without IUGR (Strauss & Dietz 1998). In addition, children with IUGR scored lower on measures of IQ and motor development. However, within sibling pairs discordant for IUGR, there were no differences on these measures (Strauss & Dietz 1998). There were differences, however, when siblings with IUGR had significant deficits in head circumference (Strauss & Dietz 1998). As a result, it appears that children with IUGR demonstrate the greatest impairment when head growth is reduced.

Infants born with low birthweight have less positive affect, are less active, and vocalize less than normal birthweight infants (Gardner et al. 2003; Grantham-McGregor et al. 1998). Low-birthweight infants are more likely to develop behavioural problems reported by both teachers and parents during adolescence than those born with a normal weight (Liu et al. 2001). Difficulties with emotion and behaviour may extend into adulthood. Adults who were conceived at the height of the Dutch Hunger Winter (1944–1945) and were thus exposed to severe malnutrition early in gestation showed a twofold greater risk of schizophrenia than those who were not exposed to famine at this early period (Susser et al. 1996). Males who experienced malnutrition during the second trimester of fetal development due to the Dutch

Hunger Winter showed a significantly increased risk of affective psychosis (Brown et al. 1995). These cognitive and affective changes are likely related to the neural circuitry developing at this specific time period, including the patterning of neurons in the embryonic period and the formation of neural structures during the fetal period.

However, evidence for long-term effects of IUGR remains mixed. For example, there were no IQ or behavioural differences reported in 6-year-old Jamaicans (Walker et al. 2010), 8-year old Brazilians (Emond et al. 2006), or 12-year-old South Africans who were with IUGR and born at a normal size (Sabet et al. 2009). In mothers from Jamaica who were generally nourished, weight before pregnancy and the amount gained during pregnancy had no association with their child's cognitive outcomes at age 7 (Walker et al. 2007). This mixed result may follow evidence from the moderately preterm infant literature that early outcomes (before age 2) are associated with prenatal biological insults, while, later into childhood and adolescence, other factors such as parenting, socio-economic status (SES), and education may be more related to long-term outcomes.

In developed countries, adolescents who had IUGR were more likely to be recommended with special education and less likely to be in the top 15% of the class than adolescents who were of normal birthweight (Strauss 2000). Adults who had IUGR had lower weekly pay, were less likely to have professional or managerial careers, and remained shorter during adulthood (Strauss 2000). As most studies in individuals with IUGR do not extend past infancy or early childhood, future longitudinal studies should follow these individuals' development throughout adulthood, with a special focus on specific neurodevelopmental outcomes in this group. Longitudinal studies of interventions to increase birthweight in at-risk infants are also needed to understand long-term cognitive/socio-emotional effects of increasing birthweight beyond improving health at birth.

2.3.3 Postnatal Growth Stunting

Worldwide, growth stunting is present in approximately a quarter of children under 5 years of age (United Nations Children's Fund 2014). Stunting can be the result of severe undernutrition, infectious disease, psychosocial stress, or a combination of these factors, and severity and duration of stunting have been used as indices of the extent of nutritional and/or social deprivation. As with IUGR, stunting rarely represents pure protein or protein–energy malnutrition. The other causes of stunting carry their own independent risks to brain development. Nevertheless, a robust finding in the literature on macronutrient deprivation is that, controlling for socio-economic status, stunting in early childhood is associated with cognitive delays, poorer scholastic performance, less likelihood of enrollment in primary school, and an increased risk of school dropout (Beasley et al. 2000; Chang et al. 2002; Daniels & Adair 2004; Martorell et al. 1992; Mendez & Adair 1999; Walker et al. 2005). In Zimbabwean adolescents, height by age 6 was linked to school grades and age at enrollment in school (Alderman et al. 2006).

Children stunted at 24 months scored 10 points lower on an IQ assessment at age 9 than non-stunted children (Berkman et al. 2002). Children with stunted growth in the first 2 years had lower test scores at ages 8 and 11 years than non-stunted children, and the effect was the largest for those who were the most stunted (Mendez & Adair 1999). There is evidence that the lower test scores in the stunted group are at least partially the result of delays in school enrollment, more absences, and repeating years of school in the stunted group (Mendez & Adair 1999). Additionally, children who were stunted at 24 months were more likely to drop out of grade school (Daniels & Adair 2004). Over time, the effect of early stunting appeared to decline, as differences between groups were stronger at age 8 than 11 (Mendez & Adair 1999). Overall, stunting that is 1 or more SD below the mean for height between the ages of 12 and 36 months is associated with 0.4–1.05 SD effect size on cognitive development (Grantham-McGregor et al. 2007), indicating that growth stunting may be used as an indicator of poor development or early risk. Duration of stunting may be particularly important for predicting cognitive outcomes, as children who were stunted between 6 and 18 months of age but then showed significant catch-up growth by 4.5–6 years did not differ in verbal and quantitative ability from never-stunted children (Crookston et al. 2010). However, children who were stunted at both time points showed significantly lower verbal and quantitative ability than children who were not stunted at either period (Crookston et al. 2010). The timing of linear growth may also be a key, as linear growth between birth and 1 year was significantly related to IQ at age 9, while growth from ages 1 to 9 was not related to IQ (Pongcharoen et al. 2012).

There has been less work examining the effects of growth stunting in young children, but current evidence from Zanzibar and Nepal suggests that children with greater height for age are more likely to be walking (Kariger et al. 2005; Siegel et al. 2005). Additionally, being stunted during infancy predicts age of walking (Cheung et al. 2001; Kuklina et al. 2004).

Although most research has focused on the cognitive outcomes for malnourished children, social and emotional functioning is also affected. Low weight for height or linear growth stunting in young children is related to less play, less positive effect, greater lethargy, and less likelihood of secure attachment compared to children without growth delay (Gardner et al. 1999; Graves 1978). These problems can translate into difficulties in school, including conduct issues, attention problems, and poorer quality relationships (Chang et al. 2002; Galler & Ramsey 1989, Richardson et al. 1972). A study of Jamaican adolescents demonstrated that stunting in childhood is related to poorer psychological functioning, including greater depression and anxiety symptoms, increased hyperactivity, and lower self-esteem (Walker et al. 2007). A group of stunted children who received psychosocial stimulation in childhood differed from the non-stunted group only in hyperactivity symptoms (Walker et al. 2007). These largely frontal lobe–mediated functions which are impacted by linear stunting are in line with structures developing in the postnatal brain, particularly connections between primary structures such as the hippocampus and striatum to the prefrontal cortex.

The effects of growth stunting can persist into adolescence and adulthood. In late adolescence, verbal, mathematical, cognitive, and general knowledge domains were all related to stunting at 36 months (Martorell et al. 1992). A recent approximation of adult income lost due to the effects of early stunting estimates a 22.2% reduction in adult income for stunted children not living in poverty and 30.1% for children stunted and in poverty (Grantham-McGregor et al. 2007). A study in the Philippines that followed stunted children into early adulthood reported that those who were stunted early in life were less likely to have formal employment between ages 20 and 22 years (Carba et al. 2009). This evidence suggests that the effect of macronutrient deprivation and stunting on later development may be greater than the independent effect of poverty.

2.3.4 Role of Catch-Up Growth in Determining Neurodevelopment

Further research has indicated that the amount of growth after macronutrient deprivation in IUGR and stunted children may predict cognitive outcomes and motor development better than just being stunted at a certain time point. This finding falls in line with the principle of sensitive periods of brain development, in which the potential for growth early in life may improve developmental outcomes if it occurs before a certain time. The infant brain in these cases often exhibits a great deal of plasticity in response to environmental inputs, even after the insult of macronutrient deprivation. A study of IUGR infants in Guatemala demonstrated delayed development for infants between 6 and 24 months of age, with greater linear growth and weight gain in the first 24 months related to better developmental outcomes at 36 months (Kuklina et al. 2006). Additionally, growth was more closely related to motor than mental development (Kuklina et al. 2006). Birthweight unadjusted for gestational age has been linked to IQ at age 5 as well as grade achieved in high school (Martorell et al. 2010; Santos et al. 2008). Consistent with other studies of early growth, weight gain in the first 2 years is related to more positive school outcomes, but growth between 24 and 36 months of age was not related to developmental outcomes (Martorell et al. 2010; Pongchareon et al. 2012). A Taiwanese study demonstrated that at age 15, small deficits were present in overall academic achievement of adolescents who were IUGR (Wang et al. 2008). There is evidence that catch-up growth following IUGR is associated with differential cognitive outcomes in an inverted J-shaped pattern during middle childhood (Pylipow et al. 2009). Infants gaining the least amount of weight by 16 weeks (1200 g) had the lowest scores on cognitive tests at the age of 7 years (15.5 points lower than the score-maximizing amount of growth; Pylipow et al. 2009). On the other hand, the highest amount of weight gain was also related to lower cognitive scores (2.4 points lower than score-maximizing growth; Pylipow et al. 2009).

In general, early nutritional support and growth are critical factors in medical and neurobehavioural outcomes in premature infants. Stunted linear growth is common in VLBW preterm infants as well, and this linear growth failure is related to poorer scores on cognitive tests at 24 months corrected age even after controlling for increases in weight and head circumference (Ramel et al. 2012). Greater linear growth in VLBW infants has been associated with improvements in cognitive and motor development at 2 years corrected age as well as a decreased likelihood of developing cerebral palsy (Latal-Hajnal et al. 2003). Faster linear growth between term and 4 months corrected age in preterm low-birthweight infants decreases the odds of having an IQ lower than one standard deviation below the mean between 8 and 18 years (Belfort et al. 2013). Linear growth between birth and hospital discharge is also related to higher language scores at 24 months corrected age

(Ramel et al. 2012), and growth after discharge is associated with improvements in motor development for infants born before 33 weeks gestation (Belfort et al. 2011). In addition to gains in height, increased fat-free mass is related to better cognitive performance and faster neural processing (Pfister et al. 2013).

An analysis of 1366 extremely premature infants demonstrated that the amount of energy intake during the first week of life mediated the association between critical illness and adverse outcomes, with greater energy intake related to a greater number of positive outcomes, including faster growth, less likelihood of death, less late-onset sepsis, and more positive neurodevelopment (Ehrenkranz et al. 2011). Providing the macronutrients for healthy development in sick infants proves to be difficult because, compared to the term infant, feeding becomes more challenging, nutritional demand changes, and both inflammatory and stress responses induce catabolic states in the infant (Ramel et al. 2014). While these adaptations may help infants survive in the short-term, long-term growth and neurodevelopment may be put at risk, especially given research on the importance of feeding and growth for healthy neurodevelopment in early postnatal life.

There is also some evidence that birthweight and postnatal growth are not related to IQ or behaviour in preterm children, but in term children both birthweight and postnatal weight gain predict IQ between the ages of 4 and 7 years (Huang et al. 2012). This may be the result of an overwhelming number of risk factors in the preterm group that is minimizing the effect of growth during childhood. An increase of 1 unit (z-score) in birthweight was related to an IQ increase of 1.6 points, and a 1 unit increase (z-score) in postnatal weight gain predicted a 0.46 point increase in IQ (Huang et al. 2012). Likewise, weight for the age of 1 year was not predictive of cognitive functioning at age 7, but the weight change from 1 to 7 years of age was predictive of later cognition, suggesting that weight gain during childhood may be more predictive of cognitive functioning than poor growth in infancy (Cheung 2006). Another study that followed women from birth to adulthood reported that although birthweight did not predict educational achievement in adulthood, greater growth between birth and 2 years predicted higher achievement, while growth after 2 years was unrelated to achievement (Li et al. 2004). Growth also appears to mediate some of the effects of poverty on IQ, along with parental education and home stimulation (Hamadani et al. 2014). In addition, in this rural poverty sample in Bangladesh, growth in the first 2 years of life was more predictive of IQ at 64 months than growth after age 2 (Hamadani et al. 2014).

2.4 SUPPLEMENTATION STUDIES

Much of the literature on growth failure or macronutrient malnutrition and neurodevelopment are observational studies, which are subject to multiple known and unknown confounding variables. However, macronutrient supplementation interventions have consistently demonstrated more positive developmental outcomes for those in the intervention group (Walker et al. 2007). Food supplementation for at-risk pregnant women, infants, and young children has been shown to improve physical, motor, and cognitive development (Behrman et al. 2004; Gillespie & Allen 2002; Pollitt et al. 1993; Schroeder et al. 1995; Walker et al. 2007). Prenatal and early postnatal interventions are more effective than interventions later on, and postnatal interventions are the most effective and of long-term if delivered during the first 2–3 years of life (Engle et al. 2007; Pollitt et al. 1993). Even during pregnancy, early supplementation may be better than later. A food supplementation study conducted in Bangladesh with undernourished pregnant women suggested that early supplementation (8–10 weeks gestation) is better for problem-solving in the infant at age 7 months than later supplementation (approximately 17 weeks gestation; Tofail et al. 2008). Importantly, food supplementation studies differ from macronutrient supplementation in that the former would include micronutrients, which also aid neurodevelopment.

Food supplementation aimed to improve nutritional status and promote growth has positive effects on cognitive development and motor development (Grantham-McGregor et al. 1991; Husaini et al. 1991; Pollitt & Schurch 2000; Pollitt et al. 1993), with effect sizes of between 6 and 13 developmental quotient points (Walker et al. 2007). The positive effects are likely due to macronutrient and micronutrient supplementation. Decreased behavioural distress and reductions in apathy have been reported for these interventions as well (Mora et al. 1979; Pollitt & Schurch 2000). Evidence is mixed for what domains macronutrient supplementation is most effective at improving. For example, a food supplementation study in Taiwan for pregnant women showed improvements in motor development of the infant at 8 months (Adair & Pollitt 1985). However, no improvements in intelligence were reported in this group at the age of 5 years (Adair & Pollitt 1985), so there may be differences by the age of assessment and domain of functioning. This could be due to the timing of supplementation in relation to the neural structures that are rapidly developing. For example, the striatum develops primarily prenatally and early in the postnatal period. However, IQ may be more influenced by myelination and neural connectivity across diffusely distributed systems, which largely occurs postnatally. Additionally, supplementing Colombian women in the third trimester and infants as old as 6 months showed no benefit on developmental levels between 6 months and 3 years of age (Waber et al. 1981). For socio-emotional and behavioural domains, children who had the largest supplement intake before age 2 showed the greatest behavioural effects between the ages of 6 and 8 years, including less anxiety and greater social interaction (Barrett et al. 1982). Although we see consistent cognitive benefits across studies, the presence of effects on behaviour is variable. However, it could be the case that trials that did not supplement during both the prenatal and early postnatal periods do not see the same effect on behaviour, which would suggest a sensitive period for certain behavioural effects. Thus, the most effective interventions should start as early as possible, particularly in the prenatal period, and supplementation in at-risk groups should aim for the prevention of macronutrient deprivation rather than only the treatment.

A comparison of two nutritional supplements given to mothers, infants, and young children in Guatemala was conducted to determine which was related to better cognitive outcomes (Pollitt et al. 1995). The first supplement, called Atole, contained 163 kcal and 11.5 g protein, and the second, named Fresco, contained 59 kcal and no protein. Both supplements were fortified with vitamins and minerals to ensure that any effects were not due to micronutrient deficiencies. Overall, findings indicated that supplementation that begins during pregnancy and continues through the first 2 postnatal years has demonstrated both cognitive and emotional benefits into adulthood (Pollitt et al. 1993). In adolescence, those who received the Atole supplement showed faster information processing and performed better on cognitive tests, including both numeracy and verbal tests, than those who received Fresco (Pollitt et al. 1995). Further, in villages receiving the Atole supplement, the typical SES disparities in cognitive outcomes were eliminated (Pollitt et al. 1995). However, in villages receiving Fresco, the expected cognitive advantages of living in a high SES versus a low SES household were observed (Pollitt et al. 1995). Overall, this study suggests that greater macronutrient supplementation, specifically one that involves protein, provides cognitive benefits above the effect of micronutrient supplementation. In a follow-up of this study, individuals receiving the Atole intervention during the first 2 years of life performed better on tests of reading comprehension and cognitive functioning between 25 and 42 years than those who were supplemented later, even after accounting for schooling (Stein et al. 2008). Men who were supplemented with Atole during their first 3 years of life received higher wages as adults (Hoddinott et al. 2008). The increase in hourly wages was approximately 46% for men who were supplemented during the first 2 years of life (Hoddinott et al. 2008). Overall, this series of studies suggests that there are lasting effects of early macronutrient intake and that there may be an early period where macronutrient supplementation is most beneficial. Future studies are needed to examine whether supplementation for mothers before pregnancy further improves birth outcomes and overall functioning throughout childhood and into adulthood.

2.5 TIMING OF MACRONUTRIENT DEPRIVATION

Long-term benefits may be dependent on the timing, duration, and execution of the intervention. For example, a follow-up study of Indonesian children who received a 3-month supplementation between the ages of 6 and 60 months did not show significant differences on a number of cognitive assessments 8 years later compared to the non-supplemented group (Pollitt et al. 1997). However, when the group is restricted to those who received supplementation before 18 months of age, significant benefits were conferred in working memory (Pollitt et al. 1997). Thus, the lack of effects could be due to the specificity of intervention during later infancy rather than during the prenatal or early postnatal periods or to the short supplementation period (3 months). Another follow-up study of 17- and 18-year-olds who participated in a supplementation trial between ages 9 and 24 months showed short-term effects but no long-term effects of the intervention (Walker et al. 2005). All long-term effects on IQ and verbal skills were the result of a psychosocial stimulation intervention rather than supplementation (Walker et al. 2005). It is likely that differences in sensitive periods for nutritional versus psychosocial interventions play a role in later outcomes. For example, nutritional supplementation may be most effective if implemented during the prenatal or early postnatal period, while psychosocial interventions may be most effective during late infancy and early childhood. Thus, multi-faceted interventions must be designed to provide components of care when they will be the most beneficial (Wachs et al. 2014).

It must be noted that the brain is not a single, homogeneous organ. Indeed, its various regions and neural networks develop at different rates across different time periods, and as a result, there are unique growth trajectories and sensitive periods during which environmental influences, including nutrition, may have a particularly large effect (Johnson 2005; Kretchmer et al. 1996). Researchers must consider what brain regions are developing the most rapidly at the time of the insult, the nutritional requirements for that period of development, and what previous insults may have occurred that produce the current phenotype. Macronutrient deficiencies appear to be the most damaging when there is peak growth, and the brain needs nutrients for basic neural metabolic processes (Wachs et al. 2014). Supplementation during or before these rapid periods of brain development is often the most likely to produce large positive effects, and supplementation after these periods often results in failure to correct brain structure and function following earlier deficits. Further, neurodevelopmental outcomes may also differ at different ages and in different domains of functioning (e.g. cognitive, social, motor). Certain macronutrients may be particularly important for the development of particular cognitive outcomes at one period but more important for social development at another time period. Conversely, a number of macronutrient deficiencies likely have impacts on the same regions of the brain, making it difficult to determine the unique contribution of each nutrient. For example, the developing hippocampus needs protein energy, iron, and zinc in order to function properly. Thus, a multilayer combination of human, animal, and cellular models will be needed to understand specific effects of micro- and macronutrient deficiencies. Additionally, there may be differences in the effect sizes of macronutrient supplementation on developmental outcomes between groups of people living in different environments. For example, for those in the Guatemalan cohort who received the Atole supplement, the greatest benefits were derived by children who were in the lowest SES groups and those who achieved higher levels of education (Pollitt et al. 1993). As a result, there can be individual differences in macronutrient needs and later development. For supplementation interventions, the knowledge of macronutrient demands, timing of brain development, and individual differences in supplementation outcomes can be used in order to optimize intervention strategies for children.

2.6 ENVIRONMENTAL INFLUENCES ON COGNITIVE DEVELOPMENT

In addition to variability in timing of macronutrient deficiency and brain development, significant variation in early stressful experiences, both infectious and psychological, can occur such that individuals experiencing macronutrient deprivation also undergo additional significant stressors in both pre- and postnatal periods. An example of a group that may experience multiple independent stressors during the prenatal and early postnatal period includes infants born prematurely. Individuals who were born prematurely often show developmental delays in motor abilities, visual motor skills, executive functioning, greater ADHD symptoms, lower IQ, and poorer school achievement than individuals born at term (reviewed in Aylward 2005). In addition, many infants born prematurely experience IUGR (reviewed in

Section 2.3.2), which is an independent risk factor for a number of poorer neurodevelopmental outcomes. Premature infants who are of normal size for gestational age (termed 'macropremie') are still at higher risk for cerebral palsy, hypoxic–ischemic–inflammatory–associated disorders, intellectual disability, hyperactivity, and poorer school achievement in a number of subjects (Amiel-Tison et al. 2002; Huddy et al. 2001), indicating that macronutrient deficiencies are not solely responsible for neurodevelopmental outcomes. Even within infants born prematurely, there is a greater neurodevelopmental risk for infants who had lower weight at birth (Aylward 2005), suggesting that macronutrient effects still account for significant variation in developmental outcomes in this high-risk group. Thus, premature birth and IUGR may be separate 'hits' to development even though they often co-occur, and future research must elucidate the mechanisms between each of these hits and neurodevelopmental outcomes and examine what factors may prevent both premature birth and IUGR to promote optimal development.

Although poor nutrient delivery is often considered to be the primary cause of growth failure, a considerable body of research documents the impact that infection, psychosocial factors, and the environment have on growth. Chronic stress and resulting behaviours can influence metabolism by impacting both feeding behaviours and nutrient absorption (Wachs et al. 2014). A primary example of a group often affected by both psychosocial deprivation and undernutrition includes children living in or adopted from institutional (e.g. orphanage) care. Children often fail to get the nutrients needed to sustain growth or the stress of the institution leads to difficulties with nutrient absorption, causing growth failure even if enough sustenance is provided (Monk et al. 2013). There is also a substantial literature documenting the negative effects of psychosocial deprivation, as is experienced in institutions that often have a high caregiver-to-child ratio and high caregiver turnaround on later physical, cognitive, or socio-emotional development (reviewed in Doom and Gunnar 2016). Internationally adopted children with lower z-scores for head circumference, height, and weight are significantly more likely to have poorer motor development and more severe cognitive and language delays (Miller et al. 1995). Recent work has started to tease apart the impacts of nutrition and psychosocial deprivation on cognitive development and has reported independent effects of nutritional status and psychosocial deprivation (e.g. Doom et al. 2014, 2015). There is even evidence that psychosocial stimulation may play an equal or larger role relative to nutrition. Indeed, after 20 years of psychosocial stimulation study in Jamaica in growth-stunted children, those in the intervention group earned wages that were comparable to non-stunted individuals (Gertler et al. 2014). Psychosocial stimulation thus has independent impacts on the development that may ameliorate later outcomes, even in the context of malnutrition. More work is needed to address independent contributions of macronutrient and psychosocial deprivation on the development of children living in adverse environments to optimize care in institutions and post-adoption. These studies serve to remind that 'supply side' economics are only one side of the coin. Consideration should be given to how nutrients are utilized by the non-stressed growing individual versus the stressed or chronically infected individual. The latter condition results in the release of pro-inflammatory cytokines (which damage the brain themselves), suppression of growth factors, and subsequent repurposing of macronutrient substrates (glucose, amino acids) for fight or flight responses. While highly necessary for survival, this repurposing is not consistent with an anabolic state and promotion of brain growth (Ramel et al. 2014).

Of course, nutritional factors are not the only determinants of neurodevelopmental outcomes. As environmental enrichment, such as living in a high-resource family, and having sensitive and responsive caregivers have been shown to support optimal cognitive development, it is possible that environmental or family factors may mask some of the effects of macronutrient deprivation. For example, living in an enriched environment with several factors that promote resilience may mitigate deficits in global development and memory. Thus, the environment of the individual must be considered when assessing recovery from macronutrient deprivation and determining what factors best promote cognitive and motor development after an early period of nutrient deprivation.

2.7 CONCLUSION

When considering many factors associated with nutrition and neurodevelopment, one might argue that macronutrient effects are instead due to co-occurring micronutrient deficiencies (e.g. iron or zinc). While most observational studies in humans do not assess all possible micronutrient deficiencies that may co-occur, preclinical studies are especially useful for determining specific effects of macronutrients. Preclinical studies allow researchers to control for micronutrient deficiencies and isolate macronutrient deprivation as the sole experimental factor different between groups, thus making an argument for the beneficial impact of macronutrient supplementation even in the absence of specific micronutrient supplementation. Thus, individuals implementing nutritional interventions in populations experiencing or at risk for prenatal and/or postnatal malnutrition should consider macronutrient supplementation, as macronutrient deficiencies are an independent risk factor for poorer developmental outcomes. With appropriate nutritional supplementation during optimal developmental periods, millions of individuals currently experiencing macronutrient deficiencies can become closer to fulfilling their developmental potential.

REFERENCES

Adair LS and Pollitt E. 1985. Outcome of maternal nutritional supplementation: A comprehensive review of the Bacon Chow study. *Am J Clin Nutr* 41: 948–978.

Alderman H, Hoddinott J, and Kinsey B. 2006. Long term consequences of early childhood malnutrition. *Oxf Econ Pap* 58: 450–474.

Amiel-Tison C, Alen MC, Leburn F et al. 2002. Macropremies: Underpriviledged newborns. *Ment Retard Dev Disabil Res Rev* 8: 281–292.

Anju TR and Paulose CS. 2015. Cortical cholinergic dysregulation as a long-term consequence of neonatal hypoglycemia. *Biochem Cell Biol* 93(1): 47–53.

Aylward GP. 2005. Neurodevelopmental outcomes of infants born prematurely. *J Dev Behav Pediatr* 26(6): 427–440.

Barrett DE, Radke-Yarrow M, and Klein RE. 1982. Chronic malnutrition and child behavior: Effects of early caloric supplementation on social and emotional functioning at school age. *Dev Psychol* 18: 541–556.

Beasley NMR, Hall A, Tomkins AM et al. 2000. The health of enrolled and non enrolled children of school age in Tanga, Tanzania. *Acta Trop* 76: 223–229.

Behrman J, Cheng Y, and Todd P. 2004. Evaluating preschool programs when length of exposure to the program varies: A nonparametric approach. *Rev Econ Stats* 86: 108–132.

Belfort MB, Gillman MW, Buka SL et al. 2013. Preterm infant linear growth and adiposity gain: Trade-offs for later weight status and intelligence quotient. *J Pediatr* 163(6): 1564–1569.e2.

Belfort MB, Rifas-Shiman SL, Sullivan T et al. 2011. Infant growth before and after term: Effects on neurodevelopment in preterm infants. *Pediatrics* 128: e899–e906.

Berkman DS, Lescano AG, Gilman RH, Lopez SL, and Black MM. 2002. Effects of stunting, diarrhoeal disease, and parasitic infection during infancy on cognition in late childhood: A follow-up study. *Lancet* 359: 564–571.

Brown AS, Susser ES, Lin SP, Neugebauer R, and Gorman JM. 1995. Increased risk of affective disorders in males after second trimester prenatal exposure to the Dutch hunger winter of 1944–45. *Br J Psychiatry* 166: 601–606.

Burns CM, Rutherford MA, Boardman JP, and Cowan FM. 2008. Patterns of cerebral injury and neurodevelopmental outcomes after symptomatic neonatal hypoglycemia. *Pediatrics* 122: 65–74.

Caprau D, Schober ME, Bass K et al. 2012. Altered expression and chromatin structure of the hippocampal IGFr gene is associated with impaired hippocampal function in the adult IUGR male rat. *J Dev Orig Health Dis* 3(2): 83–91.

Carba DB, Tan VL, and Adair LS. 2009. Early childhood length-for-age is associated with the work status of Filipino young adults. *Econ Hum Biol* 7: 7–17.

Chang SM, Walker SP, Grantham-McGregor S, and Powell CA. 2002. Early childhood stunting and later behaviour and school achievement. *J Child Psychol Psyc* 43: 775–783.

Cheung YB. 2006. Growth and cognitive function of Indonesian children: Zero-inflated proportion models. *Stat Med* 25: 3011–3022.

Cheung YB, Yip PSF, and Karlberg JPE. 2001. Fetal growth, early postnatal growth and motor development in Pakistani infants. *Int J Epidemiol* 30: 66–72.

Chockalingam UM, Murphy E, Ophoven JC, Weisdorf SA, and Georgieff MK. 1987. Cord transferrin and ferritin levels in newborn infants at risk for prenatal uteroplacental insufficiency and chronic hypoxia. *J Pediatr* 111: 283–286.

Christian P, Morgan ME, Murray-Kolb L et al. 2011. Preschool iron-folic acid and zinc supplementation in children exposed to iron-folic acid in utero confers no added cognitive benefit in early school-age. *J Nutr* 141(11): 2042–2048.

Christian P, Murray-Kolb LE, Khatry SK et al. 2010. Prenatal micronutrient supplementation and intellectual and motor function in early school-aged children in Nepal. *JAMA* 304(24): 2716–2723.

Crookston BT, Penny ME, Alder SC et al. 2010. Children who recover from early stunting and children who are not stunted demonstrate similar levels of cognition. *J Nutr* 140: 1996–2001.

Cusick SE and Georgieff MK. 2012. Nutrient supplementation and neurodevelopment: timing is the key. *Arch Pediatr Adolesc Med* 166: 481–482.

Daniels MC and Adair LS. 2004. Growth in young Filipino children predicts schooling trajectories through high school. *J Nutr* 134: 1439–1446.

Dieni S and Rees S. 2003. Dendritic morphology is altered in hippocampal neurons following prenatal compromise. *J Neurobiol* 55(1): 41–52.

Dieni S and Rees S. 2005. BDNF and TrkB protein expression is altered in the fetal hippocampus but not cerebellum after chronic prenatal compromise. *Exp Neurol* 192(2): 265–273.

Dobbing J and Sands J. 1979. Comparative aspects of the brain growth spurt. *Early Hum Dev* 3: 79–83.

Doom JR, Georgieff MK, and Gunnar MR. 2015. Institutional care and iron deficiency increase ADHD symptomology and lower IQ 2.5–5 years post-adoption. *Dev Sci* 18: 484–494.

Doom JR and Gunnar MR. 2016. Institutional care and neurobiological development in infancy. In: Sale A (ed.), *Environmental Experience and Plasticity of the Developing Brain*. Wiley, pp. 185–214.

Doom JR, Gunnar MR, Georgieff MK, Kroupina M, Frenn KA, Fuglestad AJ, and Carlson SM. 2014. Beyond stimulus deprivation: Iron deficiency and cognitive deficits in post-institutionalized children. *Child Dev* 85(5), 1805–1812.

Ehrenkranz RA, Das A, Wrage LA et al. 2011. Early nutrition mediates the influence of severity of illness on extremely LBW infants. *Pediatr Res* 69: 522–529.

Emond AM, Lira PI, Lima MC, Grantham-McGregor SM, and Ashworth A. 2006. Development and behaviour of low-birthweight term infants at 8 years in northeast Brazil: A longitudinal study. *Acta Paediatr* 95: 1249–1257.

Engle PL, Black MM, Behrman JR et al. 2007. Strategies to avoid the loss of developmental potential in more than 200 million children in the developing world. *Lancet* 369: 229–242.

Ennis K, Deelchand DK, Tkac I, Henry PG, and Rao R. 2011. Determination of oxidative glucose metabolism in vivo in the young rat brain using localized direct-detected (1)(3)C NMR spectroscopy. *Neurochem Res* 36: 1962–1968.

Ennis K, Tran PV, Seaquist ER, and Rao R. 2008. Postnatal age influences hypoglycemia-induced neuronal injury in the rat brain. *Brain Res* 1224: 119–126.

Erecinska M, Cherian S, and Silver IA. 2004. Energy metabolism in mammalian brain during development. *Prog Neurobiol* 73: 397–445.

Fretham SJB, Carlson ES, and Georgieff MK. 2011. The role of iron in learning and memory. *Adv Nutr* 2: 1–10.

Fuglestad AJ, Rao R, and Georgieff MK. 2008. The role of nutrition in cognitive development. In Nelson CA and Luciana M (eds.), *Handbook of Developmental Cognitive Neuroscience*, 2nd edn. Cambridge, MA: The MIT Press, pp. 623–637.

Fung C, Ke X, Brown AS, Yu X, McKnight RA, and Lane RH. 2012. Uteroplacental insufficiency alters rat hippocampal cellular phenotype in conjunction with ErbB receptor expression. *Pediatr Res* 72(1): 2–9.

Galler JR and Ramsey F. 1989. A follow-up-study of the influence of early malnutrition on development: Behavior at home and at school. *J Am Acad Child Adolescent Psychiat* 28: 254–261.

Gardner JM, Grantham-McGregor SM, Himes J, and Chang S. 1999. Behaviour and development of stunted and nonstunted Jamaican children. *J Child Psychol Psychiatry* 40: 819–827.

Gardner JM, Walker SP, Powell CA, and Grantham-McGregor S. 2003. A randomized controlled trial of a home-visiting intervention on cognition and behavior in term low birth weight infants. *J Pediatr* 143: 634–639.

Georgieff MK. 2007. Nutrition and the developing brain: Nutrient priorities and management. *Am J Clin Nutr* 85: 614S–620S.

Georgieff MK, Brunette KE, and Tran PV. 2015. Early life nutrition and neural plasticity. *Dev Psychopathol* 27: 411–423.

Georgieff MK and Innis S. 2005. Controversial nutrients in the perinatal period that potentially affect neurodevelopment: Essential fatty acids and iron. *Pediatr Res* 57: 99R–103R.

Gertler PJ, Heckman JJ, Zanolini A et al. 2014. Labor market returns to an early childhood stimulation intervention in Jamaica. *Science* 344: 998–1001.

Gillespie S and Allen L. 2002. What works and what really works? A review of the efficacy and effectiveness of nutrition interventions. *Public Health Nutrition* 5: 513–514.

Gluckman PD and Hanson MA. 2004. Living with the past: Evolution, development, and patterns of disease. *Science* 305(5691): 1733–1736.

Gorman KS and Pollitt E. 1992. Relationship between weight and body proportionality at birth, growth during the first year of life, and cognitive development at 36, 48, and 60 months. *Infant Behav Dev* 15: 279–296.

Gottleib SJ, Biasini FJ, and Bray NW. 1998. Visual recognition memory in IUGR and normal birthweight infants. *Infant Behav Dev* 11: 223–228.

Grantham-McGregor S. 1995. A review of studies of the effect of severe malnutrition on mental development. *J Nutr* 125: 2233S–2238S.

Grantham-McGregor S, Cheung Y, Cueto S, Glewwe P, Richter L, and Strupp L. 2007. Developmental potential in the first 5 years for child in developing countries. *Lancet* 369: 60–70.

Grantham-McGregor SM, Lira PI, Ashworth A, Morris SS, and Assuncao AM. 1998. The development of low birth weight term infants and the effects of the environment in northeast Brazil. *J Pediatr* 132: 661–666.

Grantham-McGregor SM, Powell CA, Walker SP, and Himes JH. 1991. Nutritional supplementation, psychosocial stimulation, and mental development of stunted children: The Jamaican Study. *Lancet* 338: 1–5.

Graves PL. 1978. Nutrition and infant behavior: A replication study in the Katmandu Valley, Nepal. *Am J Clin Nutr* 31: 541–551.

Hamadani JD, Tofail F, Huda SN et al. 2014. Cognitive deficit and poverty in the first 5 years of childhood in Bangladesh. *Pediatrics* 134: e1001–e1008.

Hanson MA and Gluckman PD. 2014. Early developmental conditioning of later health and disease: Physiology or pathophysiology? *Physiol Rev* 94(4): 1027–1076.

Hay WW Jr. 1994. Placental transport of nutrients to the fetus. *Horm Res* 42(4–5): 215–222.

Hay WW Jr., Raju TN, Higgins RD, Kalhan SC, and Devaskar SU. 2009. Knowledge gaps and research needs for understanding and treating neonatal hypoglycemia: Workshop report from Eunice Kennedy Shriver National Institute of Child Health and Human Development. *J Pediatr* 155: 612–617.

Hoddinott J, Maluccio JA, Behrman JR, Flores R, and Martorell R. 2008. Effect of a nutrition intervention during early childhood on economic productivity in Guatemalan adults. *Lancet* 371: 411–416.

Huang C, Martorell R, Ren A, and Li Z. 2012. Cognition and behavioural development in early childhood: The role of birth weight and postnatal growth. *Int J Epidemiol* 42: 160–171.

Huddy CLJ, Johnson A, and Hope PL. 2001. Educational and behavioural problems in babies of 32–35 weeks gestation. *Arch Dis Child Fetal Neonatal Ed* 85: F23–F28.

Husaini MA, Karyadi L, Husaini YK, Sandjaja, Karyadi D, and Pollitt E. 1991. Developmental effects of short-term supplementary feeding in nutritionally-at-risk Indonesian infants. *Am J Clin Nutr* 54: 799–804.

Jewell JL, Kim YC, Russell RC, Yu FX, Park HW, Plouffe SW, Tagliabracci VS, and Guan KL. 2015. Metabolism. Differential regulation of mTORC1 by leucine and glutamine. *Science* 347(6218): 194–198.

Johnson M. 2005. Sensitive periods in functional brain development: Problems and prospects. *Dev Psychobiol* 46: 287–292.

Kariger PK, Stoltzfus RJ, Olney D et al. 2005. Iron deficiency and physical growth predict attainment of walking but not crawling in poorly nourished Zanzibari infants. *J Nutr* 135: 814–819.

Khan JY, Rajakumar RA, McNight RA, Devaskar UP, and Devaskar SU. 1999. Developmental regulation of genes mediating murine brain glucose uptake. *Am J Physiol* 276: R892–R900.

Kretchmer N, Beard JL, and Carlson S. 1996. The role of nutrition in the development of normal cognition. *Am J Clin Nutr* 63: 997S–1001S.

Kuklina EV, Ramakrishnan U, Stein AD, Barnhart HH, and Martorell R. 2004. Growth and diet quality are associated with the attainment of walking in rural Guatemalan infants. *J Nutr* 134: 3296–3300.

Kuklina EV, Ramakrishnan U, Stein AD, Barnhart HH, and Martorell R. 2006. Early childhood growth and development in rural Guatemala. *Early Hum Dev* 82: 425–433.

Kuzawa CW. 1998. Adipose tissue in human infancy and childhood: An evolutionary perspective. *Am J Phys Anthropol* Suppl 27: 177–209.

Larque E, Ruiz-Palacios M, and Koetzko B. 2013. Placental regulation of fetal nutrient supply. *Curr Opin Clin Nutr Metab Care* 16(3): 292–297.

Latal-Hajnal B, von Siebenthal K, Kovari H et al. 2003. Postnatal growth in VLBW infants: Significant association with neurodevelopmental outcome. *J Pediatr* 143(2): 163–167.

Lee K-H, Kalikoglu A, Ye P, and D'Ercole AJ. 1999. Insulin-like growth factor-1 (1GF-1) ameliorates and 1GF binding protein-1 (1GFBP-1) exacerbates the effects of undernutrition on brain growth during early postnatal life: Studies in 1GF-1 and 1GFBP-1 transgenic mice. *Pediatr Res* 45: 331–336.

Li H, DiGirolamo AM, Barnhart HX, Stein AD, and Martorell R. 2004. Relative importance of birth size and postnatal growth for women's educational achievement. *Early Hum Dev* 76: 1–16.

Liu X, Sun Z, Neiderhiser JM, Uchiyama M, and Okawa M. 2001. Low birth weight, developmental milestones, and behavioral problems in Chinese children and adolescents. *Psychiat Res* 101: 115–129.

Low JA and Galbraith RS. 1974. Pregnancy characteristics of intrauterine growth retardation. *Obstet Gynecol* 44: 122–126.

Mallard C, Loeliger M, Copolov D, and Rees S. 2000. Reduced number of neurons in the hippocampus and the cerebellum in the postnatal guinea-pig following intrauterine growth-restriction. *Neuroscience* 100(2): 327–333.

Martorell R, Horta BL, Adair LS et al. 2010. Weight gain in the first two years of life is an important predictor of schooling outcomes in pooled analyses from five birth cohorts from low- and middle-income countries. *J Nutr* 140(2): 348–354.

Martorell R, Rivera J, Kaplowitz J, and Pollitt E. 1992. Long term consequences of growth retardation during early childhood. In: Hernandez M and Argenta J (eds.), *Human Growth: Basic and Clinical Aspects*. Amsterdam, the Netherlands: Elsevier, pp. 143–149.

Mendez MA and Adair LS. 1999. Severity and timing of stunting in the first two years of life affect performance on cognitive tests in late childhood. *J Nutr* 129: 1555–1562.

Miller LC, Kierman MT, Mathers MI et al. 1995. Developmental and nutritional status of internationally adopted children. *Arch Pediatr Adolesc Med* 149: 40–44.

Monk C, Georgieff MK, and Osterholm EA. 2013. Research review: Maternal prenatal distress and poor nutrition – Mutually influencing risk factors affecting infant neurocognitive development. *J Child Psychol Psychiatry Allied Discipl* 54: 115–130.

Moore H, Craft TK, Grimaldi LM, Babic B, Brunelli SA, and Vannucci SJ. 2010. Moderate recurrent hypoglycemia during early development leads to persistent changes in affective behavior in the rat. *Brain Behav Immun* 24: 839–849.

Mora JO, Clement JR, Christiansen NE, Ortiz N, Vuori L, and Wagner M. 1979. Nutritional supplementation, early stimulation and child development. In: Brozek J (ed.), *Behavioural Effects of Energy and Protein Deficits*. Washington, DC: DHEW NIH Pub 79–1906, pp. 255–269.

Morgane PJ, Mokler DJ, and Galler JR. 2002. Effects of prenatal protein malnutrition on the hippocampal formation. *Neurosci Biobehav Rev* 26: 471–483.

Nishijima M. 1986. Somatomedin-C as a fetal growth promoting factor and amino acid composition of cord blood in Japanese neonates. *J Perinatol Med* 14: 163–166.

Pfister KM, Gray HL, Miller NC et al. 2013. An exploratory study of the relationship of fat-free mass to speed of brain processing in preterm infants. *Pediatr Res* 74(5): 576–583.

Pinto F, Onofrj M, Mancinelli R, Garzetti GG, Masini L, and Bellati U. 1981. A follow-up electrophysiological study of rats with poor intrauterine fetal growth: The development of visual evoked responses (VERs). *Experientia* 37(7): 724–726.

Pollitt E and Gorman KS. 1994. Nutritional deficiencies as developmental risk factors. In: Nelson CA (ed.), *Threats to Optimal Development: The Minnesota Symposia on Child Psychology*, Vol. 27. Hillsdale, NJ: Erlbaum Associates, pp. 121–144.

Pollitt E, Gorman KS, Engle PL, Martorell R, and Rivera J. 1993. Early supplementary feeding and cognition: Effects over two decades. *Monogr Soc Res Child Dev* 58: 1–99.

Pollitt E, Gorman KS, Engle PL, Rivera JA, and Martorell R. 1995. Nutrition in early life and the fulfillment of intellectual potential. *J Nutr* 125(Suppl): 1111S–1118S.

Pollitt E and Schurch B. 2000. Developmental pathways of the malnourished child. Results of a supplementation trial in Indonesia. *Eur J Clin Nutr* 54 (Suppl 2): 2–113.

Pollitt E, Watkins WE, and Husaini MA. 1997. Three-month nutritional supplementation in Indonesian infants and toddlers benefits memory function 8 y later. *Am J Clin Nutr* 66: 1357–1363.

Pongcharoen T, Ramakrishnan U, DiGirolamo AM et al. 2012. Influence of prenatal and postnatal growth on intellectual functioning in school-aged children. *Arch Pediatr Adolesc Med* 166(5): 411–416.

Prins A. 2011. The brain–gut interaction: the conversation and the implications. *S Afr J Clin Nutr* 24: s8–s14.

Prins ML. 2008. Cerebral metabolic adaptation and ketone metabolism after brain injury. *J Cereb Blood Flow Metab* 28: 1–16.

Pylipow M, Spector LG, Puumala SE, Boys C, Cohen J, and Georgieff MK. 2009. Early postnatal weight gain, intellectual performance, and body mass index (BMI) at seven years of age in term infants with intrauterine growth-restriction (IUGR). *J Pediatr* 154(2): 201–206.

Ramel SE, Brown LD, and Georgieff MK. 2014. The impact of neonatal illness on nutritional requirements-one size does not fit all. *Curr Pediatr Rep* 2: 248–254.

Ramel SE, Demerath EW, Gray HL et al. 2012. The relationship of poor linear growth velocity with neonatal illness and two year neurodevelopment in preterm infants. *Neonatology* 102: 19–24.

Rao R, Ennis K, Long JD, Ugurbil K, Gruetter R, and Tkac I. 2010. Neurochemical changes in the developing rat hippocampus during prolonged hypoglycemia. *J Neurochem* 114: 728–738.

Reid MV, Murray KA, Marsh ED, Golden JA, Simmons RA, and Grinspan JB. 2012. Delayed myelination in an intrauterine growth retardation model is mediated by oxidative stress upregulating bone morphogenetic protein 4. *J Neuropathol Exp Neurol* 71(7): 640–653.

Richardson SA, Birch HG, Grabie E, and Yoder K. 1972. The behavior of children in school who were severely malnourished in the first two years of life. *J Health Soc Behav* 13: 276–284.

Sabet F, Richter LM, Ramchandani PG, Stein A, Quigley MA, and Norris SA. 2009. Low birthweight and subsequent emotional and behavioural outcomes in 12-year-old children in Soweto, South Africa: Findings from birth to twenty. *Int J Epidemiol* 38: 944–954.

Santos DN, Assis AM, Bastos AC et al. 2008. Determinants of cognitive function in childhood: A cohort study in a middle income context. *BMC Public Health* 8: 202.

Schober ME, McKnight RA, Yu X, Callaway CW, Ke X, and Lane RH. 2009. Intrauterine growth restriction due to uteroplacental insufficiency decreased white matter and altered NMDAR subunit composition in juvenile rat hippocampi. *Am J Physiol Regul Integr Comp Physiol* 296(3): R681–R692.

Schroeder D, Martorell R, Rivera J, Ruel M, and Habicht J. 1995. Age differences in the impact of nutritional supplementation on growth. *J Nutr* 125(4 Suppl): 1051S–1059S.

Sherin A, Anu J, Peeyush KT, Smijin S, Anitha M, Roshni BT, and Paulose CS. 2012. Cholinergic and GABAergic receptor functional deficit in the hippocampus of insulin-induced hypoglycemic and streptozotocin-induced diabetic rats. *Neuroscience* J202: 69–76.

Siegel EH, Stoltzfus RJ, Kariger PK et al. 2005. Growth indices, anemia, and diet independently predict motor milestone acquisition of infants in South Central Nepal. *J Nutr* 135: 2840–2844.

Spinello A, Stronati M, Ometto A et al. 1993. Infant neurodevelopmental outcome in pregnancies complicated by gestational hypertension and intra-uterine growth retardation. *J Perinat Med* 21: 195–203.

Stein AD, Wang M, DiGirolamo A et al. 2008. Nutritional supplementation in early childhood, schooling, and intellectual functioning in adulthood: A prospective study in Guatemala. *Arch Pediatr Adolesc Med* 162: 612–618.

Strauss RS. 2000. Adult functional outcome of those born small for gestational age: Twenty-six-year follow-up of the 1970 British Birth Cohort. *JAMA* 283: 625–632.

Strauss RS and Dietz WH. 1998. Growth and development of term children born with low birth weight: Effects of genetic and environmental factors. *J Pediatr* 133: 67–72.

Susser E, Neugebauer R, Hoek HW et al. 1996. Schizophrenia after prenatal famine: Further evidence. *Arch Gen Psychiatry* 53: 25–31.

Tofail F, Persson LA, El Arifeen S et al. 2008. Effects of prenatal food and micronutrient supplementation on infant development: A randomized trial from the Maternal and Infant Nutrition Interventions, Matlab (MINIMat) study. *Am J Clin Nutr* 87: 704–711.

Turner CP, Blackburn MR, and Rivkees SA. 2004. A1 adenosine receptors mediate hypoglycemia-induced neuronal injury. *J Mol Endocrinol* 32(1): 129–144.

Uauy R and Dangour AD. 2006. Nutrition in brain development and aging: Role of essential fatty acids. *Nutr Rev* 64(5 Pt 2): S24–S33; discussion S72–S91.

United Nations Children's Fund, World Health Organization, The World Bank, UNICEF-WHO-World Bank Joint Child Malnutrition Estimates, 2014.

Waber DP, Vuori-Christiansen L, Ortiz N et al. 1981. Nutritional supplementation, maternal education, and cognitive development of infants at risk of malnutrition. *Am J Clin Nutr* 34: 807–813.

Wachs TD, Georgieff M, Cusick S, and McEwen B. 2014. Issues in the timing of integrated early interventions: Contributions from nutrition, neuroscience and psychological research. *Ann NY Acad Sci* 1308: 89–106.

Walker SP, Chang SM, Powell CA, and Grantham-McGregor SM. 2004. Psychosocial intervention improves the development of term low-birth-weight infants. *J Nutr* 134: 1417–1423.

Walker SP, Chang SM, Powell CA, and Grantham-McGregor SM. 2005. Effects of early childhood psychosocial stimulation and nutritional supplementation on cognition and education in growth-stunted Jamaican children: Prospective cohort study. *Lancet* 366: 1804–1807.

Walker SP, Chang SM, Powell CA, Simonoff E, and Grantham-McGregor SM. 2007. Early childhood stunting is associated with poor psychological functioning in late adolescence and effects are reduced by psychosocial stimulation. *J Nutr* 137: 2464–2469.

Walker SP, Chang SM, Younger N, and Grantham-McGregor SM. 2010. The effect of psychosocial stimulation on cognition and behaviour at 6 years in a cohort of term, low-birthweight Jamaican children. *Dev Med Child Neurol* 52: e148–e154.

Walker SP, Wachs TD, Grantham-McGregor S et al. 2011. Inequality in early childhood: Risk and protective factors for early child development. *Lancet* 378: 1325–1338.

Wang WL, Sung YT, Sung FC, Lu TH, Kuo SC, and Li CY. 2008. Low birth weight, prematurity, and paternal social status: Impact on the basic competence test in Taiwanese adolescents. *J Pediatr* 153: 333–338.

Wiggins RC, Fuller G, and Enna SJ. 1984. Undernutrition and the development of brain neurotransmitter systems. *Life Sci* 35: 2085–2094.

Winer EK and Tejani N. 1994. Four to seven year evaluation in two groups of small for gestational age infants. In: Tejani N (ed.), *Obstetric Events and Developmental Sequelae*, 2nd edn. Boca Raton, FL: CRC Press, pp. 77–94.

Wullschleger S, Loewith R, and Hall MN. 2006. TOR signaling in growth and metabolism. *Cell* 124: 471–484.

Xie L, Antonow-Schlorke I, Schwab M, McDonald TJ, Nathanielsz PW, and Li C. 2013. The frontal cortex IGF system is down regulated in the term intrauterine growth restricted fetal baboon. *Growth Horm IGF Res* 23(5): 187–192.

Yamada KA, Rensing N, Izumi Y, De Erausquin GA, Gazit V, Dorsey DA, and Herrera DG. 2004. Repetitive hypoglycemia in young rats impairs hippocampal long-term potentiation. *Pediatr Res* 55: 372–379.

Yan H and Rivkees SA. 2006. Hypoglycemia influences oligodendrocyte development and myelin formation. *Neuroreport* 17(1): 55–59.

Yehuda S, Rabinovitz S, and Mostofsky DI. 1998. Modulation of learning and neuronal membrane composition in the rat by essential fatty acid preparation: Time-course analysis. *Neurochem Res* 23(5): 627–634.

Yehuda S, Rabinovitz S, and Mostofsky DI. 2005. Essential fatty acids and the brain: From infancy to aging. *Neurobiol Aging* 26(Suppl 1): 98–102.

Zheng X, Liang Y, He Q, Yao R, Bao W, Bao L, Wang Y, and Wang Z. 2014. Current models of mammalian target of rapamycin complex 1 (mTORC1) by leucine and glutamine. *Int J Mol Sci* 15(11): 20753–20769.

3 Long-Chain Polyunsaturated Fatty Acids and Their Influence on the Developing Brain

Lotte Lauritzen, Laurine B.S. Harsløf, Louise B. Sørensen, and Camilla T. Damsgaard

CONTENTS

3.1 INTRODUCTION

The essentiality of n-3 polyunsaturated fatty acids (PUFAs) was recognized in 1960–1980, that is, much later than the discovery of the essentiality of n-6 PUFAs. This was due to the more subtle symptoms of n-3 PUFA deficiency related to neurological outcomes, which are hard to detect and test compared to the presence of scaly skin seen with n-6 PUFA deficiency. Therefore, the study of actual functional effects of dietary n-3 PUFA has progressed slowly. Although highly promising, the field is still at a stage where we cannot draw definite conclusions about the importance of n-3 PUFA, let alone determine the ranges of optimal intakes with respect to dose and specific types of n-3 PUFA at different ages.

The first studies about the functional effects of n-3 PUFA focused on the development of visual acuity in breastfed versus formula-fed infants and on randomized controlled trials in infants that were supplied with formulas with higher or lower amounts of α-linolenic acid (18:3n-3, ALA) or with or without n-3 long-chain PUFA (LCPUFA), mainly docosahexaenoic acid (22:6n-3, DHA). The hypothesis for an effect of n-3 PUFAs on visual acuity is based on the extraordinary high DHA content in the outer disc membranes of the retina, which can be as high as 50% of the phospholipid fatty acids (FAs), and the unique existence of di-DHA phospholipids (Lauritzen et al. 2001). Also, compared to the testing of cognitive outcomes, visual acuity is relatively easy to test by means of Teller acuity cards or visual evoked potentials in the visual cortex. Meta-analyses (SanGiovanni et al. 2000a,b) and meta-regression analyses indicate a direct linear association between DHA intake and early development of visual acuity (Lauritzen et al. 2001; Uauy et al. 2003), although this has not been fully confirmed in randomized controlled trials (Birch et al. 2010). Many of the studies on visual acuity indicate that the effect is transient, that is, dietary DHA advances the development of visual acuity by a few weeks and unsupplemented infants catch up within the first year of life (Birch et al. 2007). However, few studies have done any follow-up later in childhood.

During the 1990s and the beginning of the new millennium came the testing of effects of n-3 LCPUFA on cognitive development and intelligence quotient (IQ). These studies were based on the well-recognized effect of breastfeeding on IQ (Horta & Victoria 2013) and the hypothesis that this may be at least partially due to LCPUFA in breast milk. The rationale is that there may be a specific need for dietary preformed LCPUFA in the perinatal period – that is, they are conditionally essential nutrients in infancy. Randomized controlled trials investigating the potential effects of LCPUFA addition to infant formulas were first conducted mainly in preterm infants. The assumptions were that these infants were more vulnerable as the intrauterine phase of brain and adipose tissue development is shorter and that LCPUFA synthesis is less mature. However, the latter appears not to be true, as LCPUFA synthesis in neonates has in fact been shown to decrease with increasing gestational age (Uauy et al. 2000). Furthermore, while the field evolved to test effects in term infants, the circumstances of hypothesis testing changed as increasing amounts of n-3 PUFA were now found in standard infant formulas. No studies have compared the effects of LCPUFA on neurodevelopment in preterm and term infants or the effect of LCPUFA supplementation during later stages of infancy or childhood on neurodevelopmental outcomes.

This chapter will focus on the potential effects of LCPUFA intake on cognitive, mental, and behavioural outcomes in term infants – although we will include results from large studies in preterm infants when relevant and compare results from meta-analyses in term and preterm infants. Most studies have looked at the immediate effects – that is, the effect at the end of intervention and before 2 years of age, but the major question is whether early intake has a long-term programming effect on cognitive and mental abilities past infancy. Other important issues to be addressed are the potential differential effects of arachidonic acid (20:4n-6, AA) and DHA as well as potential modifying effects of sex.

3.2 PERINATAL SUPPLY AND EFFECTS ON BRAIN FATTY ACID COMPOSITION OF DIETARY AA VERSUS DHA

The two main LCPUFAs of the n-3 and n-6 PUFA families, DHA and AA, are present in cell membranes of all tissues. However, DHA is especially high in central nervous system structures, whereas AA is more ubiquitously distributed among all tissues of the body. The LCPUFA content of membranes is affected by intake as well as endogenous synthesis of AA and DHA from linoleic acid (LA, 18:2n-6) and ALA, respectively. This synthesis is mediated via elongases and desaturases. The key regulatory and limiting enzyme in these pathways is delta-6-desaturase, which is involved twice to generate DHA but only once in the production of AA (Lauritzen et al. 2001). This difference between the two PUFA families leads to a general difference in the impact of diet on the membrane LCPUFA content – the AA content changes little with changing intake of LA or AA, whereas the DHA content varies with diet. In the early 1990s, when infant formulas contained no LCPUFA, Makrides et al. compared postnatal increases in the central nervous system LCPUFA content between breastfed and formula-fed infants. They found an increase in the brain DHA content of breastfed infants but not among formula-fed infants. In contrast, no differences between the groups were seen in brain AA content, which accumulated rapidly in both formula-fed and breastfed infants (Makrides et al. 1994).

Both DHA and AA are present in breast milk. The amounts depend on maternal diet (this mainly concerns DHA) and on genetic variation in the fatty acid desaturase (*FADS*) gene cluster, which among other encodes the delta-6-desaturase (this mainly concerns AA). Breast milk LCPUFA levels, that is, the absolute quantities of DHA and AA, seem to be quite stable throughout lactation (Marangoni et al. 2000) but with a high degree of variability in the ratio of DHA to AA in individual breast milk samples. This variability is mainly due to variations in the content of DHA in breast milk, which spans from 0.2 to 1.0 percent of the fatty acids (FA%), whereas the mean content of AA in breast milk is similar across studies and countries, typically around 0.4–0.5 FA% (Brenna et al. 2007). We supplied fish oil to lactating mothers and found positive correlations between mothers and infants in the DHA content of erythrocyte membranes (a general marker of tissue DHA status), whereas erythrocyte AA proportion showed no correlation (Lauritzen & Carlson 2011). This difference indicates a mutual dependence in mothers and infants on maternal DHA intake, whereas AA levels seem to be determined by the capacity for endogenous synthesis.

In line with this, studies on the effects of single nucleotide polymorphisms (SNPs) in the *FADS* gene cluster in mothers and infants generally find genotype-dependent AA levels in tissues and breast milk, whereas DHA is little affected. Minor allele homozygotes of various *FADS* SNPs have been shown to have lower erythrocytes and plasma levels of AA and higher levels of LA and ALA during pregnancy (Koletzko et al. 2011; Xie & Innis 2008). Findings in plasma from mothers and neonates also show strong inverse associations between the presence of minor alleles of individual *FADS* SNPs and concentrations of AA (Steer et al. 2012). These studies furthermore suggest that neonates have a greater capacity to synthesize AA compared to DHA, although some DHA synthesis was observed as well (Steer et al. 2012). Curiously, a study of 2000 cord blood samples showed that minor allele *FADS* SNPs in mothers gave rise to increased levels of LA and di-homo γ-linolenic acid, whereas minor allele SNPs in their children resulted in increased levels of AA and other n-6 LCPUFA (Lattka et al. 2013). The content of AA and DHA in colostrum has also been found to be lower in minor allele carriers of a number of *FADS* SNPs compared to wild type (Morales et al. 2011). Two recent studies confirm the different regulation of AA and DHA in mature breast milk, indicating that AA is affected by the genetic pattern in the *FADS* gene cluster (Lattka et al. 2011) and that breast milk AA is less sensitive than DHA to dietary LCPUFA supplementation (van Goor et al. 2009).

Most studies on the effect of *FADS* SNPs on the fatty acid composition of blood and breast milk have examined the effect of individual SNPs one at a time. However, it is plausible that desaturase activity will depend on the overall SNP profile in the *FADS* gene cluster. The SNPs are to some extent more or less intercorrelated and vary in frequency. It is therefore expected that analyses based on individual SNPs will reflect the effect of the most frequent SNPs with the strongest effects on desaturase activity and that statistical adjustment for these more prominent SNPs would be needed to determine the true effect of other SNPs in the *FADS* cluster. The use of tag SNPs that by high linkage disequilibrium represents several other SNPs can simplify the complexity of analyzing numerous individual *FADS* SNPs in one model. In such a multiple *FADS* SNP statistical allele model including three relatively frequent tag SNPs (rs1535, rs174448, and rs174575), we recently found that *FADS* polymorphisms contributed substantially (i.e. as much as breastfeeding and fish intake) to DHA levels in erythrocytes of 9-month-old infants (Harsløf et al. 2013). Also, contrary to the general assumption that minor alleles in *FADS* SNPs down-regulate DHA production, we found that the minor allele of rs1535 up-regulated the DHA content of erythrocytes. However, as expected, the minor alleles of all three investigated tag SNPs consistently lowered erythrocyte AA (Jensen et al. 2014). Interestingly, identical analyses did not reveal any effect of these three tag SNPs on erythrocyte DHA status at 3 years of age, which could be explained by increased residual variation in the model due to a more diverse fish intake or could be interpreted as differential determinants of DHA status at different developmental stages due to differences in the endogenous LCPUFA synthesis. Furthermore, a longitudinal study found weaker correlations of serum phospholipid n-6 LCPUFA between 2 and 6 years of age in children, who were homozygous for the major allele of various *FADS* SNPs, compared to carriers of at least one minor allele (Steer et al. 2010). In contrast, tracking of n-3 LCPUFA levels was highest in the major allele carriers.

The low dietary sensitivity of tissue AA and predominant dependence on endogenous synthesis capacity suggests that dietary AA may be of little importance in relation to cognitive development, and we will therefore in the following focus on the role of dietary DHA.

3.3 EFFECT OF DIETARY n-3 LCPUFA ON INFANT DEVELOPMENT: RESULTS OF CLINICAL TRIALS

Many observational studies have shown that the cognitive abilities of breastfed and formula-fed infants differ from the first year of life to early adulthood. Combined analyses of these studies indicate that breastfeeding is associated with an IQ benefit of around 3–4 points (Horta & Victoria 2013). There are of course numerous differences between breastfed and formula-fed infants that may explain this difference – socio-economic and biological. However, most of the studies were performed before 2000, when no LCPUFAs were added to infant formula and the lack of dietary DHA in formula could therefore in theory contribute to the cognitive differences.

Over the past three decades, a number of studies have investigated the importance of dietary DHA for the development of cognitive function in infants. The first studies compared the development in preterm infants who received infant formulas with and without added fish oil, and similar studies have subsequently been performed in term infants. These studies generally had large differences in the duration of the intervention period from only a few weeks in the neonatal ward in some of the preterm infant studies (Uauy et al. 1990) to study the entire first year of life (Birch et al. 2010). The first studies among preterm infants provided relatively large doses of n-3 LCPUFA from fish oil (i.e. EPA and DHA in concentrations of approximately 1 FA%) (Carlson et al. 1993; Uauy et al. 1990), whereas the later trials in term infants used pure DHA in combination with AA in doses of around 0.1–0.3 and 0.4–0.6 FA%, respectively (Auestad et al. 2001; Birch et al. 2010; Bouwstra et al. 2005; Morris et al. 2000). As results accumulated to indicate that early n-3 PUFA intake improved visual development and that it might also affect cognitive development, the standard infant formulas evolved towards higher n-3 PUFA contents (from 0.5 in the early studies towards 2.5 FA% [Lauritzen et al. 2001]) and addition of LCPUFA became the norm. Furthermore, a number of studies have supplied infants with DHA indirectly via fish oil or pure DHA supplements to pregnant and/or lactating mothers. These design differences along with numerous other differences between studies – including cultural background and habitual PUFA intake – complicate systematic reviews and meta-analyses. Thus, the evaluation of the overall evidence for a beneficial effect of DHA is not straightforward.

In addition to differences in dose, mode, and timing of the intervention, studies also differ with respect to how and when they assessed the potential effect on cognitive outcomes. Usually, trials assess the effect within the first 2 years of life, but a few studies have been able to follow up on effects later in childhood (Campoy et al. 2011; Cheatham et al. 2011; de Jong et al. 2011; Helland et al. 2008). Many of the studies have used clinically accepted tests of infant development such as the Bayley Scales. However, a number of experimental tests of more specific cognitive functions such as habituation, attention, and problem-solving have also been employed. The use of infant development scales such as the Bayley Scales has been debated as these were developed mainly for identifying children with developmental delays and thus may not be sensitive enough to examine differences between normally developing children (Cheatham et al. 2006). Many of the more specific tests were designed for testing differences in a certain skill at one specific age – typically the age at which the particular skill develops – and therefore cannot be used in longitudinal studies. Furthermore, there are gaps in our knowledge about infant development and the specific test can be hard to interpret in terms of their ability to predict long-term cognitive function and as to whether a certain effect is beneficial or detrimental. Moreover, although a test is designed for testing a specific function, one cannot be certain that the result actually reflects the child's ability to perform that task or if other parameters interfere. For example, language tests, which require the child to make a response to show that he or she understands, could be influenced by the child's overall willingness to interact and answer. Questions meant to determine social skills could be influenced by basic personality traits such as introversion and extroversion.

Meta-analyses of all randomized controlled trials, which have supplemented infant formulas with LCPUFA and investigated neurodevelopmental outcomes during the first 2 years of life, have not shown any statistically significant benefit on the Bayley Scales in either term or preterm infants (Schulzke et al. 2011; Simmer et al. 2011) (Table 3.1). However, a meta-analysis that combined LCPUFA formula supplementation trials in term and preterm infants found a trend for a beneficial effect on the Bayley Mental Development Index at around 12 months of age (Qawasmi et al. 2012) (Table 3.1). This meta-analysis did not find any effect of prematurity on the efficacy of LCPUFA supplementation. Nor did it find a clear effect of the dose of LCPUFA, although there was a trend towards a dose effect for DHA, but not for AA (Qawasmi et al. 2012). Meta-analyses looking at the developmental effects of n-3 LCPUFA supplementation during pregnancy and lactation have suggested some effects on infant neurodevelopment, but this was based on very few studies (Delgado-Noguera et al. 2010; Gould et al. 2013). It should be noted that the age of neurodevelopmental examination varied across trials, and the effects in the first years of life may differ from the effects later in childhood. Such methodological aspects may contribute to the lack of firm conclusions regarding the effects of dietary DHA on neurodevelopmental outcomes in these meta-analyses. However, a very large Australian trial with maternal DHA supplementation, the DINO trial in preterm infants (Makrides et al. 2009), showed reductions in the proportion of children with mental delays, which was also shown after prenatal maternal supplementation in the DOMInO trial (Makrides et al. 2010). In the DINO trial, the effect was most pronounced in infants with low birthweight. A 2.5-year follow-up of the DOMInO trial also showed a beneficial of DHA on the number of looks away from toys in a multiple object attention test (Gould et al. 2014), thus indicating that early DHA supply might have long-term impact.

3.4 STUDIES OF FATTY ACID DESATURASE POLYMORPHISM AND COGNITIVE OUTCOMES IN CHILDREN

Applying current knowledge about the genetic control of LCPUFA synthesis is an alternative way to derive information about the potential effects of dietary preformed LCPUFA in the perinatal period on cognitive development. It is hypothesized that minor allele carriers of SNPs in the fatty acid desaturase (*FADS*) gene cluster are carriers of the mutant genotype with impaired desaturase activity and thus lower LCPUFA synthesis – in line with the results of most studies that examine blood LCPUFA levels, as previously described. Few studies have investigated the effect of *FADS* SNPs on cognitive development, emotions, and behaviour. One study explored associations between attention-deficit hyperactivity disorder (ADHD) and polymorphisms in the *FADS* genes and found a significant association between ADHD and the SNP (Brookes et al. 2006). Two other *FADS* SNPs were associated with ADHD in the context of prenatal alcohol exposure.

TABLE 3.1
Effect of Early Dietary Long-Chain Polyunsaturated Fatty Acids on Cognitive Development in Infants: Results from Large Individual Randomized Controlled Trials and Meta-Analyses of Randomized Controlled Trials

References	RCT Type	Infants	DHA (FA%)	AA (FA%)	Results
Schulzke et al. (2011)	*Meta-analysis* Formula ± LCPUFA	n = 858 Preterm (7 RCT)	0.05–0.76 versus 0	0.04–1.10 (1 RCT 0) versus 0	No significant difference in Bayley MDI at 12 months (4 RCT) or 18 months (3 RCT), but heterogeneity (I^2 = 71%) at 12 months.
Simmer et al. (2011)	*Meta-analysis* Formula ± LCPUFA	n = 986 Term (9 RCT)	0.13–0.35 versus 0	0.34–0.72 (1 RCT 0 and 2 RCT also 0) versus 0	No significant difference in Bayley MDI at 3 months (1 RCT), 6 months (2RCT), 12 months (3 RCT), 18 months (4 RCT) or 24 months (1 RCT), but heterogeneity (I^2 = 75%) at 18 months.
Qawasmi et al. (2012)	*Meta-analysis* Formula ± LCPUFA	n = 1802 Term and preterm (6 + 6 RCT)	0.05–0.50	0.04–0.72 (2 RCT also 0)	No Bayley MDI difference ~12 months (WMD = 1.1 [−0.1;2.4], p = 0.06). Heterogeneity (I^2 = 54%), but efficacy was not affected by prematurity or LCPUFA dose (dose–response analysis DHA: β = 8.9 and AA: β = −0.3).
Makrides et al. (2009)	Maternal n-3 LCPUFA supplement (from birth to term date)	n = 657 Preterm	1.0 versus 0.2–0.3 in breast milk (or formula)	0.6 in breast milk (unchanged)	No overall difference in MDI at 18 months, but in girls ↑ and mental delay (score < 85) ↓.
Delgado-Noguera et al. (2010)	*Meta-analysis* Maternal n-3 LCPUFA supplement (mainly postnatal, but 1 RCT also prenatal)	n = 939 Term (4 RCT)	0.4–1.3 versus 0.2–0.4 in breast milk	0.3–0.5 versus 0.4–0.5 in breast milk	No significant difference in IQ or problem-solving at 12 months (2 RCT, I^2 = 37%) or 24 months (2 RCT, I^2 = 88%), Bayley MDI at 2 years (2 RCT, I^2 = 47%), language development after 2 years (2RCT, I^2 = 60%), but a significant effect on attention after 2 years (1 RCT).

(*Continued*)

TABLE 3.1 (*Continued*)
Effect of Early Dietary Long-Chain Polyunsaturated Fatty Acids on Cognitive Development in Infants: Results from Large Individual Randomized Controlled Trials and Meta-Analyses of Randomized Controlled Trials

References	RCT Type	Infants	DHA (FA%)	AA (FA%)	Results
Gould et al. (2013)	*Meta-analysis* Maternal n-3 LCPUFA supplement (during pregnancy and most trials also lactation)	n = 5272 (8 RCT)	0.2–2.2 g/day (n-3 LCPUFA in total 0.3–3.3 g/day)	None supplied	No significant effect on standardized scales of IQ 1, 1–2, or 7 years, but a significant improvement at 2–5 years (WMD = 3.9[0.8;7.1], $p = 0.01$, $I^2 = 0\%$) (1–2 RCT per age)

Notes: AA, arachidonic acid; DHA, docosahexaenoic acid; FA%, % of fatty acids in infant formula or breast milk; IQ, intelligence (developmental) quotient; MDI, Mental Developmental Index on the Bayley Scales; RCT, randomized controlled trial; WMD, weighted mean difference.

Several studies have shown that infant *FADS* genotype, examined by the use of different individual SNPs, modifies the effect of breastfeeding on IQ-like neurodevelopmental outcomes in childhood (Caspi et al. 2007; Martin et al. 2011; Morales et al. 2011; Steer et al. 2010) (Table 3.2). Although results are somewhat inconsistent, the highest IQ scores were obtained in children that were breastfed, and in the case of differences between breastfed children, the highest IQ scores were found in those with at least one major allele. Furthermore, across all the studies those with the lowest IQ score were formula-fed children, but only two of the studies (Martin et al. 2011; Steer et al. 2010) found the lowest scores in the homozygote minor allele carriers. In the study by Morales et al. (2011), formula-fed infants who were homozygous minor allele carriers had higher IQ than homozygous major allele carriers, and in the study by Caspi et al. (2007), they had higher IQ than the heterozygotes. In the study by Caspi et al., the difference between breastfed and formula-fed major allele carriers was seen between the two largest groups (with around 1500 individuals each). In contrast, the significant feeding group difference in the studies by Steer et al. (2010) and Morales et al. (2011) was based on a small group of formula-fed heterozygote minor and major allele carriers, respectively (with <100 subjects), resulting in an increased risk of type-2 errors. Given the variation in the year of birth of the subjects in these studies, it is reasonable to assume that there could have been differences in the PUFA composition of the formulas and presumably also in maternal fish intake, and thus the DHA content of the breast milk of the study populations. Furthermore, the studies used different *FADS* SNPs and, as indicated by the previous study from our group, they may not all down-regulate the endogenous DHA

TABLE 3.2
Results of Studies of Potential Effect Modification of the Association between Breastfeeding and Cognitive Performance Later in Life by Single Nucleotide Polymorphisms in the Fatty Acid Desaturase Gene Cluster

References	Population	Exposure *FADS* SNP and Outcome	Groups with Mean Cognition Equal to 100	Interactions between Breastfeeding and *FADS* SNP
Caspi et al. (2007)	Born in NZ 1972–1973, 57% BF (n = 1037) and UK 1994–1995, 49% BF (n = 2232)	rs174575 Wechsler IQ scale (WICS) at 7–13 years and 5 years, respectively	BF and FF mm Non-significantly higher means in BF and lower in FF MM + Mm	6–7 IQ-point increase in BF versus FF MM + Mm adj. for among other birthweight, maternal SES, and IQ ($p < 0.001$ for both and $p_{interaction} = 0.035$ and 0.018, respectively)
Steer et al. (2010)	Born in the United Kingdom 1990–1992, 83% BF (n = 5934)	rs174575 and rs1535 in infant (and mother) WICS at 8 years	BF irrespective of *FADS* genotype Non-significantly lower in FF, most pronounced in mm	4 IQ-point lower in rs174575 FF mm versus MM + Mm and 6 IQ-point reduction in FF versus BF mm adj. for among other sex, birthweight, maternal education, and SES ($p_{interaction} = 0.009$); less effect of rs1535 and no effect of maternal SNP
Steer et al. (2013)	Same as previous (n = 4403 due to missing maternal SNPs)	Multiple *FADS* SNP models including 17 maternal SNPs WICS at 8 years		Opposing effects of rs3834458 and rs174574 (in strong disequilibrium with each other) which increased IQ by 4.2 ($p = 0.002$) and decreased it by 3.7 ($p = 0.008$) IQ-points, respectively
Morales et al. (2011)	Born in Spain 1997–1998 or 2004–2006, 81% BF (n = 400 and 340, respectively)	11 *FADS* SNPs in infant (and mother) Cognitive index from McCarthy Scales of Children's Abilities at 4 years and Bayley Scale at 14 months, respectively	BF and FF mm + mM Similar or non-significantly higher in BF MM and lower in FF MM	8–9 IQ-point reduction in FF versus BF rs174468 MM adj. for among others sex, age, and maternal education ($p_{interaction} = 0.077$ and 0.020, respectively); no other replicated BF–*FADS* SNP interactions

(Continued)

TABLE 3.2 (*Continued*)
Results of Studies of Potential Effect Modification of the Association between Breastfeeding and Cognitive Performance Later in Life by Single Nucleotide Polymorphisms in the Fatty Acid Desaturase Gene Cluster

References	Population	Exposure *FADS* SNP and Outcome	Groups with Mean Cognition Equal to 100	Interactions between Breastfeeding and *FADS* SNP
Martin et al. (2011)	Adolescent twins born in AU around 1996 (n = 700)	rs174575, rs1535, and rs174583 in infant (and mother) Full-scale IQ by Multidimensional Aptitude Battery at 16 years	FF mm Non-significantly higher in all other groups	No BF–*FADS* SNP interactions (mm versus mM + MM) on IQ adj. for sex, age, birthweight, parental SES, and education (rs174575 p = 0.26).

Notes: BF, breastfed; FF, formula fed; mm, minor allele homozygotes; mM, heterozygotes; MM, major allele homozygotes; IQ, intelligence quotient; SES, socio-economic status.

synthesis in the infants (Harsløf et al. 2013). This could contribute to the observed variable associations with different *FADS* SNPs. Interestingly, Steer et al. (2013) reported the opposing effects of rs174574 and rs3834458, which in our study was found to be linked to rs1535 and to increased erythrocyte DHA levels in infants (Harsløf et al. 2013).

3.5 POTENTIAL SEX SPECIFICITY IN THE EFFECT OF DHA ON BRAIN FUNCTION

In our recent study among 3-year-olds (Jensen et al. 2014), we found that *FADS* SNPs rs1535 and rs174448 were associated with problem-solving and communication skills, assessed by the Ages and Stages Questionnaire (ASQ), in opposing directions. Moreover, the effects were found to be modified by sex. Few of the previous studies and none of the meta-analyses have examined whether the effect of n-3 LCPUFA supplementation in the perinatal period depends on sex. To our knowledge, we were the first to report sex–treatment interaction effects on cognitive outcomes in our trial of maternal fish oil supplementation during lactation (Lauritzen et al. 2005). However, when we followed up the children in later childhood, these effects were less clear (Cheatham et al. 2011). To our knowledge, only two other studies, the DINO and DOMInO trials, have differentiated between boys and girls in their statistical analyses. These too indicate that an increased early DHA supply can exert different effects on cognitive outcomes in girls and boys (Table 3.3). Interestingly, the different effects of increased DHA supply – whether provided by dietary supplementation during pregnancy or lactation or being a result of *FADS* polymorphisms – on various outcomes in girls and boys all appear to counteract the normally observed gender differences in behaviour. It could, however, appear as if there is a tendency towards

TABLE 3.3
Results of Studies with Potential Effect Modification by Sex of the Effect of Perinatal DHA Supply on Cognitive Outcomes

References	Study Design	Outcome	Control Girls	Control Boys	+DHA Girls	+DHA Boys	DHA–Gender Interaction
Jensen et al. (2014)	Healthy infants (n = 244) *FADS* SNPs rs1535, rs174448, and rs174575 combined to one variable of DHA-increasing alleles 2–3 (control) and 4–5 (+DHA)	Problem-solving	60[50,60][a]	50[45,60]	55[45,60]	55[50,60]	p = 0.013
		Communication	50[50,55]	50[50,59]	50[50,55]	50[50,50]	p = 0.005
	ASQ at 3 years – 5 outcomes (problem-solving, communication, personal and social abilities, and fine and gross motor function)	Fine motor function	55[50,60]	50[50,50]	50[50,55]	50[50,59]	p = 0.xxx in analyses with DHA-increasing alleles as a continuous variable
DOMInO Makrides et al. (2010)	Maternal supplementation with 800 mg DHA/d *vs.* vegetable oil from week 21 of pregnancy to birth Term and preterm infants (n = 726)	Cognitive score and score <85 (%)	104 ± 11[b] 3.5[2,7]	100 ± 13 9.6[7,14]	103 ± 10 1.9[1,5] RR versus control 0.5[0.2–1.5]	101 ± 12 3.5[2,7] RR versus control 0.4[0.2–0.8]	p = 0.23 p = 0.59

(Continued)

TABLE 3.3 (*Continued*)
Results of Studies with Potential Effect Modification by Sex of the Effect of Perinatal DHA Supply on Cognitive Outcomes

References	Study Design	Outcome	Control Girls	Control Boys	+DHA Girls	+DHA Boys	DHA–Gender Interaction
	Bayley MDI at 18 months – five scales (cognitive, language, motor, socio-emotional, and adaptive behaviour)	Language score and score <85	103 ± 13 7.0[5,11]	93 ± 16 27.4[23,33]	99 ± 14 12.8[9,18] RR versus control 1.8[1.1–3.1]	94 ± 13 23.2[19,29] RR versus control 0.8[0.6–1.1]	$p < 0.001$ $p = 0.009$
		Adaptive behaviour	105 ± 14	97 ± 14	101 ± 14	97 ± 13	$p = 0.020$
DINO Makrides et al. (2009)	Maternal and/or formula n-3 LCPUFA supplementation (approximate milk DHA 1 versus 0.3 FA%) from birth to term date (8–11 weeks) Preterm infants (n = 657) Bayley MDI score at 18 months	Cognitive score and score <85 (%)	94 ± 18[c] 26.0	92 ± 17 27.8	99 ± 14 11.0 RR versus control 0.4[0.2–0.8]	91 ± 17 27.4 RR versus control 1.0[0.7–1.5]	$p = 0.04$ $p = 0.02$
Lauritzen et al. (2005)	Maternal supplementation with 1.5 g/day n-3 LCPUFA versus olive oil for the first 4 months of lactation	Intention score in problem test (0–12)	3.7 ± 2.5[d]	4.9 ± 3.6	5.7 ± 2.7	3.9 ± 3.1	$p = 0.026$

(*Continued*)

TABLE 3.3 (*Continued*)
Results of Studies with Potential Effect Modification by Sex of the Effect of Perinatal DHA Supply on Cognitive Outcomes

References	Study Design	Outcome	Control Girls	Control Boys	+DHA Girls	+DHA Boys	DHA–Gender Interaction
	Term infants (n = 150)	Comprehension at 1 year (no. of words)	64 ± 42	77 ± 47	68 ± 37	44 ± 34	p = 0.034
	Problem-solving by infant planning test at 9 months (2 outcome), Communication by MacArthur CDI at 1 and 2 years (6 and 7 outcomes, respectively)	Sentence complexity at 2 years (0–33)	3.0[0–10]	4.5[0–10]	4.0[1–13]	0.5[0–3]	p = 0.072
	SDQ (five scales) at 7 years (Cheatham et al. 2011)	Prosocial score at 7 years (0–15)	8.5[5–10]	9.0[5–10]	9.0[6–10]	7.9[5–9]	p = 0.100

Notes: ASQ, Ages and Stages Questionnaire; MDI, Mental Developmental Index on the Bayley Scales; SDQ, Strength and Difficulty Questionnaire; RR, relative risk.

[a] Results from the ASQ are given as median (25,75 percentile) for this and all other outcomes from this study. Statistical analyses were adjusted for parental education, older siblings, birthweight, total duration of breastfeeding, and erythrocyte DHA at 3 years.

[b] Mean ± standard deviation and % (95% confidence interval) for these and all other similar values from this study. Statistical analyses were adjusted for centre, parity, maternal education, and smoking status.

[c] Mean ± standard deviation and % of the infants in the group for these and all other similar values from this study. Statistical analyses were adjusted for gestational age at delivery, maternal education, and birth order.

[d] Values from this study are given as mean ± standard deviation or median (25–75 percentile). The statistical analyses were adjusted for age, mean parental education, and number of older siblings.

benefits in girls and adverse effects in boys in two postnatal interventions (Lauritzen et al. 2005; Makrides et al. 2009), whereas the prenatal trial and the genotype study (Jensen et al. 2014; Makrides et al. 2010) tended to show negative effects in girls and positive in boys. However, more studies are needed in order to determine the exact nature of the differential effects of n-3 LCPUFA supplementation in girls and boys.

Should we really interpret these results as beneficial in one sex and adverse in the other? The brain of boys and girls obviously works differently under different conditions, which we culturally have come to perceive as normal, but these differences appear to be diminished by an increased DHA supply to the brain. So what do these results tell us about the actual effect of DHA in the brain? Could the long-term effects of DHA – that is indicated by the DHA–breastfeeding interaction on later IQ – be a secondary effect to some other effect of DHA in the brain?

Interestingly, in our maternal fish oil supplementation trial, we also found treatment–sex interactions on parameters that are not normally defined as cognitive outcomes – namely blood pressure (Asserhøj et al. 2009). The assessment of blood pressure in adults is well known to be affected by anxiety – the so-called white coat syndrome. The blood pressure measurement is therefore influenced by cognitive and emotional components in terms of how the subjects react to have their blood pressure measured. This may be of specific relevance in the assessment of blood pressure in young children, who cannot comprehend the necessity of the assessment procedure. We found a treatment–sex interaction on both diastolic blood pressure and mean arterial blood pressure ($p = 0.03$) at 7 years of age in the children whose mothers were randomized to fish oil or olive oil during the first 4 months of lactation (Asserhøj et al. 2009). When this interaction was explored in sex-stratified analyses, it turned out that the mean arterial blood pressure in girls and boys in the fish oil group was 79 ± 6 and 78 ± 5 mmHg, respectively, whereas it was 78 ± 4 and 72 ± 5 mmHg, respectively, in the control group (Asserhøj et al. 2009). This indicates that early DHA intake increases blood pressure in boys to levels comparable to those in girls. We also found that the intervention had effects on energy intake and physical activity at 7 years of age (Asserhøj et al. 2009), and this again tended to level out sex differences. Overall energy intake was under-reported in the study (i.e. 1.5 ± 0.9 kJ lower than the estimated daily energy expenditure), but the reported energy deficit in the daughters and sons of the fish oil–supplemented mothers was -1.5 ± 0.6 and -1.3 ± 0.8 kJ/day, respectively, whereas in the control group it was -1.2 ± 1.1 and -2.3 ± 1.1 kJ/day in girls and boys, respectively ($p = 0.01$ for sex–treatment interaction). These results indicate that early DHA intake could have long-term health consequences which might be mediated via effects in the brain and lifestyle choices.

3.6 POTENTIAL CRITICAL PERIODS WITH RESPECT TO OPTIMAL n-3 LCPUFA SUPPLY FOR BRAIN FUNCTION

The current prevailing hypothesis is that there is a window of vulnerability for DHA in the early period of brain development – that is, the perinatal period. This view is built on the high rate of DHA accretion in the brain during late pregnancy and early postnatal life. However, brain DHA accretion continues until childhood, and although the accretion rate declines, the incorporation of DHA is still high during this phase. Breast milk has been shown to be a main contributor to DHA content at least in erythrocytes (Harsløf et al. 2013) and complementary feeding usually supplies less DHA, which results in decreasing DHA status after infancy (Rise et al. 2013). Furthermore, the intake of n-3 LCPUFA has been shown to be low in a number of studies in children (Rahmawaty et al. 2013), and European children have been shown to have whole blood n-3 LCPUFA levels consistently below 2.5 FA% between 3 and 8 years of age (Wolters et al. 2014). Therefore, it is plausible that DHA supplementation could lead to improvements in young children – both with respect to their status and their brain function. However, few studies have tested potential cognitive effects of fish oil interventions later in infancy or childhood or even in healthy young adults. The lack of studies makes it hard to evaluate if the hypothesis regarding a potential early window of vulnerability is correct, but from few studies which have been performed, n-3 LCPUFA supplementation appears to have potential effects on cognitive, emotional, or behavioural outcomes later in childhood.

Very few studies have examined the effects of fish oil supplementation in toddlers. A single pooling study that combined data from three trials that randomized to infant formula with LCPUFA (both DHA and AA) immediately after birth or after breastfeeding for 6 weeks or 4–6 months and that continued supplementation to the end of the first year of life found significant beneficial effects on infant problem-solving at 9 months but only in the two studies that started intervention early (Drover et al. 2009). However, one study has examined the effects of DHA-enriched baby food, which supplied 83 mg DHA per day from 6 to 12 months of age (Hoffman et al. 2004). This apparently improved cognitive outcomes, but the results have only been published in a patent certificate (Birch et al. 2005). It is an old tradition of the Nordic countries to give cod liver oil to children from around 1 month of life and throughout childhood. The main rationale for this supplementation is that cod liver oil is an excellent source of vitamin D, which is critical for bone development. We have tested the effect of one teaspoonful of cod liver oil free from vitamins A and D (providing approximately 1.1 g n-3 LCPUFA/day) compared with no supplement from 9 to 12 months of age. In that trial, we found that the supplemented children had an increased number of looks away from the toy in a free play test at 12 months of age (Harbild et al. 2013). The effect was most pronounced in boys – which is in agreement with the effect that was observed at 2.5 years of follow-up in the DOMInO trial. The free play test measures voluntary attention and the ability to hold and maintain attention – and the results therefore indicate that the intake of DHA in early and late infancy can affect attention. However, the development of attention is complex and attention in the context of toy play has been shown to change across the development (Wainwright & Colombo 2006), so the interpretation of these results is not straightforward in terms of whether the effect is beneficial or not.

Results from studies among schoolchildren in low-income countries show relatively convincing cognitive effects of fish oil supplementation. In 3- to 13-year-old Australian children, Parletta et al. (2013) found no effect on reading or spelling but found improved performance in a test of cognitive maturity after 20 weeks of fish oil supplementation (174 mg DHA and 558 mg EPA per day on school days). Interestingly, the effect was strongest in the indigenous children, who typically have a number of health problems associated with malnutrition and consume very little n-3 PUFA (Parletta et al. 2013). Dalton et al. found improvements in three out of five cognitive outcomes in a randomized trial that supplied bread with 192 mg DHA and 82 mg EPA on most school days during a 6-month period in 7- to 9-year-old South African children. These children also had low socio-economic status and a very low fish intake. The same research group found no overall cognitive effects after fish oil supplementation (420 mg DHA and 80 mg EPA per day for 4 days per week during 8.5 months) of 6 to 11-year-old South African children with poor iron and n-3 LCPUFA status (Baumgartner et al. 2012). They did, however, identify an adverse effect of fish oil on memory in children with iron-deficiency anaemia and in girls. The authors suggested that the adverse effect might be related to disruption of neurotransmitter balance in a situation where the brain had adapted to chronic deficiency (Baumgartner et al. 2012).

Little research has been performed on the effects of n-3 LCPUFA on brain functions in school-aged children from high-income countries. One functional magnetic resonance imaging study showed that supplementation with DHA (400 or 1200 mg/day) for 8 weeks is associated with increased activation of the prefrontal cortex and reaction time during sustained attention in healthy 8 to 10-year-old boys (McNamara et al. 2010). Some observational studies have also observed a positive association between dietary intake of n-3 LCPUFA and cognitive performance, and a study of 4000 American children found that the association was stronger in girls than in boys (Eilander et al. 2007). We have recently performed a large crossover intervention trial in more than 800 schoolchildren, where we found that healthy school meals rich in fish improved children's reading performance and reduced attention scores (Sørensen et al. 2015). We have identified four randomized trials in high-income countries that have supplied schoolchildren specifically with n-3 LCPUFA. Three of these found some beneficial effects on cognition or school performance. The study which did not find any effect on cognitive performance, reading, or mathematical reasoning was a large study, performed in 396 South Australian 6 to 10-year-old children, which supplied a low dose of n-3 LCPUFA (88 mg DHA plus 22 mg EPA) in a daily fortified drink for 12 months compared to a control drink with no oil supplement (Osendarp et al. 2007). The other trials found only few effects out of multiple tested outcomes, so these may have been chance findings. One study was conducted in 90 British 10 to 12-year-old children and found a beneficial effect of 400 mg DHA per day for 8 weeks on word recognition but slower performance in children supplemented with 1000 mg DHA per day (Kennedy et al. 2009). They did, however, find that children supplemented with DHA (both 400 and 1000 mg/day) had a more relaxed mood compared to controls. A 16-week randomized trial with fish oil capsules (400 mg DHA and 56 mg EPA per day plus vitamins A, C, D, and E) versus olive oil in 450 healthy 8 to 10-year-old children also indicated a lack of cognitive effects (IQ, reading, spelling, working memory, visual attention, and attention). However, the fish oil apparently affected behaviour and mood in the form of not only an overall increased rating of social difficulties but also a reduction in impulsivity and antisocial behaviour in the fish oil group (Kirby et al. 2010). The last trial supplied 600 mg DHA per day for 16 weeks in 74 children aged 7–9 years and showed improvement in parent-rated behaviour in 8 out of 14 outcomes, but no effects on teacher-rated behaviour or working memory (Richardson et al. 2012). Behavioural effects were also observed in one of the South African studies, which showed that the fish oil supplement resulted in decreased physical activity during school hours, which was correlated with less oppositional behaviour, inattention, and scores on an ADHD rating scale (Smuts et al. 2015). The use of different tests, doses, and duration makes the results difficult to compare, but comparable behavioural effects have been indicated, although not firmly proven, in children with ADHD (Rytter et al. 2015).

As was the case in the studies on the effects of DHA in the perinatal period, a sex–treatment effect was observed on mean arterial blood pressure after fish oil supplementation from 9 to 18 months of age in healthy Danish infants ($p = 0.020$), which just as in the previously mentioned maternal fish oil supplementation study was mostly affected in boys (Harsløf et al. 2014). In this case, blood pressure was reduced in boys, which however was still counteracting the observed gender difference in the control group (89 ± 19 mmHg in girls and 93 ± 17 mmHg in boys), resulting in mean arterial blood pressure in girls and boys of the fish oil–supplemented group of 88 ± 19 and 85 ± 16 mmHg, respectively (Harsløf et al. 2014). A similar effect was observed in a study where we supplied infants with fish oil versus no fish oil (Damsgaard et al. 2006), where the systolic blood pressure was 105 ± 10 and 104 ± 9 mmHg in fish oil–supplemented girls and boys, respectively, versus 104 ± 9 and 112 ± 11 mmHg, respectively, in the unsupplemented group. The observed changes in systolic blood pressure were found to be correlated with the previously mentioned changes in toy attention in the free play test (Harbild et al. 2013), which could indicate a common emotional component.

The studies in toddlers and schoolchildren indicate that not only early but also later fish oil supplementation can affect cognitive and other brain-mediated or brain-modulated functions in children and that these effects may depend on sex. Only few studies have examined if fish oil supplementation can affect brain functions in healthy young adults. Recently, in a randomized controlled crossover trial in young adults, we observed a sex-specific effect of fish oil supplementation after a 3-week intervention on the sensation of appetite that abolished gender differences observed in the soy oil control period (Damsbo-Svendsen et al. 2013). This suggests that the effects may not be confined to early life and motivates further studies that challenge the hypothesis about specific effects during a window of opportunity in early life. Furthermore, studies on potential programming effect, as well as those on acute effect later in life, clearly indicate the necessity of sex differentiation in the analysis of the results on cognitive and behavioural outcomes in n-3 LCPUFA supplementation trials.

3.7 POTENTIAL MECHANISMS FOR EFFECTS OF n-3 LCPUFA ON BRAIN FUNCTION

The intrauterine development of sexual dimorphism is mainly driven by testosterone, and in its absence, the fetus will develop female characteristics, both in the somatic and in the behavioural phenotype. In the perinatal period, testosterone is produced by the developing testis, during the so-called early androgen surge or mini-puberty. This testosterone production starts within the first weeks of pregnancy, and its levels remain within a pubertal range for a few months postnatally before it, from around 6 months of age, decreases to barely detectable childhood levels (Kuiri-Hanninen et al. 2014) with only brief testicular activations (Chemes 2001). Testosterone is converted to oestrogen by aromatase which, partly due to substrate availability, is up-regulated in the brain – most pronouncedly in the amygdala and in the limbic and hypothalamic areas (Beyer 1999). The produced oestrogen plays a key role in brain development and the sexual differentiation of the brain (Beyer 1999), which is also affected by environmental cues and other sex-determining genes – for example, tyrosine hydroxylase, a rate-limiting enzyme in the synthesis of dopamine (Arnold 2012). The sexual dimorphism of the brain includes differences in the distribution and function of monoaminergic neurons, specifically in the dopaminergic system (Beyer 1999), which is involved in the regulation of cognitive and emotional functions. Early testosterone levels have been shown to program the sensitivity of the brain's reward system (Lombardo et al. 2012) and thus may play a role in predicting the risk of sex-skewed neuropsychiatric conditions like ADHD.

Gender differences, for example in school performance, may be related to sociocultural differences because school lessons are less likely to include elements that are compatible with male preferences like physical activity, competition, hierarchy, and status. Such differences could also lead to differences in the responses of boys and girls to intervention studies as well as their responses to the testing of effects. Gender differences exist in several cognitive domains, for example, boys tend to have better visuospatial skills and girls tend to perform better in verbal tasks and in episodic memory performance (Herlitz et al. 2013). Gender differences in academic performance are also well known – girls are generally better at reading and boys are better at mathematics (Stoet & Geary 2013). A main explanation of the gender differences seems to be that boys experience lower engagement and less joy from reading (OECD 2014). The gender difference in mathematics has been proposed to be related to girls having lower confidence in their skills, who are more apprehensive, and who are less motivated for mathematics (OECD 2014). The gender differences are probably explained not only by biological differences but also by children's responses to social expectations.

Traditionally, girls have faster psychomotor development than boys in most domains, which is also apparent in the cognitive scores, communication, and adaptive behaviour in the control groups, as given in Table 3.3. Many of the described results indicate that these differences are diminished by an increase in the DHA supply – both by supplementation during gestation and lactation and by polymorphisms in the *FADS* gene cluster which gives rise to increased DHA status in infancy. We have shown that the association between DHA-increasing *FADS* alleles and problem-solving in boys and girls may be modulated by the Pro12Ala SNP in the gene that encodes peroxisome proliferator–activated receptor gamma (*PPARG*) (Jensen et al. 2014). This may indicate that PPAR-γ to some extent mediates the effect of DHA in the brain. As PPAR-γ has been shown to be involved in the regulation of aromatase, and as the *PPARG* Pro12Ala polymorphism has been shown to be associated with a less-efficient aromatase transcription (Memisoglu et al. 2002), DHA regulation of PPAR-γ could be hypothesized to explain the observed sex specificity in some of the DHA-induced effects on brain functions. Also, DHA-induced PPAR-γ regulation of aromatase could be speculated to reduce the sexual differentiation of the brain through a reduced conversion of testosterone to oestrogen.

Animal studies, mainly in rodents, have shown that n-3 PUFA deprivation results in reduced brain DHA incorporation and impaired learning (Lauritzen et al. 2001) as well as poor performance in a number of cognitive and behavioural tests (McCann & Ames 2005). Dietary n-3 PUFA deficiency has also been shown to permanently increase motor activity (Fedorova & Salem 2006; McNamara & Carlson 2006) and to affect emotional outcomes such as depression, anxiety, and aggression in rodents, and this too appear to be unchanged by later n-3 LCPUFA supplementation (Lavialle et al. 2010; McNamara & Carlson 2006). n-3 PUFA–deficient adult mice showed signs of higher levels of anxiety and aggression under stressful conditions like unpredictability, whereas no effects were seen under normal conditions (Lavialle et al. 2010). In rats, decreased brain DHA accrual early in life in combination with parental neglect has also been shown to result in increased impulsivity, depression-like syndrome, and stress-induced anxiety (Lavialle et al. 2010). Conversely, both pre- and postnatal dietary regimes rich in n-3 LCPUFA have been seen to reduce stress vulnerability and responses to corticosterone (Hennebelle et al. 2014). Fish oil supplementation of adult male lemurs showed that n-3 LCPUFA can lower anxiety, reduce locomotor activity, and improve learning, also in primates (Vinot et al. 2011).

Many maternal n-3 PUFA–modulating studies in rodents have only examined effects in either male or female offspring. However, a few studies have used offspring of both sexes and found apparent differential effects in these. A study that varied dietary DHA during pregnancy and lactation showed that decreased brain DHA was associated with reduced locomotor activity (Levant et al. 2006). The effect was most pronounced in post-adolescent males, whereas no association was observed in females. In the spontaneously hypertensive rat model with ADHD, supplementation of dams with n-3 LCPUFA during pregnancy resulted in two distinct types of changes in ADHD-like behaviours in the offspring: a reduction in general locomotor activity in both sexes and reduced levels of reinforcer-controlled activity, impulsivity, and inattention in male offspring, with no or opposite effects in female offspring. The change in general locomotor activity appeared to correlate with sex-independent changes in brain glycine and glutamate, whereas the other behavioural changes were associated with enhanced neostriatal dopamine and serotonin turnover, predominantly in the male offspring (Dervola et al. 2012).

The suggested effects are in line with the fact that many of the previously described DHA-affected brain functions can be linked to monoaminergic neurotransmitter pathways – for example, ADHD-related behaviours, attention, and physical activity, as well as anxiety and appetite. Early n-3 fatty acid deficiency has furthermore been shown to result in persistently reduced stimulated extracellular levels of serotonin and dopamine in the rat brain (McNamara & Carlson 2006). Extensive evidence indicates that decreased DHA levels result in reduced levels of phosphatidylserine in membranes, including neuronal membranes. Phosphatidylserine is a negatively charged phospholipid that plays an important role in membrane processes such as signal transduction and vesicular trafficking (McNamara & Carlson 2006). This could be a potential mechanism for the effects of DHA on serotonin and dopamine concentrations, as these are released into the synapse from secretory vesicles upon stimulation.

Perinatal n-3 PUFA deficiency has also been associated with increased hypothalamic–pituitary–adrenal axis activity in rodents, and this could partly be due to increases in blood–brain barrier permeability, for example, to corticosterone (Hennebelle et al. 2014), which could be speculated to be a way in which DHA could affect the stress response. The stress-reducing response to n-3 LCPUFA could also be related to their anti-inflammatory effects mediated by the conversion of EPA and DHA to resolvins and neuroprotectins, as stress responses have been shown to involve brain inflammation (Hennebelle et al. 2014). Low dietary n-3 PUFA regimes have furthermore been shown to reduce the expression of brain-derived neurotrophic factor (Hennebelle et al. 2014), which plays an important role in neuron survival, growth, differentiation, and synaptogenesis, specifically in areas vital to learning and memory. Glutamate neurotransmission, which plays a key role in memory and learning, has been shown to be modulated by stress in several brain regions (Hennebelle et al. 2014), so the reported changes in learning and stress sensitivity could be linked. PUFAs have also been shown to affect a range of nuclear receptors (transcription factors), including PPARs, retinoid X receptor, liver X receptor, and sterol regulatory element–binding protein 1, all of which are expressed in the brain (Kitajka et al. 2004). Thus, all of the 'usual' n-3 LCPUFA mechanisms could be important in explaining the effects of DHA on brain function – including effects on membrane fatty acid composition, eicosanoid action, and gene expression, which could result in changes in brain structure, membrane function, electrical signaling, and neurotransmitter systems.

3.8 CONCLUSION

Both AA and DHA are accumulated in the brain during early life, but only the accumulation of DHA appears to be determined mainly by the dietary intake. It is therefore not likely that dietary AA should have any pronounced functional effects on brain development, but few studies have been performed to distinguish between the effects of different LCPUFA. From the evidence presented, specifically the latest studies, it appears that DHA could play a role in brain development in a sex-specific way. Presently, it is not easy to interpret whether early DHA supply results in improved brain function or merely a change in the development. More evidence from well-designed randomized controlled trials in children is obviously needed. However, based on the results thus far, we would question whether we are currently at a stage where we should conduct large randomized controlled trials in order to prove the potential beneficial effects of DHA on one specific outcome or whether we should rather spend more time exploring what the relevant effects to test might be. It is possible that DHA may affect not only intellectual abilities as such but also some basic aspects of brain function related to how we interact with the world – for example, personality traits, monoaminergic-controlled emotions, or stress vulnerability, which links up to potential effects on ADHD-like outcomes. An accumulating amount of evidence indicates that DHA intake may counteract the development of gender differences, but this needs to be explored in more detail. Interestingly, gender-equalizing effects have also been observed in studies that supply n-3 LCPUFA in toddlers, schoolchildren, and young adults. This challenges the hypothesis that DHA mainly affects the brain during early development and raises a need for studies which compare the effects of n-3 LCPUFA supplementation in different age groups, in addition to studies which follow up on the effect of early supplementation in later childhood. This approach would help determine whether the effects of DHA and n-3 LCPUFA in young children are transient or in fact result in real programming effects on brain function later in life.

REFERENCES

Arnold, AP. 2012. The end of gonad-centric sex determination in mammals. *Trends in Genetics* 28(2), 55–61.

Asserhøj, M, Nehammer, S, Matthiessen, J, Michaelsen, KF, & Lauritzen, L. 2009. Maternal fish oil supplementation during lactation may adversely affect long-term blood pressure, energy intake, and physical activity of 7-year-old boys. *Journal of Nutrition* 139(2), 298–304.

Auestad, N, Halter, R, Hall, RT et al. 2001. Growth and development in term infants fed long-chain polyunsaturated fatty acids: A double-masked, randomized, parallel, prospective, multivariate study. *Pediatrics* 108(2), 372–381.

Baumgartner, J, Smuts, CM, Malan, L et al. 2012. Effects of iron and n-3 fatty acid supplementation, alone and in combination, on cognition in school children: A randomized, double-blind, placebo-controlled intervention in South Africa. *American Journal of Clinical Nutrition* 96(6), 1327–1338.

Beyer, C. 1999. Estrogen and the developing mammalian brain. *Anatomy and Embryology* 199(5), 379–390.

Birch, EE, Carlson, SE, Hoffman, DR et al. 2010. The DIAMOND (DHA Intake And Measurement Of Neural Development) Study: A double-masked, randomized controlled clinical trial of the maturation of infant visual acuity as a function of the dietary level of docosahexaenoic acid. *American Journal of Clinical Nutrition* 91(4), 848–859.

Birch, EE, Cool, MB, Harvey, RA, Hoffman, DR, Rocklin, TL, San, FV, Shaul, GE, Theuer, RC, & BEECH-NUT NUTRITION CORP. 2005. Improvement of cognitive ability in infant involves feeding the infant with shelf-stable semi-solid baby-food composition containing specified amount of docohexaenoic acid. US Patent 053713–A1; 7413759–B2.

Birch, EE, Garfield, S, Castaneda, Y, Hughbanks-Wheaton, D, Uauy, R, & Hoffman, D. 2007. Visual acuity and cognitive outcomes at 4 years of age in a double-blind, randomized trial of long-chain polyunsaturated fatty acid-supplemented infant formula. *Early Human Development* 83(5), 279–284.

Bouwstra, H, Dijck-Brouwer, DAJ, Boehm, G, Boersma, ER, Muskiet, FAJ, & Hadders-Algra, M. 2005. Long-chain polyunsaturated fatty acids and neurological developmental outcome at 18 months in healthy term infants. *Acta Paediatrica* 94(1), 26–32.

Brenna, JT, Varamini, B, Jensen, RG, Diersen-Schade, DA, Boettcher, JA, & Arterburn, LM. 2007. Docosahexaenoic and arachidonic acid concentrations in human breast milk worldwide. *American Journal of Clinical Nutrition* 85(6), 1457–1464.

Brookes, KJ, Chen, W, Xu, X, Taylor, E, & Asherson P. 2006. Association of fatty acid desaturase genes with Attention-Deficit/Hyperactivity Disorder. *Biological Psychiatry* 60(10), 1053–1061.

Campoy, C, Escolano-Margarit, MV, Ramos, R et al. 2011. Effects of prenatal fish-oil and 5-methyl-tetrahydro-folate supplementation on cognitive development of children at 6.5 y of age. *American Journal of Clinical Nutrition* 94(6), 1880S–1888S.

Carlson, SE, Werkman, SH, Rhodes, PG, & Tolley, EA. 1993. Visual acuity development in healthy preterm infants: Effect of marine-oil supplementation. *American Journal of Clinical Nutrition* 58, 35–42.

Caspi, A, Williams, B, Kim-Cohen, J et al. 2007. Moderation of breastfeeding effects on the IQ by genetic variation in fatty acid metabolism. *Proceedings of the National Academy of Sciences of the United States of America* 104(47), 18860–18865.

Cheatham, CL, Colombo, J, & Carlson, SE. 2006. n-3 fatty acids and cognitive and visual acuity development: Methodologic and conceptual considerations. *American Journal of Clinical Nutrition* 83(6), 1458S–1466S.

Cheatham, CL, Nerhammer, AS, Asserhøj, M, Michaelsen, KF, & Lauritzen, L. 2011. Fish oil supplementation during lactation: Effects on cognition and behavior at 7 years of age. *Lipids* 46(7), 637–645.

Chemes, HCE. 2001. Infancy is not a quiescent period of testicular development. *International Journal of Andrology* 24(1), 2–7.

Damsbo-Svendsen, S, Rønsholdt, MD, & Lauritzen, L. 2013. Fish oil-supplementation increases appetite in healthy adults: A randomized controlled cross-over trial. *Appetite* 66, 62–66.

Damsgaard, CT, Schack-Nielsen, L, Michaelsen, KF, Fruekilde, MB, Hels, O, & Lauritzen, L. 2006. Fish oil affects blood pressure and the plasma lipid profile in healthy Danish infants. *Journal of Nutrition* 136(1), 94–99.

de Jong, C, Boehm, G, Kikkert, HK, & Hadders-Algra, M. 2011. The Groningen LCPUFA Study: No effect of short-term postnatal long-chain polyunsaturated fatty acids in healthy term infants on cardiovascular and anthropometric development at 9 years. *Pediatric Research* 70(4), 411–416.

Delgado-Noguera, MF, Calvache, JA, & Cosp, XB. 2010. Supplementation with long chain polyunsaturated fatty acids (LCPUFA) to breastfeeding mothers for improving child growth and development. *Cochrane Database of Systematic Reviews* (12), art. CD007901. doi: 10.1002/14651858.CD007901.pub2.

Dervola, KS, Roberg, BÅ, Wøien, G et al. 2012. Marine omega-3 polyunsaturated fatty acids induce sex-specific changes in reinforcer-controlled behaviour and neurotransmitter metabolism in a spontaneously hypertensive rat model of ADHD. *Behavioral and Brain Functions* 8(1), art. 56. http://www.behavioralandbrainfunctions.com/content/8/1/56.

Drover, J, Hoffman, DR, Castaneda, YS, Morale, SE, & Birch, EE. 2009. Three randomized controlled trials of early long-chain polyunsaturated fatty acid supplementation on means-end problem solving in 9-month-olds. *Child Development* 80(5), 1376–1384.

Eilander, A, Hundscheid, DC, Osendarp, SJ, Transler, C, & Zock, PL. 2007. Effects of n-3 long chain polyunsaturated fatty acid supplementation on visual and cognitive development throughout childhood: A review of human studies. *Prostaglandins Leukotrienes and Essential Fatty Acids* 76(4), 189–203.

Fedorova, I & Salem, N. 2006. Omega-3 fatty acids and rodent behavior. *Prostaglandins Leukotrienes and Essential Fatty Acids* 75(4–5), 271–289.

Gould, JF, Makrides, M, Colombo, J, & Smithers, LG. 2014. Randomized controlled trial of maternal omega-3 long-chain PUFA supplementation during pregnancy and early childhood development of attention, working memory, and inhibitory control. *American Journal of Clinical Nutrition* 99(4), 851–859.

Gould, JF, Smithers, LG, & Makrides, M. 2013. The effect of maternal omega-3 LCPUFA supplementation during pregnancy on early childhood cognitive and visual development: A systematic review and meta-analysis of randomized controlled trials. *American Journal of Clinical Nutrition* 97(3), 531–544.

Harbild, HL, Harsløf, LBS, Christensen, JH, Kannass, KN, & Lauritzen, L. 2013. Fish oil-supplementation from 9 to 12 months of age affects infant attention in a free-play test and is related to change in blood pressure. *Prostaglandins Leukotrienes and Essential Fatty Acids* 89(5), 327–333.

Harsløf, LB, Damsgaard, CT, Hellgren, LI, Andersen, AD, Vogel, U, & Lauritzen, L. 2014. Effects on metabolic markers are modified by PPARG2 and COX2 polymorphisms in infants randomized to fish oil. *Genes and Nutrition* 9(3), art. 396. doi:10.1007/s12263-014-0396-4.

Harsløf, LB, Larsen, LH, Ritz, C et al. 2013. FADS genotype and diet are important determinants of DHA status: A cross-sectional study in Danish infants. *American Journal of Clinical Nutrition* 97(6), 1403–1410.

Helland, IB, Smith, L, Blomen, B, Saarem, K, Saugstad, OD, & Drevon, CA. 2008. Effect of supplementing pregnant and lactating mothers with n-3 very-long-chain fatty acids on children's IQ and body mass index at 7 years of age. *Pediatrics* 122(2), E472–E479.

Hennebelle, M, Champeil-Potokar, G, Lavialle, M, Vancassel, S, & Denis, I. 2014. Omega-3 polyunsaturated fatty acids and chronic stress-induced modulations of glutamatergic neurotransmission in the hippocampus. *Nutrition Reviews* 72(2), 99–112.

Herlitz, A, Reuterskiold, L, Loven, J, Thilers, PP, & Rehnman, J. 2013. Cognitive sex differences are not magnified as a function of age, sex hormones, or puberty development during early adolescence. *Developmental Neuropsychology* 38(3), 167–179.

Hoffman, DR, Theuer, RC, Castaneda, YS et al. 2004. Maturation of visual acuity is accelerated in breast-fed term infants fed baby food containing DHA-enriched egg yolk. *Journal of Nutrition* 134(9), 2307–2313.

Horta, BL & Victoria, CG. 2013. Long-term effects of breastfeeding: A systematic review. WHO, http://www.who.int/maternal_child_adolescent/documents/breastfeeding_long_term_effects/en/. Accessed on February 2, 2015.

Jensen, HAR, Harsløf, LBS, Nielsen, MS et al. 2014. FADS single-nucleotide polymorphisms are associated with behavioral outcomes in children, and the effect varies between sexes and is dependent on PPAR genotype. *American Journal of Clinical Nutrition* 100(3), 826–832.

Kennedy, DO, Jackson, PA, Elliott, JM et al. 2009. Cognitive and mood effects of 8 weeks' supplementation with 400 mg or 1000 mg of the omega-3 essential fatty acid docosahexaenoic acid (DHA) in healthy children aged 10–12 years. *Nutritional Neuroscience* 12(2), 48–56.

Kirby, A, Woodward, A, Jackson, S, Wang, Y, & Crawford, MA. 2010. A double-blind, placebo-controlled study investigating the effects of omega-3 supplementation in children aged 8–10 years from a mainstream school population. *Research in Developmental Disabilities* 31(3), 718–730.

Kitajka, K, Sinclair, AJ, Weisinger, RS et al. 2004. Effects of dietary omega-3 polyunsaturated fatty acids on brain gene expression. *Proceedings of the National Academy of Sciences of the United States of America* 101(30), 10931–10936.

Koletzko, B, Lattka, E, Zeilinger, S, Illig, T, & Steer, C. 2011. Genetic variants of the fatty acid desaturase gene cluster predict amounts of red blood cell docosahexaenoic and other polyunsaturated fatty acids in pregnant women: Findings from the Avon Longitudinal Study of Parents and Children. *American Journal of Clinical Nutrition* 93(1), 211–219.

Kuiri-Hanninen, T, Sankilampi, U, & Dunkel, L. 2014. Activation of the hypothalamic-pituitary-gonadal axis in infancy: Minipuberty. *Hormone Research in Paediatrics* 82(2), 73–80.

Lattka, E, Koletzko, B, Zeilinger, S et al. 2013. Umbilical cord PUFA are determined by maternal and child fatty acid desaturase (FADS) genetic variants in the Avon Longitudinal Study of Parents and Children (ALSPAC). *British Journal of Nutrition* 109(7), 1196–1210.

Lattka, E, Rzehak, P, Szabo, E et al. 2011. Genetic variants in the FADS gene cluster are associated with arachidonic acid concentrations of human breast milk at 1.5 and 6 mo postpartum and influence the course of milk dodecanoic, tetracosenoic, and trans-9-octadecenoic acid concentrations over the duration of lactation. *American Journal of Clinical Nutrition* 93(2), 382–391.

Lauritzen, L & Carlson, SE. 2011. Maternal fatty acid status during pregnancy and lactation and relation to newborn and infant status. *Maternal and Child Nutrition* 7, 41–58.

Lauritzen, L, Hansen, HS, Jørgensen, MH, & Michaelsen, KF. 2001. The essentiality of long-chain *n*-3 fatty acids in relation to development and function of the brain and retina. *Progress in Lipid Research* 40(1–2), 1–94.

Lauritzen, L, Jørgensen, MH, Olsen, SF, Straarup, EM, & Michaelsen, KF. 2005. Maternal fish oil supplementation in lactation: Effect on developmental outcome in breast-fed infants. *Reproduction Nutrition Development* 45(5), 535–547.

Lavialle, M, Denis, I, Guesnet, P, & Vancassel, S. 2010. Involvement of omega-3 fatty acids in emotional responses and hyperactive symptoms. *Journal of Nutritional Biochemistry* 21(10), 899–905.

Levant, B, Ozias, MK, & Carlson, SE. 2006. Sex-specific effects of brain LCPUFA composition on locomotor activity in rats. *Physiology & Behavior* 89(2), 196–204.

Lombardo, MV, Ashwin, E, Auyeung, B et al. 2012. Fetal programming effects of testosterone on the reward system and behavioral approach tendencies in humans. *Biological Psychiatry* 72(10), 839–847.

Makrides, M, Gibson, RA, & McPhee, AJ. 2010. Effect of DHA supplementation during pregnancy on maternal depression and neurodevelopment of young children: A randomized controlled trial. *Journal of the American Medical Association* 304(15), 1675–1683.

Makrides, M, Gibson, RA, McPhee, AJ et al. 2009. Neurodevelopmental outcomes of preterm infants fed high-dose docosahexaenoic acid: A randomized controlled trial. *Obstetrical & Gynecological Survey* 64(5), 297–298.

Makrides, M, Neumann, MA, Byard, RW, Simmer, K, & Gibson, RA. 1994. Fatty acid composition of brain, retina, and erythrocytes in breast- and formula-fed infants. *American Journal of Clinical Nutrition* 60(2), 189–194.

Marangoni, F, Agostoni, C, Lammardo, AM, Giovannini, M, Galli, C, & Riva, E. 2000. Polyunsaturated fatty acid concentrations in human hindmilk are stable throughout 12-months of lactation and provide a sustained intake to the infant during exclusive breastfeeding: An Italian study. *British Journal of Nutrition* 84(1), 103–109.

Martin, NW, Benyamin, B, Hansell, NK et al. 2011. Cognitive function in adolescence: Testing for interactions between breast-feeding and FADS2 polymorphisms. *Journal of the American Academy of Child and Adolescent Psychiatry* 50(1), 55–62.

McCann, JC & Ames, BN. 2005. Is docosahexaenoic acid, an n-3 long-chain polyunsaturated fatty acid, required for development of normal brain function? An overview of evidence from cognitive and behavioral tests in humans and animals. *American Journal of Clinical Nutrition* 82(2), 281–295.

McNamara, RK, Able, J, Jandacek, R et al. 2010. Docosahexaenoic acid supplementation increases prefrontal cortex activation during sustained attention in healthy boys: A placebo-controlled, dose-ranging, functional magnetic resonance imaging study. *American Journal of Clinical Nutrition* 91(4), 1060–1067.

McNamara, RK & Carlson, SE. 2006. Role of omega-3 fatty acids in brain development and function: Potential implications for the pathogenesis and prevention of psychopathology. *Prostaglandins Leukotrienes and Essential Fatty Acids* 75(4–5), 329–349.

Memisoglu, A, Hankinson, SE, Manson, JE, Colditz, GA, & Hunter, DJ. 2002. Lack of association of the codon 12 polymorphism of the peroxisome proliferator-activated receptor gamma gene with breast cancer and body mass. *Pharmacogenetics* 12(8), 597–603.

Morales, E, Bustamante, M, Gonzalez, JR et al. 2011. Genetic variants of the FADS gene cluster and ELOVL gene family, colostrums LCPUFA levels, breastfeeding, and child cognition. *PLoS One* 6(2), art. e17181. doi: 10.1371/journal.pone.0017181.

Morris, G, Moorcraft, J, Mountjoy, A, & Wells, JCK. 2000. A novel infant formula milk with added long-chain polyunsaturated fatty acids from single-cell sources: A study of growth, satisfaction and health. *European Journal of Clinical Nutrition* 54(12), 883–886.

OECD. 2014. *PISA 2012 Results: What Students Know and Can Do – Student Performance in Mathematics, Reading and Science*. OECD Publishing, Paris, France. http://dx.doi.org/10.1787/9789264201118-en.

Osendarp, SJM, Baghurst, KI, Bryan, J et al. 2007. Effect of a 12-mo micronutrient intervention on learning and memory in well-nourished and marginally nourished school-aged children: 2 parallel, randomized, placebo-controlled studies in Australia and Indonesia. *American Journal of Clinical Nutrition* 86(4), 1082–1093.

Parletta, N, Cooper, P, Gent, DN, Petkov, J, & O'Dea, K. 2013. Effects of fish oil supplementation on learning and behaviour of children from Australian Indigenous remote community schools: A randomised controlled trial. *Prostaglandins Leukotrienes and Essential Fatty Acids* 89(2–3), 71–79.

Qawasmi, A, Landeros-Weisenberger, A, Leckman, JF, & Bloch, MH. 2012. Meta-analysis of long-chain polyunsaturated fatty acid supplementation of formula and infant cognition. *Pediatrics* 129(6), 1141–1149.

Rahmawaty, S, Charlton, K, Lyons-Wall, P, & Meyer, BJ. 2013. Dietary intake and food sources of EPA, DPA and DHA in Australian children. *Lipids* 48(9), 869–877.

Richardson, AJ, Burton, JR, Sewell, RP, Spreckelsen, TF, & Montgomery, P. 2012. Docosahexaenoic acid for reading, cognition and behavior in children aged 7–9 years: A randomized, controlled trial (the DOLAB Study). *PLoS One* 7(9), art. e43909. doi: 10.1371/journal.pone.0043909.

Rise, P, Tragni, E, Ghezzi, S et al. 2013. Different patterns characterize Omega 6 and Omega 3 long chain polyunsaturated fatty acid levels in blood from Italian infants, children, adults and elderly. *Prostaglandins Leukotrienes and Essential Fatty Acids* 89(4), 215–220.

Rytter, MJH, Andersen, LBB, Houmann, T et al. 2015. Diet in the treatment of ADHD in children: A systematic review of the literature. *Nordic Journal of Psychiatry* 69(1), 1–18.

SanGiovanni, JP, Berkey, CS, Dwyer, JT, & Colditz, GA. 2000a. Dietary essential fatty acids, long-chain polyunsaturated fatty acids, and visual resolution acuity in healthy fullterm infants: A systematic review. *Early Human Development* 57(3), 165–188.

SanGiovanni, JP, Parra-Cabrera, S, Colditz, GA, Berkey, CS, & Dwyer, JT. 2000b. Meta-analysis of dietary essential fatty acids and long-chain polyunsaturated fatty acids as they relate to visual resolution acuity in healthy preterm infants. *Pediatrics* 105(6), 1292–1298.

Schulzke, SM, Patole, SK, & Simmer, K. 2011. Long-chain polyunsaturated fatty acid supplementation in preterm infants. *Cochrane Database of Systematic Reviews* (2), art. CD000375. doi:10.1002/14651858.CD000375.pub4.

Simmer, K, Patole, SK, & Rao, SC. 2011. Long-chain polyunsaturated fatty acid supplementation in infants born at term *Cochrane Database of Systematic Reviews* (12), art. CD000376. doi:10.1002/14651858.CD000376.pub3.

Smuts, CM, Greeff, J, Kvalsvig, J, Zimmermann, M, & Baumgartner, J. 2015. Long-chain n-3 polyunsaturated fatty acid supplementation decrease physical activity during class in iron deficient South African school children. *British Journal of Nutrition* 113(2), 212–224.

Sørensen, LB, Dyssegaard, CB, Damsgaard, CT et al. 2015. The effect of Nordic school meals on concentration and school performance in 8 to 11 year-old children in the OPUS School Meal Study: A cluster-randomized controlled cross-over trial. *British Journal of Nutrition* 113(8), 1280–1291.

Steer, CD, Hibbeln, JR, Golding, J, & Smith, GD. 2012. Polyunsaturated fatty acid levels in blood during pregnancy, at birth and at 7 years: Their associations with two common FADS2 polymorphisms. *Human Molecular Genetics* 21(7), 1504–1512.

Steer, CD, Lattka, E, Koletzko, B, Golding, J, & Hibbeln, JR. 2013. Maternal fatty acids in pregnancy, FADS polymorphisms, and child intelligence quotient at 8 y of age. *American Journal of Clinical Nutrition* 8(6), 1575–1582.

Steer, CD, Smith, GD, Emmett, PM, Hibbeln, JR, & Golding, J. 2010. FADS2 polymorphisms modify the effect of breastfeeding on child IQ. *PLoS One* 5(7), art. e11570. doi: 10.1371/journal.pone.0011570.

Stoet, G & Geary, DC. 2013. Sex differences in mathematics and reading achievement are inversely related: Within- and across-nation assessment of 10 years of PISA data. *PLoS One* 8(3), art. e57988. doi: 10.1371/journal.pone.0057988.

Uauy, R, Hoffman, DR, Mena, P, Llanos, A, & Birch, EE. 2003. Term infant studies of DHA and ARA supplementation on neurodevelopment: Results of randomized controlled trials. *Journal of Pediatrics* 143(Suppl. 4), S17–S25.

Uauy, RD, Birch, DG, Birch, EE, Tyson, JE, & Hoffman, DR. 1990. Effect of dietary omega-3 fatty acids on retinal function of very-low-birth-weight neonates. *Pediatric Research* 28(5), 485–492.

Uauy, RD, Mena, P, Wegher, B, Nieto, S, & Salem, N Jr. 2000. Long chain polyunsaturated fatty acid formation in neonates: Effect of gestational age and intrauterine growth. *Pediatric Research* 47(1), 127–135.

van Goor, SA, Dijck-Brouwer, DAJ, Hadders-Algra, M et al. 2009. Human milk arachidonic acid and docosahexaenoic acid contents increase following supplementation during pregnancy and lactation. *Prostaglandins Leukotrienes and Essential Fatty Acids* 80(1), 65–69.

Vinot, N, Jouin, M, Lhomme-Duchadeuil, A et al. 2011. Omega-3 fatty acids from fish oil lower anxiety, improve cognitive functions and reduce spontaneous locomotor activity in a non-human primate. *PLoS One* 6(6), art. e20491. doi: 10.1371/journal.pone.0020491.

Wainwright, PE & Colombo, J. 2006. Nutrition and the development of cognitive functions: Interpretation of behavioral studies in animals and human infants. *American Journal of Clinical Nutrition* 84(5), 961–970.

Wolters, M, Schlenz, H, Foraita, R et al. 2014. Reference values of whole-blood fatty acids by age and sex from European children aged 3–8 years. *International Journal of Obesity* 38(Suppl. 2), S86–S98.

Xie, L & Innis, SM. 2008. Genetic variants of the FADS1-FADS2 gene cluster are associated with altered n-6 and n-3 essential fatty acids in plasma and erythrocyte phospholipids in women during pregnancy and in breast milk during lactation. *Journal of Nutrition* 138(11), 2222–2228.

4 The Antioxidant Vitamins A, C, and E and the Developing Brain

Stephanie A. Dillon and Heather Ohly

CONTENTS

4.1 INTRODUCTION

Antioxidant vitamins are important dietary components sourced from a diverse range of foods. Vitamins A, C, and E have important roles to play during the growth and development of the brain and nervous system during embryogenesis and fetal and postnatal periods. The antioxidant effects of these vitamins become particularly important during these periods of intense growth and development when there is an increased production of reactive oxygen/nitrogen species (ROS/RNS). These reactive species also have important physiological roles during the growth and development but can be problematic if their production is excessive and antioxidant defences are insufficient. This chapter will initially provide a brief overview of the metabolism and functions of the antioxidant vitamins A, C, and E and will then consider their specific roles during the growth and development of the brain from conception through to childhood. The impact of deficiency and interventions during critical periods will also be discussed in relation to cognitive function and development of motor skills.

4.1.1 Metabolism and Functions of Vitamin A

Since its discovery in 1913 by Elmer McCollum, fat-soluble vitamin A has been implicated in the functioning of the central nervous system (CNS) initially from the identification of its role in vision followed by the discovery of its role in the development of the eye and brain during embryogenesis (Shearer et al. 2012). Vitamin A and its active metabolites, the retinoids (retinol, retinal, and retinoic acid), are derived from animal sources and are readily absorbed in the intestine. There are also plant sources of vitamin A named the carotenoids, some of which can be converted to vitamin A. It is important to appreciate that the efficiency of absorption from the intestine and conversion to vitamin A is dependent on the particular carotenoid, and not all carotenoids possess vitamin A activity (Tang 2014). β-Carotene is the most studied to date and has the highest vitamin A conversion efficiency of the carotenoids with 12 μg β-carotene equivalent to 1 μg vitamin A. The efficacy of conversion varies even for a particular carotenoid and is dependent on the food source, vitamin A status, and age (conversion efficiency decreases with increasing age) (Tang 2014). The conversion between the vitamin A metabolites retinol and retinal is reversible, in contrast to the formation of retinoic acid which is irreversible (see Figure 4.1). Any discussion of the antioxidant activity of vitamin A relates primarily to carotenoids, in particular β-carotene, as to date there is no evidence which supports the direct antioxidant activity of vitamin A.

In addition to its antioxidant functions, vitamin A plays an important role in supporting vision, protein synthesis, reproduction, growth, and development. It is essential for the production of rhodopsin in the retina, and deficiency of this vitamin is

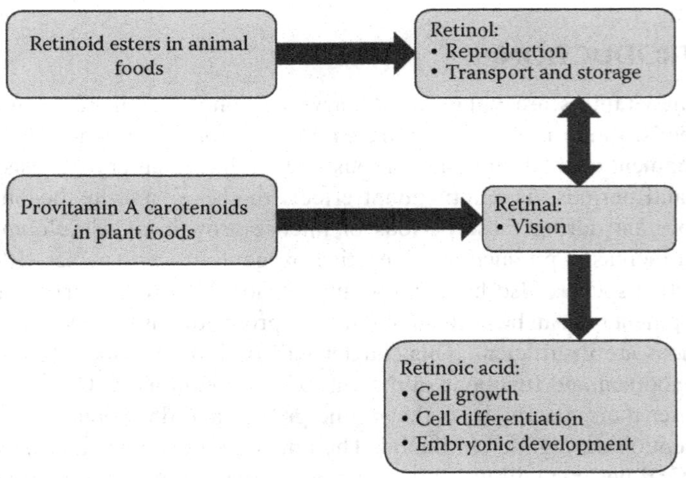

FIGURE 4.1 Conversion of vitamin A compounds derived from animal and plant sources. The retinoid esters from animal sources are well absorbed in the gut and are converted to retinol and reversibly converted to retinal. The provitamin A carotenoids (primarily β-carotene) are less well absorbed in the gut, and the extent of conversion to retinal is variable. Retinal derived from retinol or β-carotene can be irreversibly converted to retinoic acid.

a major cause of preventable blindness in children in developing countries (World Health Organization 2002). The WHO also recognizes vitamin A deficiency as a major cause of illness in developing countries, and outcomes potentially associated with vitamin A deficiency include fetal loss, low birthweight, preterm birth, and infant mortality; and populations most at risk of vitamin A deficiency are preschool children and women of childbearing age (World Health Organization 2002). Adverse health consequences related to vitamin A consumption are also observed when intake is excessive, particularly in the form of supplements or from animal sources. A recent meta-analysis of prospective studies has identified a U-shaped dose–response relationship between blood vitamin A levels and risk of hip fracture in ageing populations (Wu et al. 2014). The teratogenic effects of excessive vitamin A intake are evident in the developing embryo, resulting in significant neurological and physiological birth defects (Maden 2001).

4.1.2 Metabolism and Functions of Vitamin C

In Oslo, in 1907, Holst and Frolich developed an animal model of scurvy by manipulating the diet of guinea pigs; subsequently, they identified vitamin C (ascorbic acid) as the antiscorbutic factor of various fruit and vegetables originally termed hexuronic acid by the biochemist and Nobel Prize winner Laureate Albert Szent-Gyorgyi (Baron 2009). Vitamin C consists of two interconverting compounds, L-ascorbic acid and L-dehydroascorbic acid, both of which are biologically active compounds. Like glucose, vitamin C is a 6-carbon compound, and while most plants and animals can synthesize vitamin C from glucose, humans, primates, guinea pigs, and some birds lack this ability, so dietary intake is essential to prevent deficiency (Lykkesfeldt et al. 2014). The most notable signs of vitamin C deficiency (known as scurvy) reflect its role in collagen formation maintaining the integrity of blood vessels: the gums bleed easily around the teeth and small haemorrhages under the skin can be observed due to ruptured capillaries. Severe symptoms include further haemorrhaging, muscle degeneration, softening of bones, and inadequate wound healing. Conversely, too much vitamin C can cause gastrointestinal distress and diarrhoea. As such, vitamin C levels in the body are tightly controlled using a number of mechanisms, which include saturable transporters that can prevent absorption and promote excretion of vitamin C and enzymes that recycle oxidized vitamin C.

The actions of vitamin C can be conveniently allocated to two roles: the role of vitamin C as an antioxidant and the role of vitamin C as a cofactor for enzymes involved in collagen and neurotransmitter synthesis. The importance of vitamin C as a water-soluble antioxidant is clear, as it is the major water-soluble antioxidant in plasma and plays an important role in recycling lipid-soluble antioxidants such as vitamin E (see Figure 4.2). Vitamin C also promotes iron absorption and release of iron from ferritin stores. Paradoxically, this released iron is able to participate in fenton-type reactions resulting in the generation of reactive species, suggesting that under certain conditions, this water-soluble antioxidant may take on a pro-oxidant role (Lane & Richardson 2014).

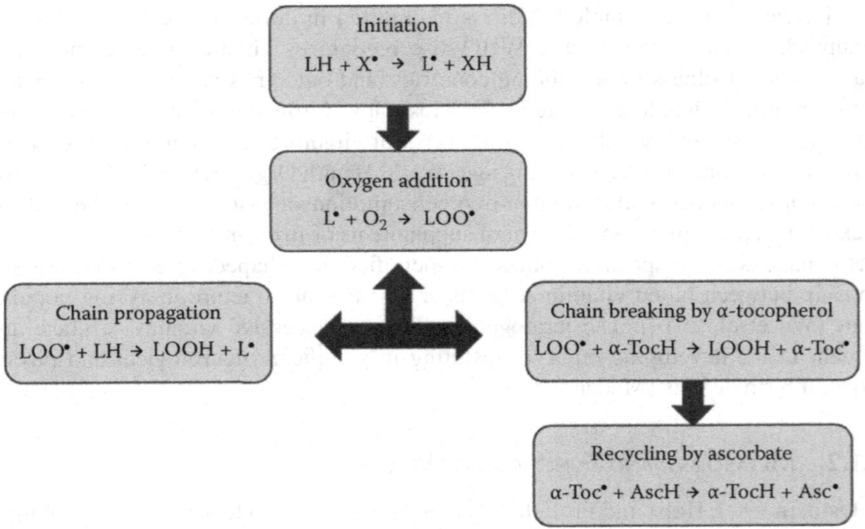

FIGURE 4.2 The elementary reactions of lipid peroxidation highlighting the roles played by vitamin E (α-tocopherol, α-TocH) and vitamin C (ascorbate, AscH). Lipid peroxidation is initiated when an unstable ROS/RNS reacts with a lipid containing an unsaturated fatty acid (LH). This generates an unstable lipid radical (L•) that reacts very quickly with available oxygen, resulting in the formation of a lipid peroxyl radical (LOO•). The lipid peroxyl radical can then react with neighbouring lipids containing unsaturated fatty acids propagating a lipid peroxidation chain reaction unless α-tocopherol is present to prevent the peroxidation process. The ability of α-tocopherol to exert this effect is prolonged in the presence of ascorbate which is capable of recycling the α-tocopherol radical (α-Toc•) thereby becoming a reactive species itself (Asc•). (Modified from Halliwell, B. & Gutteridge, J.M.C., *Free Radicals in Biology and Medicine*, 4th edn., Chapter 4, Oxford University Press, Oxford, UK, 2007.)

4.1.3 Metabolism and Functions of Vitamin E

Vitamin E (α-tocopherol) was discovered more than 90 years ago when it was identified that an adequate vitamin E intake was required for rats to achieve full-term pregnancies (Evans & Bishop 1922). Vitamin E itself is not a single compound but describes a number of tocopherols and tocotrienols, with α-tocopherol being recognized as the most biologically important form. Vitamin E is the most important fat-soluble antioxidant and plays an essential role in protecting unsaturated fatty acids from damage and hence protects the structural integrity of cell membranes and lipoproteins. This importance is demonstrated in cases of severe deficiency where the requirement for vitamin E cannot be replaced by other antioxidants (Ingold et al. 1987). Vitamin E is needed to maintain the normal neurological structure and function, and severe and prolonged deficiency leads to progressive neurological degeneration (Muller 2010; Muller & Goss-Sampson 1989). As vitamin E is fat soluble, its absorption from foods is dependent on the uptake of dietary fats, and its transport around the body is dependent on the transport of lipids in chylomicrons and lipoproteins (very-low-, low-, and high-density lipoproteins [VLDL, LDL, and HDL]). This dependency on dietary fat intake to increase absorption and distribution of vitamin E means that any drug or condition that impairs fat absorption from the gut can result in low circulating levels of vitamin E. This is exemplified in disorders such as cystic fibrosis and cholestatic liver disease, where bile synthesis/secretion is impaired and when lipase inhibitors are used to reduce fat absorption in the intestine (Floreani et al. 2000; Melia et al. 1996; Rana et al. 2014; Sokol et al. 1985). The metabolism of vitamin E occurs in the liver, where it is incorporated into lipoproteins and enters the circulation or in times of excess can be conjugated and excreted, and this ensures that vitamin E does not accumulate to toxic levels in the liver (Traber 2013).

The primary function of vitamin E relates to its ability to protect fatty acids from oxidative damage, and it is the unsaturated fatty acids (polyunsaturated [PUFA] and monounsaturated [MUFA]) that are susceptible to damage by ROS/RNS due to the presence of one or more double bonds in the carbon chain. PUFAs which have more than one double bond are more susceptible than MUFAs (Hargrove et al. 2001). This damage (termed lipid peroxidation) is a chain-propagating process which requires an effective chain-breaking antioxidant such as vitamin E (α-tocopherol) (Figure 4.2). The α-tocopherol radical is formed as a consequence of its chain-breaking activity; however, there is evidence to suggest that water-soluble vitamin C (ascorbate) plays an important synergistic role in recycling the α-tocopherol radical, thereby permitting its antioxidant activity to continue (May et al. 1998). In addition to its antioxidant function, it is thought that vitamin E has other specific functions in the nervous system such as influencing enzyme activities and gene regulation (Muller 2010).

4.2 THE ROLE OF ANTIOXIDANT VITAMINS A, C, AND E ON THE DEVELOPING BRAIN

Brain growth and development during embryogenesis, the fetal period, and early postnatal life is heavily influenced by nutritional status, and certain nutrients appear particularly influential (Georgieff 2007). While brain growth and development can be affected during the period of nutrient deprivation, it is becoming clear that longer lasting and permanent effects may occur (Wachs et al. 2014). To add further complexity, the developing brain is not a homogeneous tissue and different regions of the brain will have specific critical/sensitive periods for particular nutrients (Georgieff 2007; Wachs et al. 2014).

Periods of rapid brain growth and development are subject to increased production of reactive oxygen/nitrogen species (ROS/RNS) (Halliwell 2006). ROS in particular are generated as a normal by-product of mitochondrial respiration in all cells of the developing brain and when tightly controlled play an important role in directing cell growth, proliferation, differentiation, and apoptosis (programmed cell death) during all stages of embryogenesis and fetal development (Agarwal et al. 2008; Halliwell 2006). Along with this cellular capacity to generate ROS/RNS are antioxidant defence systems capable of preventing possible damage induced by the excessive production of ROS/RNS. These antioxidant defence systems consist of endogenous enzymatic and nonenzymatic antioxidants; the actions of which are both strongly influenced by nutritional status and supported by the intake of dietary antioxidants, such as vitamins A, C, and E.

As shown in Figure 4.3, if antioxidant defences are impaired, this may result in an imbalance, favouring oxidative stress. If this imbalance occurs during a crucial stage of embryonic, fetal, and placental growth and development, it can impact negatively on reproductive outcomes (Al-Gubory et al. 2010; Jauniaux et al. 2006). The expression and activity of endogenous antioxidant systems increase with gestational age and may be suboptimal during early embryogenesis (Jauniaux et al. 2000), and this may be a crucial period where the availability of dietary antioxidants such as vitamins A, C, and E may be of importance.

Oxidative stress is characterized by the excessive production of ROS/RNS coupled with inadequate antioxidant defences, and the link between increased oxidative stress and poor birth outcomes, such as miscarriage, has been reported in a number of studies (Hempstock et al. 2003; Hseih et al. 2012; Shamim et al. 2015). Additionally, increased oxidative stress has also been implicated in the pathogenesis of intrauterine growth restriction (IUGR) and pre-eclampsia (Biri et al. 2007; Redman & Sargent 2005). Biri et al. (2007) reported higher levels of malondialdehyde (a marker of oxidative stress) and lower levels of antioxidants in the plasma, placenta, and umbilical cords in patients with IUGR compared to controls.

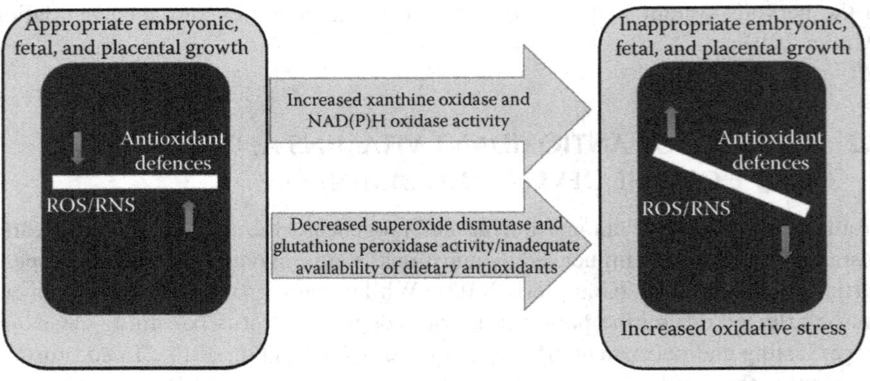

FIGURE 4.3 Growth and development of the embryo, fetus, and the placenta depend on a critical balance between the generation of reactive oxygen and nitrogen species (ROS/RNS) and endogenous cellular and dietary antioxidant defences. Cellular enzymes are key players in this process either by generating reactive species such as superoxide (xanthine and NAD(P)H oxidases) or by scavenging reactive species as observed with antioxidant enzymes such as superoxide dismutases and glutathione peroxidases. The availability of dietary antioxidants supports cellular antioxidant defences and may be more important during the early stages of embryogenesis when the activity of antioxidant enzymes is not optimal. This delicate balance is important at all stages of growth and development of the central nervous system and when disturbed results in poor pregnancy outcomes. (Modified from Craenenbroek, E.M.V. & Conraads, V.M., *Microvasc. Res.*, 79, 184, 2010, doi: 10.1016/j.mvr.2009.12.009.)

In addition, increased oxidative stress in developing organs (including the brain) has been linked to prenatal alcohol exposure (Chu et al. 2007; Dembele et al. 2006). Consistent with the role of alcohol-induced oxidative stress in prenatal brain development, dietary antioxidant treatment in animal models of fetal alcohol spectrum disorders (FASDs) attenuates the increase in oxidative stress induced by alcohol exposure (Brocardo et al. 2011; Shirpoor et al. 2009). Thus, dietary antioxidants are important in protecting cells from ROS/RNS-induced damage and, in combination with cellular antioxidant enzymes, ensure that defences are adequate. More specifically, dietary antioxidants such as vitamins A, E, and C are essential, and an adequate supply is needed during crucial periods of embryogenesis, fetal development, and early childhood for the normal development of the brain, supporting the development of cognitive and motor skills throughout childhood and into adulthood.

4.2.1 Vitamin A and the Developing Brain

It is important to note that in the body vitamin A is oxidized to its active metabolite, namely retinoic acid (RA), and it is the binding of RA to the retinoic acid receptor (RAR) that is directly responsible for the transcriptional regulatory actions of vitamin A during the growth and development of the fetal CNS. RA induces neuronal differentiation and patterning during embryogenesis and more recently has been shown to play a pivotal role in the formation of the blood–brain barrier (Maden 2007; Mizee et al. 2013). After birth, RA is also a key nutrient that shapes the brain and regulates neuroplasticity in the hippocampus, olfactory bulb, and hypothalamus/pituitary axis (Shearer et al. 2012). The effects of RA are concentration dependent in the developing embryo, and disruption can occur when RA levels are too low (deficiency) or too high (teratogenicity).

The 2010 review by Jane Adams provides a history of research on the neurobehavioural teratology of retinoids (Adams 2010). Neurobehavioural teratology is defined as the abnormal development of the CNS, resulting from exposure to exogenous agents during prenatal development. Animal studies in the 1970s and 1980s showed that behavioural effects were caused by lower doses of vitamin A (retinol and all-*trans*-retinoic acid) than were necessary to affect the growth. However, the effects of humans were unclear until the drug Accutane (active ingredient 13-*cis*-retinoic acid) became available in 1982 for the treatment of acne. Previous animal studies on this active ingredient in rats have not shown adverse effects compared to other retinoids. However, therapeutic doses in humans were associated with the increased risk of spontaneous abortion, perinatal mortality, premature birth, and other major malfunctions (Lammer et al. 1985). Longitudinal studies showed that by age 5, children's mental ability scores bordered on intellectual development disorder (Adams & Lammer 1993). This tragedy led to further animal studies in the 1990s to better understand species differences and mechanisms of retinoid neurobehavioural teratology. In summary, these studies showed that 11–13 days was the most sensitive period for lethal and, at lower doses, negative behavioural outcomes (Adams 2010). Since 2000, the scope of research has broadened to the role of retinoids in neural differentiation and patterning and influences on CNS functioning and motor system development.

Animal studies have shown that vitamin A deficiency leads to cognitive decline, and vitamin A supplementation has positive effects on learning and memory (in rats) and vocal learning (in songbirds) (Olson & Mello 2010). This combined evidence base provides strong support for the role of vitamin A (retinoic acid) in brain development and ageing process.

Vitamin A deficiency is one of the most common forms of malnutrition in human populations. It is strongly associated with an increased risk of mortality, morbidity, wasting, and stunting in children (Benton 2008). For example, a case–control study of 996 pregnant women with uncomplicated pregnancies found that retinol was positively associated with small-for-gestational-age (SGA) birth, whereas carotenoids were negatively associated with SGA (Cohen et al. 2015). Further research is needed to understand the mechanisms linking oxidative stress and fetal growth.

4.2.2 Vitamin C and the Developing Brain

All animal species have high vitamin C levels in the brain, tightly controlled by homeostatic mechanisms, even when other organs may be depleted (Adlard et al. 1974; Zalani et al. 1989). The developing brain depends on the SVCT2 transporter to distribute vitamin C around it, and studies have shown that mice born without functional SVCT2 do not survive birth due to cerebral haemorrhages (Harrison et al. 2010). This evidence supports the crucial role of vitamin C during brain development, and vitamin C deficiency can result in increased oxidative stress and impaired neurological development as summarized in Figure 4.4 (Hansen et al. 2014).

Animal studies have been used to investigate the impact of vitamin C deficiency in pregnancy and early life. Prolonged maternal vitamin C deficiency in guinea pigs was associated with intrauterine growth retardation of fetuses and their corresponding placentas, suggesting that vitamin C has a critical role in fetal development (Schjoldager et al. 2014). Furthermore, guinea pigs exposed to vitamin C deficiency

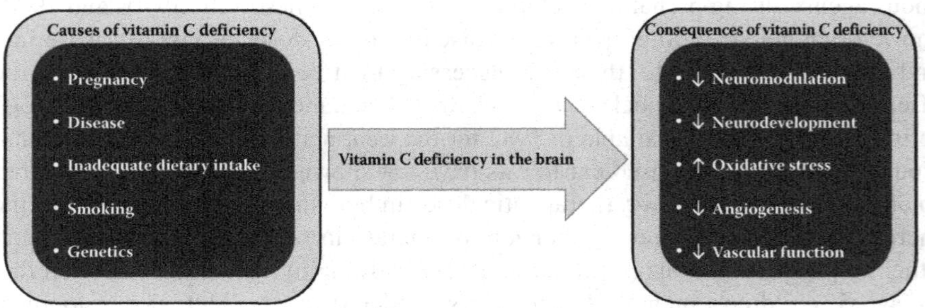

FIGURE 4.4 Potential causes and consequences of vitamin C deficiency in the brain. (Modified from Hansen, S.N. et al., *Nutrients*, 6(9), 3818, 2014, doi: 10.3390/nu6093818.) Dietary intake of vitamin C is key in determining overall vitamin C status, but requirements may be increased during intense periods of growth (pregnancy) or excessive stress (disease/smoking). The functions of vitamin C relate to its antioxidant activity, involvement in neurotransmitter synthesis/action (neuromodulation), support of angiogenesis and vascular function, and finally, development, maturation, and differentiation of neurons.

in early life showed significantly impaired spatial memory and reduced hippocampal volume compared to controls, but these experiments did not allow conclusions regarding the effects on cognitive performance (Hansen et al. 2014).

Despite the relatively high prevalence of hypovitaminosis C, particularly in high-income countries (Wrieden et al. 2000), there are few studies which have investigated the relationship between vitamin C and cognitive development and function in humans. Subpopulations at particular risk of low vitamin C are smokers and low-socio-economic groups. Maternal pre-eclampsia has also been linked to reduced levels of vitamin C and impaired cognitive performance in children, but RCTs have shown inconclusive effects of vitamin C supplementation (Hansen et al. 2014).

4.2.3 Vitamin E and the Developing Brain

Clinical vitamin E deficiency is rare but has been identified in premature infants, and low intakes have been associated with chronic degenerative conditions such as cardiovascular disease and some cancers. The landmark study by Evans and Bishop using rats identified that adequate vitamin E intake was required for rats to achieve full-term pregnancies (Evans & Bishop 1922). Although the precise reason why resorption of the embryo during early pregnancy occurs was not identified, subsequent studies using zebra fish models have highlighted the importance of α-tocopherol in embryonic development, the role of an α-tocopherol transfer protein (TTP) in regulating the delivery of α-tocopherol to the developing embryo, and the importance of this delivery system in targeting α-tocopherol to critical sites such as the developing brain (Miller et al. 2012a,b). TTP is also postulated to play an important role in human embryogenesis, as it is expressed in both human yolk sacs and placental trophoblast cells (Jauniaux et al. 2004; Kaempf-Rotzoll et al. 2003). This pattern of expression of TTP during early embryogenesis highlights a specific need for targeted vitamin E delivery across the placenta to the fetus and the developing brain. The developing brain will have a high requirement for unsaturated fatty acids to support neurogenesis, suggesting an important role of α-tocopherol in protecting fatty acids from oxidation.

A review of nutritional therapies for children with neurodevelopmental disorders presented the scientific rationale to support the use of vitamin E supplementation, in combination with omega-3 fatty acids (Gumpricht & Rockway 2014). Children with neurodevelopmental disorders, such as autism, have reduced the levels of vitamin E (Frustaci et al. 2012) and often present the same neurologic symptoms as patients with chronic lipid malabsorption states, such as children with cystic fibrosis and abetalipoproteinemia. Lower cognitive scores with low plasma α-tocopherol (<300 μg/dL) have been reported in patients with cystic fibrosis compared with α-tocopherol-sufficient control subjects (Koscik et al. 2004). Early diagnosis and minimizing the duration of vitamin E deficiency with nutritional therapy have been shown to result in better cognitive functioning in such children (Koscik et al. 2005). Children with fetal alcohol spectrum disorders (FASD) also tend to have lower intakes of vitamin E, among other nutrients, because of their social circumstances and behavioural challenges. A small study of children under the age of 5 years with FASD ($n = 31$) found that 74% had below the recommended intakes of vitamin E (Fuglestad et al. 2013) and many of the children also had below the recommended intakes of fibre, n-3 fatty acids, vitamin D, vitamin E, vitamin K, choline, and calcium. Research has shown that nutritional supplementation during pregnancy may attenuate ethanol's teratogenic effects. In animal models, pregnant rats given with nutrients high in antioxidants (e.g. vitamin C, vitamin E, omega-3 fatty acids) during the time they are also given alcohol gave birth to offspring with reduced oxidative stress and cell loss and fewer behavioural impairments (Brocardo et al. 2011; Patten et al. 2013). Although antioxidant treatments in animal models are promising, research on humans has been problematic. A clinical trial utilizing high doses of vitamins C and E in women with alcohol-exposed pregnancies was prematurely terminated after reports that high levels of vitamin C and E may lead to low birthweight among women with pre-eclampsia (Goh et al. 2007).

Longitudinal studies of humans have investigated associations between vitamins A and E status during pregnancy and intellectual development during early childhood. A study of 150 mother–child pairs in China found positive correlations between cord serum levels of vitamins A and E and certain indicators of development at age 2 (after adjusting for potential confounders such as parent's educational level, passive smoking exposure, and child's sex) (Chen et al. 2009). There was no association with vitamin C status. Evidence from a small intervention study supports the role of vitamin E in human brain development in early infancy. Supplementation in extremely low-birthweight (>1000 g) babies in Japan with α-tocopherol for longer than 6 months has been shown to be associated with improved mental development, performance IQ in particular, at 8 years of age compared to a control group (Kitajima et al. 2015).

In the absence of long-term studies of vitamin E supplementation in children, animal studies have demonstrated neuroprotective effects leading to improved cognitive function (Gumpricht & Rockway 2014). For example, a study of vitamin E–deficient rats showed improvements in the growth and neural and visual functions after 20 weeks of supplementation (Hayton et al. 2006). A more recent study of maternal vitamin E supplementation in rats showed anatomical changes in the hippocampus of offspring that lasted into adulthood, confirming long-lasting effects in the adult brain (Salucci et al. 2014). This study used high doses of vitamin E, up to 100 times the standard recommendation. Halliwell states that α-tocopherol levels in the brain are tightly regulated, and it takes many weeks or months to alter brain levels through dietary deficiency or supplementation (Halliwell 2006). This is why studies designed to assess the effects of vitamin E supplementation require large doses over long periods of time, which helps to explain the lack of human studies.

A study using a mouse model of Down syndrome (Ts65Dn) found that, following high doses of α-tocopherol during pregnancy and throughout the lifespan of the offspring, supplemented mice displayed signs of reduced anxiety and improved spatial learning compared to controls (Shichiri et al. 2011). The levels of 8-isoprostaglandin $F_{2\alpha}$, a marker of lipid peroxidation and oxidative stress, were higher in the Ts65Dn mice hippocampus and cortex brain tissues compared to control mice and the levels decreased following supplementation with α-tocopherol. In another study, mice which lacked the tocopherol transfer protein (TTP) and fed a vitamin E–deficient diet demonstrated increased cerebellar oxidative stress and compromised performance in motor coordination tests, compared to mice which had received dietary vitamin E supplementation (Ulatowski et al. 2014). These animal studies provide support for the essential role of vitamin E in CNS function, and further studies are needed to understand the potential impact of supplementation in humans with neurological and neurodevelopmental disorders.

As oxidative stress is considered to be a major contributor to neurodegeneration and hypothesized to contribute to the development of dementia, there have been several studies investigating the use of antioxidants such as vitamin E in both the ageing population and Alzheimer's disease patients. Inconsistent outcomes, however, have been reported in the literature, and the benefit of vitamin E as a treatment for neurodegenerative disorders remains under debate. For a review of current evidence, see Fata et al. (2014).

4.3 CONCLUSION

Adequate nutrition is necessary for normal brain development, and evidence suggests that the antioxidant vitamins A, C, and E have specific effects on the developing brain. The consequences of a deficiency in any one of these vitamins is dependent on the brain's requirement at a particular developmental stage and an inadequate supply may result in altered function/dysfunction which may not be recoverable even after repletion/supplementation. In excess, the toxic effects of some nutrients such as vitamin A add further complexity. The effects of deficiency for a particular nutrient on the developing brain can be studied simply *in vivo* in animal models where diets can be strictly controlled and brain tissue can be studied at all developmental stages. The major limitation to this is that in reality, nutrient deficiencies do not occur in isolation, which means translation to human brain development and the associated behavioural effects is very difficult to ascribe to a single nutrient. This can also be a problem with supplementation studies. Some studies have investigated the effects of multiple micronutrient supplements (antioxidants in combination with iron, zinc, iodine, etc.) on cognitive function in children, with some evidence of positive effects (Khor & Misra 2012; Manger et al. 2008; Van Stuijvenberg et al. 1999). However, it is not possible to determine the effects of single antioxidant nutrients from these studies.

REFERENCES

Adams, J. (2010). The neurobehavioral teratology of retinoids: A 50-year history. *Birth Defects Research. Part A, Clinical and Molecular Teratology*, 88(10), 895–905.

Adams, J. & Lammer, E. J. (1993). Neurobehavioral teratology of isotretinoin. *Reproductive Toxicology*, 7(2), 175–177.

Adlard, B. F. S., De Souza, S. W., & Moon, S. (1974). Ascorbic acid in the fetal human brain. *Archives of Disease in Childhood*, 49, 278–282.

Agarwal, A., Gupta, S., Sekhon, L., & Shah, R. (2008). Redox considerations in female reproductive function and assisted reproduction: From molecular mechanisms to health implications. *Antioxidants and Redox Signaling*, 10(8), 1375–1403.

Al-Gubory, K. H., Fowler, P. A., & Garrel, C. (2010). The roles of cellular reactive oxygen species, oxidative stress and antioxidants in pregnancy outcomes. *International Journal of Biochemistry and Cell Biology*, 42(10), 1634–1650.

Baron, J. H. (2009). Sailors' scurvy before and after James Lind – A reassessment. *Nutrition Reviews*, 67(6), 315–332.

Benton, D. (2008). Micronutrient status, cognition and behavioral problems in childhood. *European Journal of Nutrition*, 47(Suppl. 3), 38–50.

Biri, A., Bozkurt, N., Turp, A., Kavutcu, M., Himmetoglu, O., & Durak, I. (2007). Role of oxidative stress in intrauterine growth restriction. *Gynecologic and Obstetric Investigation*, 64(4), 187–192.

Brocardo, P. S., Gil-Mohapel, J., & Christie, B. R. (2011). The role of oxidative stress in fetal alcohol spectrum disorders. *Brain Research Reviews*, 67(1–2), 209–225.

Chen, K., Zhang, X., Wei, X. P., Qu, P., Liu, Y. X., & Li, T. Y. (2009). Antioxidant vitamin status during pregnancy in relation to cognitive development in the first two years of life. *Early Human Development*, 85(7), 421–427.

Chu, J., Tong, M., & de la Monte, S. M. (2007). Chronic ethanol exposure causes mitochondrial dysfunction and oxidative stress in immature central nervous system neurons. *Acta Neuropathology*, 113, 659–673.

Cohen, J. M., Kahn, S. R., Platt, R. W., Basso, O., Evans, R. W., & Kramer, M. S. (2015). Small-for-gestational-age birth and maternal plasma antioxidant levels in mid-gestation: A nested case-control study. *BJOG: An International Journal of Obstetrics and Gynaecology*, 122(10), 1313–1321.

Craenenbroek, E. M. V. & Conraads, V. M. (2010). Endothelial progenitor cells in vascular health: Focus on lifestyle. *Microvascular Research*, 79, 184–192.

Dembele, K., Yao, X.-H., Chen, L., & Gregoire Nyomba, B. L. (2006). Intrauterine ethanol exposure results in hypothalamic oxidative stress and neuroendocrine alterations in adult rat offspring. *American Journal of Physiology: Regulatory, Integrative and Comparative Physiology*, 291(3), R796–R802.

Evans, H. M. & Bishop, K. S. (1922). On the existence of a hitherto unrecognized dietary factor essential for reproduction. *Science*, 56(1458), 650.

Fata, G., Weber, P., & Mohajeri, M. H. (2014). Effects of vitamin E on cognitive performance during ageing and in alzheimer's disease. *Nutrients*, 6(12), 5453–5472.

Floreani, A., Barragiota, A., Martines, D., Naccarato, R., & D'Odorico, A. (2000). Plasma antioxidant levels in chronic cholestatic liver diseases. *Alimentary Pharmacology and Therapeutics*, 14(3), 353–358.

Frustaci, A., Neri, M., Cesario, A., Adams, J. B., Domenici, E., Dalla Bernardina, B., & Bonassi, S. (2012). Oxidative stress-related biomarkers in autism: Systematic review and meta-analyses. *Free Radical Biology and Medicine*, 52(10), 2128–2141.

Fuglestad, A. J., Fink, B. A., Eckerle, J. K., Boys, C. J., Hoecker, H. L., Kroupina, M. G., & Wozniak, J. R. (2013). Inadequate intake of nutrients essential for neurodevelopment in children with fetal alcohol spectrum disorders (FASD). *Neurotoxicology and Teratology*, 39, 128–132.

Georgieff, M. K. (2007). Nutrition and the developing brain: Nutrient priorities and measurement. *American Journal of Clinical Nutrition*, 85(2), 614S–620S.

Goh, Y. I., Ungar, W., Rover, J., & Koren, G. (2007). Mega-dose vitamin C and E in preventing FASD: The decision to terminate the study prematurely. *Journal of FAS International*, 5, e3.

Gumpricht, E. & Rockway, S. (2014). Can ω-3 fatty acids and tocotrienol-rich vitamin E reduce symptoms of neurodevelopmental disorders? *Nutrition*, 30(7–8), 733–738.

Halliwell, B. (2006). Oxidative stress and neurodegeneration: Where are we now? *Journal of Neurochemistry*, 97(6), 1634–1658.

Halliwell, B. & Gutteridge, J. M. C. (2007). Chapter 4. *Free Radicals in Biology and Medicine*, 4th edn. Oxford University Press, Oxford, UK.

Hansen, S. N., Tveden-Nyborg, P., & Lykkesfeldt, J. (2014). Does vitamin C deficiency affect cognitive development and function? *Nutrients*, 6(9), 3818–3846.

Hargrove, R. L., Etherton, T. D., Pearson, T. A., Harrison, E. H., & Kris-Etherton, P. M. (2001). Low and high fat monounsaturated diets decrease human low density lipoprotein oxidative susceptibility in vitro. *Journal of Nutrition*, 131, 1758–1763.

Harrison, F. E., Dawes, S. M., Meredith, M. E., Babaev, V. R., Li, L., & May, J. M. (2010). Low vitamin C and increased oxidative stress and cell death in mice that lack the sodium-dependent vitamin C transporter SVCT2. *Free Radical Biology and Medicine*, 49(5), 821–829.

Hayton, S. M., Kriss, T., Wade, A., & Muller, D. P. R. (2006). Effects on neural function of repleting vitamin E-deficient rats with a-tocopherol. *Journal of Neurophysiology*, 95(4), 2553–2559.

Hempstock, J., Jauniaux, E., Greenwold, N., & Burton, G. J. (2003). The contribution of placental oxidative stress to early pregnancy failure. *Human Pathology*, 34(12), 1265–1275.

Hseih, T.-T., Chen, S.-F., Lo, L.-M., Li, M.-J., Yeh, Y.-L., & Hung, T.-H. (2012). The association between maternal oxidative stress at mid-gestation and subsequent pregnancy complications. *Reproductive Sciences*, 19(5), 505–512.

Ingold, K. U., Webb, A. C., Witter, D., Burton, G. W., Metcalf, T. A., & Muller, D. P. R. (1987). Vitamin E remains the major lipid-soluble, chain-breaking antioxidant in human plasma even in individuals suffering severe vitamin E deficiency. *Archives of Biochemistry and Biophysics*, 259(1), 224–225.

Jauniaux, E., Cindrova-Davies, T., Johns, J., Dunster, C., Hempstock, J., Kelly, F. J., & Burton, G. J. (2004). Distribution and transfer pathways of antioxidant molecules inside the first trimester human gestational sac. *Journal of Clinical Endocrinology and Metabolism*, 89(3), 1452–1458.

Jauniaux, E., Poston, L., & Burton, G. J. (2006). Placental-related diseases of pregnancy: Involvement of oxidative stress and implications in human evolution. *Human Reproduction Update*, 12(6), 747–755.

Jauniaux, E., Watson, A.L., Hempstock, J., Bao, Y.-P., Skepper, J.N., & Burton, G.J. (2000). Onset of maternal arterial blood flow and placental oxidative stress. A possible factor in human early pregnancy failure. *American Journal of Pathology*, 157(6), 2111–2122.

Kaempf-Rotzoll, D. E., Horiguchi, M., Hashiguchi, K., Aoki, J., Tamai, H., Linderkamp, O., & Arai, H. (2003). Human placental trophoblast cells express a-tocopherol transfer protein. *Placenta*, 24(5), 439–444.

Khor, G. L. & Misra, S. (2012). Micronutrient interventions on cognitive performance of children aged 5–15 years in developing countries. *Asia Pacific Journal of Clinical Nutrition*, 21(4), 476–486.

Kitajima, H., Kanazawa, T., Mori, R., Hirano, S., Ogihara, T., & Fujimura, M. (2015). Long-term alpha-tocopherol supplements may improve mental development in extremely low birthweight infants. *Acta Paediatrica, International Journal of Paediatrics*, 104(2), e82–e89.

Koscik, R. L., Farrell, P. M., Kosorok, M. R., Zaremba, K. M., Laxova, A., Lai, H. C. et al. (2004). Cognitive function of children with cystic fibrosis: Deleterious effect of early malnutrition. *Pediatrics*, 113(6 I), 1549–1558.

Koscik, R. L., Lai, H. J., Laxova, A., Zaremba, K. M., Kosorok, M. R., Douglas, J. A. et al. (2005). Preventing early, prolonged vitamin E deficiency: An opportunity for better cognitive outcomes via early diagnosis through neonatal screening. *Journal of Pediatrics*, 147(3 Suppl.), S51–S56.

Lammer, E. J., Chen, D. T., Hoar, R. M., Agnish, N. D., Benke, P. J., Braun, J. T. et al. (1985). Retinoic acid embryopathy. *New England Journal of Medicine*, 313(14), 837–841.

Lane, D. R. J. & Richardson, D. R. (2014). The active role of vitamin C in mammalian iron absorption: Much more than just enhanced iron absorption! *Free Radical Biology and Medicine*, 75, 69–83.

Lykkesfeldt, J., Michels, A. J., & Frei, B. (2014). Vitamin C. *Advances in Nutrition*, 5, 16–18.

Maden, M. (2001). Vitamin A and the developing embryo. *Postgraduate Medical Journal*, 77, 489–491.

Maden, M. (2007). Retinoic acid in the development, regeneration and maintenance of the nervous system. *Nature Reviews Neuroscience*, 8(10), 755–765.

Manger, M. S., McKenzie, J. E., Winichagoon, P., Gray, A., Chavasit, V., Pongcharoen, T. et al. (2008). A micronutrient-fortified seasoning powder reduces morbidity and improves short-term cognitive function, but has no effect on anthropometric measures in primary school children in northeast Thailand: A randomized controlled trial. *American Journal of Clinical Nutrition*, 87(6), 1715–1722.

May, J. M., Qu, Z. C., & Mendiratta, S. (1998). Protection and recycling of a-tocopherol in human erythrocytes by intracellular ascorbic acid. *Archives of Biochemistry and Biophysics*, 349(2), 281–289.

Melia, A. T., Koss-Twardy, S. G., & Zhi, J. (1996). The effect of orlistat, an inhibitor of dietary fat absorption, on the absorption of vitamins A and E in healthy volunteers. *Journal of Clinical Pharmacology*, 36(7), 647–653.

Miller, G. W., Labut, E. M., Lebold, K. M., Floeter, A., Tanguay, R. L., & Traber, M. G. (2012a). Zebrafish (danio rerio) fed vitamin E-deficient diets produce embryos with increased morphologic abnormalities and mortality. *Journal of Nutritional Biochemistry*, 23(5), 478–486.

Miller, G. W., Ulatowski, L., Labut, E. M., Lebold, K. M., Manor, D., Atkinson, J. et al. (2012b). The a-tocopherol transfer protein is essential for vertebrate embryogenesis. *PLoS ONE*, 7(10), e47402.

Mizee, M. R., Wooldrik, D., Lakeman, K. A. M., van het Hof, B., Drexhage, J. A. R., Geerts, D. et al. (2013). Retinoic acid induces blood-brain barrier development. *Journal of Neuroscience*, 33(4), 1660–1671.

Muller, D. P. R. (2010). Vitamin E and neurological function. *Molecular Nutrition and Food Research*, 54(5), 710–718.

Muller, D. P. R. & Goss-Sampson, M. A. (1989). Role of vitamin E in neural tissue. *Annals of the New York Academy of Sciences*, 570, 146–155.

Olson, C. R. & Mello, C. V. (2010). Significance of vitamin A to brain function, behavior and learning. *Molecular Nutrition and Food Research*, 54(4), 489–495.

Patten, A. R., Brocardo, P. S., & Christie, B. R. (2013). Omega-3 supplementation can restore glutathione levels and prevent oxidative damage caused by prenatal ethanol exposure. *Journal of Nutritional Biochemistry*, 24(5), 760–769.

Rana, M., Wong-See, D., Katz, T., Gaskin, K., Whitehead, B., Jaffe, A. et al. (2014). Fat-soluble vitamin deficiency in children and adolescents with cystic fibrosis. *Journal of Clinical Pathology*, 67(7), 605–608.

Redman, C. W. & Sargent, I. L. (2005). Latest advances in understanding preeclampsia. *Science*, 308, 1592–1594.

Salucci, S., Ambrogini, P., Lattanzi, D., Betti, M., Gobbi, P., Galati, C. et al. (2014). Maternal dietary loads of alpha-tocopherol increase synapse density and glial synaptic coverage in the hippocampus of adult offspring. *European Journal of Histochemistry*, 58(2), 120–126.

Schjoldager, J. G., Paidi, M. D., Lindblad, M. M., Birck, M. M., Kjærgaard, A. B., Dantzer, V. et al. (2014). Maternal vitamin C deficiency during pregnancy results in transient fetal and placental growth retardation in guinea pigs. *European Journal of Nutrition*, 54(4), 667–676.

Shamim, A. A., Schulze, K., Merrill, R. D., Kabir, A., Christian, P., Shaikh, S. et al. (2015). First-trimester plasma tocopherols are associated with risk of miscarriage in rural bangladesh. *American Journal of Clinical Nutrition*, 101(2), 294–301.

Shearer, K. D., Stoney, P. N., Morgan, P. J., & McCaffery, P. J. (2012). A vitamin for the brain. *Trends in Neurosciences*, 35(12), 733–741.

Shichiri, M., Yoshida, Y., Ishida, N., Hagihara, Y., Iwahashi, H., Tamai, H., & Niki, E. (2011). A-tocopherol suppresses lipid peroxidation and behavioral and cognitive impairments in the Ts65Dn mouse model of down syndrome. *Free Radical Biology and Medicine*, 50(12), 1801–1811.

Shirpoor, A., Salami, S., Khadem-Ansari, M. H., Minassian, S., & Yegiazarian, M. (2009). Protective effect of vitamin E against ethanol-induced hyperhomocysteinemia, DNA damage, and atrophy in the developing rat male brain. *Alcoholism: Clinical and Experimental Research*, 33(7), 1181–1186.

Sokol, R. J., Balistreri, W. F., Hoofnagle, J. F., & Jones, E. A. (1985). Vitamin E deficiency in adults with chronic liver disease. *American Journal of Clinical Nutrition*, 41(1), 66–72.

Tang, G. (2014). Vitamin A value of plant food provitamin A – Evaluated by the stable isotope technologies. *International Journal for Vitamin and Nutrition Research*, 84, 25–29.

Traber, M. G. (2013). Mechanisms for the prevention of vitamin E excess. *Journal of Lipid Research*, 54(9), 2295–2306.

Ulatowski, L., Parker, R., Warrier, G., Sultana, R., Butterfield, D. A., & Manor, D. (2014). Vitamin E is essential for purkinje neuron integrity. *Neuroscience*, 260, 120–129.

Van Stuijvenberg, M. E., Kvalsvig, J. D., Faber, M., Kruger, M., Kenoyer, D. G., & Benadé, A. J. S. (1999). Effect of iron-, iodine-, and ß-carotene-fortified biscuits on the micronutrient status of primary school children: A randomized controlled trial. *American Journal of Clinical Nutrition*, 69(3), 497–503.

Wachs, T. D., Georgieff, M., Cusick, S., & Mcewen, B. S. (2014). Issues in the timing of integrated early interventions: Contributions from nutrition, neuroscience, and psychological research. *Annals of the New York Academy of Sciences*, 1308, 89–106.

World Health Organization. (2002). The world health report 2002 – Reducing risks, promoting healthy life. Retrieved from http://www.who.int/whr/2002/en. Accessed on June 1, 2015.

Wrieden, W. L., Hannah, M. K., Bolton-Smith, C., Tavendale, R., Morrison, C., & Tunstall-Pedoe, H. (2000). Plasma vitamin C and food choice in the third Glasgow MONICA population survey. *Journal of Epidemiology and Community Health*, 54(5), 355–360.

Wu, A.-M., Huang, C.-Q., Lin, Z.-K., Tian, N.-F., Ni, W.-F., Wang, X.-Y., Zu, H.-Z., & Chi, Y.-L. (2014). The relationship between vitamin A and risk of fracture: Meta-analysis of prospective studies. *Journal of Bone and Mineral Research*, 29(9), 2032–2039.

Zalani, S., Rajalakshmi, R., & Parekh, L. J. (1989). Ascorbic acid concentration of human fetal tissues in relation to fetal size and gestational age. *British Journal of Nutrition*, 61, 601–606.

5 The Influence of the B Vitamins and Choline on the Developing Brain

Victoria Hall Moran

CONTENTS

5.1 INTRODUCTION

The B vitamins are a class of water-soluble vitamins, many of which are involved in several significant metabolic processes within the brain and whose deficiency have been shown to exert negative cognitive effects. The B vitamins, which consist of thiamin (B_1), riboflavin (B_2), niacin (B_3), pantothenic acid (B_5), B_6, biotin (B_7), folate (B_9), and cobalamin (B_{12}), are an interrelated group of essential nutrients that are not synthesized in the body, and thus, they need to be obtained from food and require ongoing replenishment. Although choline is not by strict definition a vitamin, it is also an essential nutrient. Choline and several B vitamins (i.e. folate, vitamin B_2, vitamin B_6, and vitamin B_{12}) are cofactors in the one-carbon metabolism pathway (Figure 5.1). In this ATP-driven reaction, methionine is converted into *S*-adenosylmethionine (SAM), the universal cellular methyl donor. DNA methyltransferases (DNMTs) covalently attach methyl groups from SAM to the carbon-5 position of cytosine bases, generating 5-methylcytosine thus methylating DNA (Anderson et al. 2012).

The B vitamins are found in plentiful amounts in whole unprocessed foods. Processed foods, such as refined grains and white flour, contain lower levels of vitamin B than their unprocessed equivalents. The milling process, for example, removes 65%–80% of thiamin, riboflavin, and niacin from cereals and flours. For this reason,

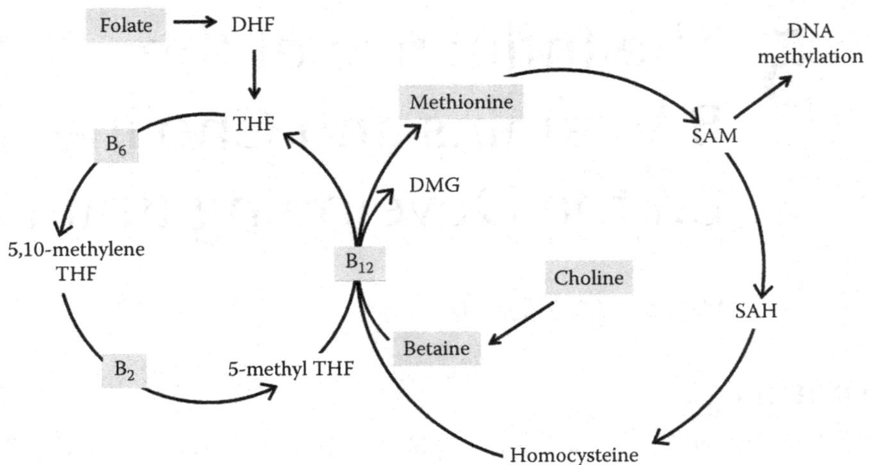

FIGURE 5.1 Involvement of the B vitamins and choline in one-carbon metabolism. Substrates obtained via diet are highlighted in gray. (1) Vitamin B_6 is a cofactor to serine hydroxymethyltransferase in the conversion of tetrahydrofolate (THF) to 5,10-methylene THF. (2) Vitamin B_2 is a precursor to FAD, which is a cofactor to methylenetetrahydrofolate reductase (MTHFR) in the conversion of 5,10-methylene THF to 5-methyl THF. (3) Vitamin B_{12} is a precursor to methionine synthase, and is involved in the production of methionine from homocysteine and betaine. (Abbreviations: Dihydrofolate [DHF], flavin adenine dinucleotide [FAD], dimethylglycine [DMG], methylenetetrahydrofolate reductase [MTHFR], *S*-adenosylhomocysteine [SAH], tetrahydrofolate [THF]). (From Anderson, O.S., Sant, K.E., & Dolinoy, D.C., *J. Nutr. Biochem.*, 23(8), 853, 2012.)

there is a long history of adding B vitamins to cereals (including wheat and maize flours) and rice grains in both low-income and high-income countries. It has been estimated that about 30% of industrially milled wheat flour, 48% of maize flour, and 1% of rice are fortified globally (Food Fortification Initiative 2014). However, wide variations in fortification practices are evident, with estimates for wheat flour fortification ranging from 97% in the Americas, 31% in Africa, 44% in Eastern Mediterranean, 21% in Southeast Asia, 6% in Europe and 4% in the Western Pacific regions (WHO 2009). The enrichment of flours and cereals has made, and continues to make, a major contribution to meeting the recommended intake of these vitamins, even in high-income countries (Allen et al. 2006). In response to the high prevalence of vitamin B_{12} deficiency worldwide, it has been proposed that vitamin B_{12} is included in food fortification programmes, particularly in countries with implemented folic acid fortification programmes, due to the interdependent metabolic roles of folate and vitamin B_{12} and the potential for exacerbation of vitamin B_{12} deficiency symptoms associated with high folic acid intake. The World Health Organization has released recommendations for food fortification programmes to include vitamin B_{12} (WHO 2009), which has been adopted by some countries, such as Tanzania and Cameroon (Sight & Life 2012).

The B vitamins are likely to have a number of influences on brain development, mediated through their central role in cell proliferation, myelination, synapse function, and neurotransmitter synthesis and functioning, as well as brain energy metabolism. For example, folate, vitamin B_6, and vitamin B_{12} are thought to influence cognitive performance through their roles in the central nervous system (CNS). Two interrelated neurochemical mechanisms have been suggested: the hypomethylation hypothesis and the homocysteine hypothesis (Bryan et al. 2004). The hypomethylation hypothesis suggests that folate, with vitamin B_{12} or B_6 as a catalyzing cofactor, may have a direct and possibly acute effect on the central nervous system (CNS) through its role in the one-carbon cycle, which is essential for many transmethylation reactions in the CNS. Low levels of folate lead to hypomethylation, inhibiting the synthesis of methionine and *S*-adenosylmethionine (SAM). This in turn inhibits methylation reactions throughout the CNS, involving proteins, membrane phospholipids, DNA, the metabolism of neurotransmitters such as the monoamines (e.g. dopamine, noradrenaline, serotonin), and melatonin, all of which have an impact on neurologic and psychological status (Calvaresi & Bryan 2001). The homocysteine hypothesis proposes an indirect, and possibly longer-term, effect of vitamin B_{12}, vitamin B_6, and folate on brain functioning by affecting the cerebral vasculature, as high levels of homocysteine, which are largely attributable to low blood levels of these vitamins are associated with an increased risk of vascular disease. Therefore, these vitamins act indirectly to support cognitive development and functioning through the prevention of vascular disease and preservation of the integrity of the CNS (Bryan et al. 2004).

This chapter will discuss the current evidence of the role of the B vitamins and choline in the developing brain. For many B vitamins, while there is strong biological plausibility for their influence on brain development due to their integral role in the CNS, there have been few studies conducted. Therefore, this chapter will focus particularly on the vitamins which have the strongest evidence base, namely thiamin, folate, and vitamin B_{12}.

5.2 B_1 (THIAMIN)

An adequate intake of thiamin is important for the metabolism of carbohydrates, lipids, and amino acids in brain tissue. While free thiamin has no known physiological role, thiamin diphosphate (ThDP) is an essential cofactor in key metabolic reactions involved in the conversion of pyruvate to acetyl coenzyme A (CoA), and alpha-ketoglutarate to succinyl CoA in carbohydrate metabolism, and reactions catalyzed by transketolase in the pentose phosphate pathway (see Figure 5.2). The pyruvate dehydrogenase enzyme that converts pyruvate to acetyl CoA seems particularly sensitive to thiamin deficiency. Thiamin deficiency leads to an inability to metabolize carbohydrate aerobically, so pyruvate and lactate accumulate in the blood and tissues. The disruption of the pentose phosphate pathway restricts the production of reduced NADP that is essential for lipid biosynthesis, including the synthesis of myelin. Other phosphorylated derivatives of thiamin, such as adenosine thiamine triphosphate (AThTP) and adenosine thiamin diphosphate, are also known to exist, but their biological roles remain unclear (Bates 2006; Bettendorff 2012).

Thiamin is found in most foods, but there are particularly rich sources such as whole grains (where it is concentrated in the bran and germ layers), meat, fish, pulses,

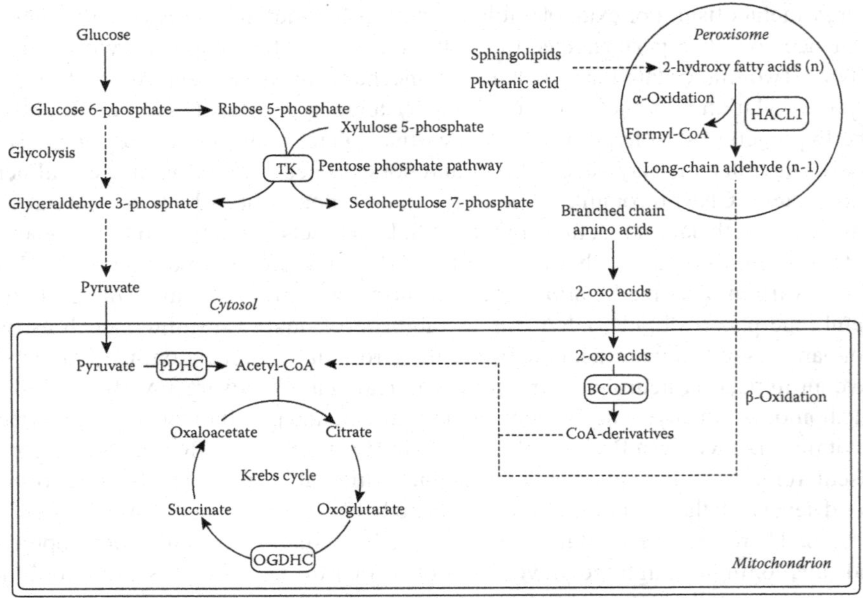

FIGURE 5.2 Cofactor role of thiamin diphosphate (ThDP). (TK, transketolase; PDHC, pyruvate dehydrogenase complex; OGDHC, oxoglutarate dehydrogenase complex; BCODC, branched-chain 2-oxo acid dehydrogenase; HACL 1,2-hydroxyacyl-CoA lyase.) (From Bettendorff, L. & Thiamin, in: Erdman, J.W., Macdonald, I.A., & Zeisel, S.H., eds., *Present Knowledge in Nutrition*, 10th edn., International Life Sciences Institute, Ames, IA, 261, 2012.)

and yeast. Vegetables contain two to three times less thiamin than meat per unit weight (Bettendorff 2012). While thiamin is stable on storage, food processing such as milling has a significant impact on the thiamin content. White flour is particularly low in thiamin, and as a consequence, it is fortified with thiamin in many parts of the world. Many other processed foods such as cereals, bread, dairy products, and infant formula are also enriched with thiamin. As thiamin is heat labile, heating, overcooking, and pasteurization may result in a considerable loss of the vitamin (Bettendorff 2012).

Thiamin requirements are linked to energy metabolism and are calculated on the basis of the total energy intake, assuming that the average diet provides 40% of energy from fat. For diets that are lower in fat, and hence higher in carbohydrate and protein, thiamin requirements will be higher. Increased intakes of thiamin are recommended in the third trimester of pregnancy and during lactation to accompany the suggested increase in energy intake. Breast milk concentrations of thiamin and subsequent infant status are strongly dependent on maternal intake and status, and maternal supplementation has been shown to rapidly improve the vitamin concentration in breast milk and the thiamin status of the breastfed infant (Allen 2012).

Thiamin deficiency is rare in high-income countries due to the enrichment of food with the vitamin, and in the United Kingdom, there is little evidence of low thiamin status in the general population (Bates et al. 2014). In this context, deficiency is often associated with chronic alcoholism, HIV–AIDS, or gastrointestinal conditions that impair vitamin absorption (Butterworth 2003). Thiamin deficiency is more prevalent in low-income populations, including many areas of rural Southeast Asia, where diets are high in refined or unfortified grains and low in animal source foods and legumes.

Thiamin deficiency is the primary cause of two conditions; beriberi and Wernicke–Korsakoff syndrome. Beriberi is characterized by lactic acidosis; peripheral neuropathy in dry beriberi, leading to loss of motor function, muscle wasting, and paralysis; and heart failure and oedema in wet beriberi. No single mechanism accounts for the thiamin deficient–induced neurologic damage, although elevated lactic acid concentrations in the brain and associated acidosis, mitochondrial damage, alterations in the levels of several neurotransmitters, induction of apoptosis, and neuronal cell death due to oxidative stress have all been implicated (Singleton & Martin 2001). Wernicke–Korsakoff syndrome is the neurological and psychiatric manifestation of thiamin deficiency. The syndrome is a combined manifestation of two disorders: one being characterized by an acute/subacute confusional state and often reversible findings of Wernicke encephalopathy (a type of delirium) and the other by persistent and irreversible findings of Korsakoff dementia.

Animal studies have demonstrated that thiamin deficiency has a negative impact on the developing brain. In studies on rats, thiamin deficiency has been shown to produce behavioural changes ranging from mild cognitive deficits to severe learning and memory impairments. The associated pathologic damage to the brain following a period of thiamin deficiency also varies from neuronal loss in select thalamic nuclei to tissue loss in large regions of the thalamus, mammillary bodies, and cortex, and the degree of cortical and diencephalic damage is closely related to these deficits in learning and memory (Langlais & Savage 1995). Evidence of the effect of thiamin deficiency on the human infant brain, however, is limited, with most cases being infants breastfed by mothers who were thiamin deficient themselves or given non-dairy formula low in thiamin (Vasconcelos et al. 1999; Wyalt et al. 1987). A magnetic resonance imaging (MRI) study of six infants aged 2–10 months with encephalopathy fed only with thiamin-deplete soy-based formula from birth found that thiamin deficiency was characterized by lesions in the periaqueductal region, thalami, and the mammillary bodies of the brain and abnormalities in the frontal lobes and basal ganglia (Kornreich et al. 2005).

An unfortunate event in Israel in 2003 provided an opportunity to study the impact of thiamin deficiency in infants. In November 2003, thiamin deficiency was diagnosed in several infants in Israel; all had been fed the same brand of soy-based formula, specifically manufactured for the Israeli market. It was subsequently discovered that the manufacturer had mistakenly stopped adding thiamin to its infant formula in early 2003, and this was estimated to have been fed to 1500–5000 children (Fattal-Valevski et al. 2005). Fattal-Valevski and colleagues (2009) conducted a small case–control study evaluating the language development of 20 children who had been exposed to the defective formula and who were followed up regularly at paediatric outpatient services. The children showed delayed language development at 5 years of age, even though the affected children had been considered 'asymptomatic' with no abnormal neurological symptoms during the thiamin deficiency period. Together, these studies suggest that thaimin deficiency may exert its effects on the brain development of children in the absence of overt clinical symptoms.

Low thiamin status has been reported to be common in critically ill children. Lima et al. (2011) demonstrated that 13.4% of 778 infants admitted to a hospital in Brazil without clinical signs of thiamin deficiency showed biochemical signs of deficiency based on blood analyses. It is less clear, however, whether the thiamin deficiency was a cause, an effect, or in fact unrelated to the specific critical illness suffered by these children, and further research is necessary in order to assess whether it is a significant contributor to mortality in sick children from other parts of the world (Kauffman et al. 2011).

5.3 VITAMIN B_2 (RIBOFLAVIN)

Riboflavin is widely distributed throughout the plant and animal kingdom and plays a central role as a coenzyme in energy-yielding metabolism. The major coenzyme forms of riboflavin function as prosthetic groups of numerous holoenzymes that catalyze diverse and often essential one- and two-electron redox reactions. Flavin mononucleotide (FMN) accounts for approximately 10% of the total flavin in cells, while flavin adenine dinucleotide (FAD) comprises nearly 90% (McCormick 2012). Flavin oxidases make a significant contribution to the oxidant stress of the body because the reoxidation of reduced flavin coenzymes is the major source of oxygen free radicals in the body. Riboflavin is also capable of generating reactive oxygen species non-enzymatically. As a consequence, and to protect the body, there is very strict control over the body content of riboflavin with limited absorption and rapid excretion of any excess.

Free riboflavin is not commonly found in food, other than milk and eggs, instead most of the vitamin in foods is present as flavin coenzymes (riboflavin phosphate and FAD) and good sources include liver, meat, fish, and some green leafy vegetables. Western diets commonly obtain 25%–30% of their riboflavin from milk. It is recommended in the United Kingdom that average riboflavin intake should increase by 0.3 mg/day (to a total of 1.4 mg/day) throughout pregnancy.

The global prevalence of riboflavin deficiency is uncertain as there is no clear deficiency disease but it is likely to be high because intake depends primarily on animal source food and green vegetable consumption (Allen 2012). There is evidence to suggest that even in high-income countries, including the United States, France, and the United Kingdom, riboflavin status is suboptimal. The UK National Diet and Nutrition Surveys (NDNSs) have revealed a high prevalence of biochemical riboflavin deficiency, as determined by measuring erythrocyte glutathione reductase activation coefficient (EGRAC), in 41% of free-living elderly people and in 95% of adolescent girls (Finch et al. 1998; Gregory & Lowe 2000; Ruston et al. 2004). Maternal riboflavin deficiency rapidly results in low breast milk concentrations of the vitamin (Allen 2012), and riboflavin concentrations can be moderately increased by supplementation of the mother when natural intake is low (Bates et al. 1985). More recently, administration of a 2 or 4 mg riboflavin supplement for 8 weeks has been shown to elicit a significant dose–response improvement in riboflavin status, as determined by EGRAC, in women aged 19–25 years (Powers et al. 2011). In addition, the improvement of riboflavin status led to an increase in the number of circulating red blood cells and haemoglobin concentrations, with greater haemoglobin concentrations observed in those with the poorest riboflavin status, highlighting the important role of riboflavin in iron metabolism.

Evidence of the influence of riboflavin on the developing brain is limited to animal models. Research on 21-day-old weanling rats that had been maintained on riboflavin-deficient diets revealed a 20% lower brain weight than those of rats on control diets (Ogunleye & Odutuga 1989), with the myelin lipids undergoing a proportional reduction. Since riboflavin plays a role in the metabolism of essential fatty acids in brain lipids, its deficiency has been considered similar to that of essential fatty acid deficiency, causing an impairment in brain development and maturation, although direct evidence to support this assumption in humans is lacking (Ramakrishna 1999).

Recent research has suggested that riboflavin supplementation can ameliorate the progression of the rare neurodegenerative condition Brown–Vialetto–Van Laere (BVVL) syndrome which affects infants, children, and young adults. BVVL is a genetic disorder, and at least one gene has been identified as its cause. The SLC52A3 gene encodes the intestinal (hRFT2) riboflavin transporter and mutations of this gene, leading to defective intestinal riboflavin transport, have uncovered the aetiology in a large proportion of cases with BVVL syndrome. Riboflavin therapy has been found to result in a rapid clinical and biochemical improvement in patients (Bosch et al. 2012). Mutations in the SLC52A2 gene coding for another human riboflavin transporter (hRFT3) have also been associated with BVVL syndrome, and in these cases, high-dose oral riboflavin supplements have again proved beneficial (Foley et al. 2014).

5.4 VITAMIN B_3 (NIACIN)

Niacin, which commonly refers to nicotinic acid or nicotinamide, is a dietary precursor of nicotinamide adenine dinucleotide (NAD), which can be phosphorylated (NADP) and reduced (NADH and NADPH). NAD and NADP serve as hydrogen acceptors and donators in numerous oxidation and reduction reactions in human biochemical pathways. It is during the reoxidation of the reduced NAD, produced during the oxidation of food, that most of the ATP yielded by aerobic metabolism is produced in the mitochondria. Over 400 enzymes require the niacin coenzymes NAD and NADP, which are thus involved in more reactions than any other vitamin-derived molecule. NAD usually functions in energy-producing reactions involving the catabolism of proteins, carbohydrates, fats, and alcohol, whereas NADP functions more often in anabolic reactions, such as in the synthesis of macromolecules, including fatty acids and cholesterol (Cervantes-Laurean et al. 1999). Organs with high energy requirements (e.g. in the brain) or high turnover rate (e.g. in the gut and skin) are usually the most susceptible to their deficiency (Ishii & Nishihara 1981).

Niacin is found in red meat, liver, pulses, milk, fish, and whole-grain cereals, although much of the vitamin naturally present in cereals may be in a bound form that is not readily available to humans. Niacin is also added to white flour and many breakfast cereals and can also be obtained indirectly by the conversion of tryptophan in dietary protein to niacin, although the efficiency of conversion is low in humans and affected by deficiencies in other nutrients.

Niacin deficiency results in the disease pellagra, the symptoms of which are often referred to as the 3 Ds – dermatitis, diarrhoea, and dementia. Neurologic symptoms of pellagra include headache, fatigue, apathy, depression, ataxia, poor concentration, delusions, and hallucinations, which can lead to confusion, memory loss, psychosis, and eventual death (Hegyi et al. 2004). Pellagra has been historically associated with poverty and consumption of a diet predominantly based on maize, which is low in tryptophan and bioavailable niacin (Park et al. 2000). Introduction of maize from the Americas has been associated with major epidemics of niacin deficiency in parts of the world where it became established as the dominant staple (e.g. North and South Africa, and southern Europe). The condition is now much less common, but it can occur in chronic alcoholics and those with malabsorption syndromes (Hegvi et al. 2004).

Some studies suggest a beneficial effect of supplemental niacin on cognitive function, risk of dementia, and neurological damage. Improvements in cognitive test scores (Herrmann et al. 1997), memory (Loriaux et al. 1985), and overall function (Battaglia et al. 1989) have been reported in trials of pharmacological preparations which include nicotinic acid. An increase in dietary niacin from 15 to 40 mg/day has been correlated with a 70% reduction in the likelihood of Alzheimer's disease in a U.S. study of 6158 patients over 65 years of age (Morris et al. 2004). More recently, it has been reported that niacin treatment of stroke promotes synaptic plasticity and axon growth in rats, which greatly improved neurological function after a stroke (Cui et al. 2010). Research on niacin's role on brain development and cognitive function, however, is lacking.

5.5 VITAMIN B_5 (PANTOTHENIC ACID)

The main role of pantothenic acid (vitamin B_5) is to act as a substrate for the synthesis of coenzyme A (CoA), a coenzyme needed for the oxidative metabolism of glucose and fatty acids, and for the biosynthesis of fatty acids, cholesterol, steroid hormones, melatonin, and the neurotransmitter acetylcholine. In the form of 4′-phosphopantetheine, pantothenic acid plays a key role in acyl carrier protein (ACP), which is needed for the synthesis of fatty acids, including phospholipids and sphingolipids. Phospholipids are important structural components of cell membranes, and the sphingolipid, sphingomyelin, is a component of the myelin sheath that enhances nerve transmission.

Pantothenic acid is found in many foods of both plant and animal origin. Particularly rich sources of the vitamin include chicken, beef, liver and other organ meats, whole grains, potatoes, and tomatoes. Due to its thermal lability and susceptibility to oxidation, significant amounts of pantothenic acid are lost from highly processed food, including refinement (resulting in a 37%–47% loss in grains), canning (20%–35% loss in meats, fish, and dairy products and 46%–78%

loss in vegetables), and freezing (37%–57% loss in frozen vegetables) (Miller & Ruckner 2012).

During pregnancy and lactation, recommended intakes of pantothenic acid are increased (adequate intake increase by 1 and 2 mg/day, respectively), accounting for the additional secretion of the vitamin in human milk (1.7 mg/day). This is likely the result of efficient sequestering of the vitamin in human milk (Miller & Ruckner 2012), estimated to be 0.4 mg for every 1 mg pantothenic acid consumed during lactation (Song et al. 1984).

Pantothenic acid is an essential nutrient, and in deficiency, many physiological systems are affected, due to the diversity of metabolic functions in which CoA and ACP participate. Neurological, immunological, haematological, reproductive, and gastrointestinal pathologies have been reported. Because pantothenic acid is such a ubiquitous component of food, naturally occurring pantothenic acid deficiency is very rare and has been observed only in cases of severe malnutrition (Iesofsky-Vig 1999). As deficiency is therefore associated with multiple micronutrient deficiencies, it is difficult to distinguish the effects specific to the lack of pantothenic acid (Gibson & Blass 1999). Given pantothenic acid's prevalence among living organisms, supplementation of this vitamin has been the subject of many health claims, including improvements in mood, memory, and brain function, yet most have little or no scientific basis (Miller & Ruckner 2012).

5.6 VITAMIN B_6

Vitamin B_6 is a family of related compounds comprising pyridoxine (PN), pyridoxal (PL), and pyridoxamine (PM), and their phosphorylated forms. The primary vitamin B_6 coenzymatic form, pyridoxal-5′-phospate (PLP), is an essential cofactor in over 140 human enzymatic reactions, principally in the metabolism of amino acids, but also of carbohydrate and lipid. PLP is also an essential coenzyme for the biosynthesis of several neurotransmitters, including noradrenaline, serotonin, GABA, and dopamine (Heller 2005). Levels of vitamin B_6 in the brain are about 100 times higher than circulating blood concentrations (Gibson & Blass 1999).

Vitamin B_6 is commonly found in many foods of plant and animal origin. Meat, fish, whole grains, and bananas are particularly good sources. While whole wheat flour is a good source of the vitamin, white flour is low which reflects the relative lack of vitamin B_6 in the endosperm. Unlike thiamin, niacin, riboflavin, and folic acid, vitamin B_6 is not added to enriched flour and other enriched gain products, although breakfast cereals fortified with PN constitute an important dietary source. Glycosylated forms of PN, particularly PNG, are found in some plant sources, which exhibit only about 50% bioavailability in humans and exert weak antagonistic effects on the utilization of non-glycosylated PN. Despite the potential for lower bioavailability of vitamin B_6 in certain plant foods, there is little evidence of insufficiency in a varied vegetarian diet. However, individuals with marginal intake of total vitamin B_6 may be more vulnerable to suboptimal nutritional status due to its low bioavailability (da Silva et al. 2012).

The global prevalence of vitamin B_6 deficiency is very uncertain, as status is rarely measured (Allen 2012). Prevalence of vitamin B_6 deficiency in children has been estimated to be between 10% and 40% of children in urban and rural areas of Indonesia, respectively (Setiawan et al. 2000). In the early 1950s, an error in the manufacture of infant formula caused some infants to develop convulsive seizures as a result of severe vitamin B_6 deficiency. These were alleviated by PN supplementation and prompted the routine fortification of infant formulas with PN (Mackey et al. 2006). Chronic alcoholics are also thought to be at risk due to low dietary intakes and impaired metabolism of the vitamin.

The predominant form of vitamin B_6 in breast milk is pyridoxal (75%), with smaller amounts of pyridoxal phosphate (9%), pyridoxamine, and pyridoxine (Morrison & Driskell 1985). The evidence is limited, but available data suggest that breast milk concentrations and infant status reflect maternal intake and status and that maternal supplementation rapidly increases the amount in breast milk (Allen 2012). Associations between levels of vitamin B_6 in human breast milk and infant behaviour have been suggested. A small study of Egyptian mothers reported that a low concentration of vitamin B_6 in breast milk (<415 nmol/L) was associated with less consolability, inappropriate build-up to a crying state, and poorer response to aversive stimuli in their infants (McCullough et al. 1990). A subsequent study also carried out in Egyptian mother–infant pairs reported a significant relationship between maternal dietary quality during lactation and infant drowsiness, and this was linked to certain B vitamin intakes (particularly vitamin B_6, niacin, and riboflavin) and/or bioavailability of the nutrients (Rahmanifar et al. 1993). A study in the United States of 25 lactating women whose vitamin B_6 intake was greater than the group median had infants whose habituation and autonomic stability scores on the Brazelton Neonatal Assessment Scale were positively correlated with their breast milk vitamin B_6 content (Boylan et al. 2002). All studies were small however, and further work needs to be done to investigate whether these findings can be replicated in other contexts.

5.7 VITAMIN B_7 (BIOTIN)

Biotin is required as a cofactor for five carboxylase enzymes that catalyze key steps in the metabolism of fatty acids, glucose, and amino acids. Biotin also regulates gene expression, mediated by biotinylation of lysine residues in histones H2A, H3, and H4 and by various transcription factors.

Biotin is widely distributed in many foods and is synthesized by the intestinal flora (Bender 2005). Foods rich in biotin include egg yolk, liver, peanuts, and some vegetables. Biotin deficiency sufficient to cause clinical signs is very rare but has been documented in individuals consuming high amounts of raw egg white that contains avidin, which binds biotin and prevents its absorption in patients on prolonged parenteral nutrition without biotin supplementation and in those with the hereditary disorder biotinidase deficiency (Bender 2005).

There is increasing evidence that suboptimal biotin status may be relatively common. Up to half of women in the first trimester of pregnancy have abnormal increases of 3-hydroxyisovaleric acid, which reflects reduced status of biotin, suggesting that marginal status may be widespread and a possible contributing factor to the aetiology of some birth defects, such as cleft palate (Higdon 2003). Such women respond well to biotin supplementation.

There is little information concerning biotin requirements and no evidence on which to base recommendations. Adequate intakes (AIs) of biotin have been recommended at 30 μg/day (United States) and dietary biotin intake in Western populations has been estimated to be 15–70 μg/day (143–287 nmol/day) (Zempleni & Mock 1999). Lactation may create an increased demand for biotin and consequently AI recommendations increase. At 8 days post-partum, biotin in human milk is approximately 8 nmol/L and by 6 weeks, the biotin concentration increases to around 30 nmol/L.

5.8 VITAMIN B_9 (FOLATE)

Folate is a generic term that includes naturally occurring food folate and synthetic folic acid found in supplements and fortified foods. Folate plays an essential role as a cofactor in one-carbon metabolism, during which it promotes the re-methylation of homocysteine – a cytotoxic sulphur–containing amino acid that can induce the DNA strand breakage, oxidative stress, and apoptosis. Folate provides the methyl group for the conversion of methionine to *S*-adenosylmethionine (SAM), the major methyl donor for most methyltransferase reactions for the methylation of lipid (PC-DHA to PE-DHA), DNA, and proteins (histones). When folate levels are low, SAM is depleted, resulting in a reduction in the methylation of DNA and thereby enhancing gene transcription and DNA strand breakage and can impair DNA repair resulting in genetic mutations or triggering apoptosis.

Folate deficiency is common in many parts of the world and is often associated with undernutrition and socio-economic disadvantage. The main cause of folate deficiency is the low intake of folate-rich food sources, such as legumes and green leafy vegetables. Food folates are relatively unstable and up to 80% can be lost when vegetables and legumes are boiled. Other risk factors for poor folate status are pregnancy, lactation, and chronic alcoholism (Allen 2008).

Pregnancy places an increased demand on the supply of folate for the synthesis of DNA and other one-carbon transfer reactions, and as a consequence, pregnant women are at increased risk of developing a folate deficiency. At particular risk of deficiency include those pregnant women who do not take the recommended amount of folic acid supplements, women on restricted diets (chronic dieters), women with lower socio-economic status, and those with limited or uncertain availability of nutritionally adequate and safe food (Morse 2012). A number of pregnancy complications and birth outcomes, including placental abruption, pre-eclampsia, spontaneous abortion, stillbirths, fetal growth restriction, low birthweight (LBW), and prematurity, have been inversely associated with impaired folate status and linked to high homocysteine levels, although data are inconclusive and definitive conclusions have yet to be drawn (Bailey & Caudill 2012). Analysis conducted in the United States of over five million birth records after initiation of the folic acid fortification programme indicated significant reductions in rates of LBW, very low birthweight, and preterm birth, which lends support to this concern (Shaw et al. 2004a).

An adequate supply of folate during the first 4 weeks of pregnancy is necessary for the normal development of the fetal spine, brain, and skull and for protection against neural tube defects (NTDs), which include anencephaly, spina bifida, and encephalocele (IOM 1998). NTDs are among the most common congenital malformations in neonates contributing to infant mortality and serious disability. The United Kingdom has the highest level of NTDs in Europe, with a prevalence rate ranging from 0.8 to 1.5 per 1000 births, depending on ethnic, geographic, and nutritional factors (European Surveillance of Congenital Abnormalities 2009). Two randomized controlled trials (RCTs) (Czeizel & Dudas 1992; MRC Vitamin Study Research Group 1991) and several observational studies have shown that 50% or more of NTDs can be prevented if women consume a folic acid–containing supplement before and during the early weeks of pregnancy in addition to folate in their diet. Recent evidence syntheses and meta-analyses reporting associations between folic acid supplementation and reduced incidence of NTDs support these recommendations (De-Regil et al. 2010; Wilson & Genetics Committee 2015; Wolff et al. 2009).

Based on these findings, it is recommended that all women planning a pregnancy, or capable of conceiving, should take a supplement containing 400 μg/day of folic acid to reduce the risk of NTDs, and these recommendations are endorsed around the world. Some countries provide additional recommendations such as those in New Zealand where even women at low risk of a neural tube defect who plan to become pregnant are recommended to take 800 μg of folic acid daily for at least 4 weeks prior to conception and for 12 weeks after conceiving to reduce the risk (New Zealand Ministry of Health 2006).

There is increasing evidence that even with the introduction of government policies, clinical recommendations, and health education campaigns, the decrease in the incidence of NTDs has been lower than anticipated (Busby et al. 2005; CDC 2004). One contributing factor may be a high number of unplanned pregnancies and associated lack of compliance, particularly in the preconception period. One in six pregnancies in the United Kingdom is unplanned, and 1 in 60 women (1.5%) experience an unplanned pregnancy in a year, according to the National Survey of Sexual Attitudes and Lifestyles (Wellings et al. 2013). A systematic review including studies from 50 countries found that, in many countries, fewer than 50% of women take periconceptional folic acid supplements (Ray et al. 2004). In the United Kingdom, a recent cross-sectional study of almost 500,000 women found that only 31% of women reported taking folic acid before pregnancy. Those least likely to take folic acid supplements were women under 20 years of age and non-Caucasian women (Bestwick et al. 2014).

Research has demonstrated that lack of awareness of folic acid supplementation is common among women of childbearing age. Research conducted in many different contexts, for example, Pakistan (Hisam et al. 2014), Nigeria (Rabiu et al. 2012), Qatar (Bener et al. 2006), China (Ren et al. 2006), and Thailand (Nawapun & Phupong 2007), demonstrates that the knowledge of the importance of periconceptional folic acid supplementation is low. A recent study of 603 pregnant women in the United Kingdom found that, although nearly 98% of the women had heard of folic acid, only 40% of women knew that they should take it before pregnancy,

42%–52% knew the medical condition it protects against, and between 36% and 46% knew the dietary sources of folate (Maher & Keriakos 2014). A large survey of nearly 23,000 women of childbearing age in Europe confirmed that 83% were unaware that periconceptional folic acid supplementation reduces the risk of birth defects (Bitzer et al. 2013).

Steps to achieve folate sufficiency have included the mandatory fortification of staple foods in more than 50 countries around the world, such as the United States, Canada, Chile, Costa Rica, and New Zealand. It has been reported that fortification of staple food stuff with folic acid may reduce the number of births complicated by NTDs by up to 50% (Herrmann & Obeid 2011). The United Kingdom has been cautious in recommending fortification as folic acid supplementation may mask the haematologic changes caused by vitamin B_{12} deficiency, may have an adverse effect on zinc absorption, and could lead to delayed diagnosis and treatment of neurological symptoms (Cuskelly et al. 2007). Intervention and observational studies have suggested that raised folate status may also increase the risk of breast cancer (Charles et al. 2005), prostate cancer (Figueiredo et al. 2009), and colon cancer (Lonn et al. 2006). A recent meta-analysis of 10 RCTs, however, found only a borderline significant increase in the incidence of overall cancer in populations taking folic acid supplements ≥400 μg/day compared to controls, and prostate cancer was the only cancer type where an increased risk was shown for folic acid supplements. There is limited evidence to indicate that more people have developed nerve damage as a result of vitamin B_{12} deficiency in countries with mandatory folic acid flour fortification (BDA 2013). Further, several absorption and supplementation studies have investigated the potential adverse effect of folic acid on zinc absorption, but results remain inconclusive (Fekete et al. 2010).

The safety of high, and possibly even physiological, doses of supplemental folic acid in malaria-endemic areas has been called into question as these supplements may favour the growth of *Plasmodium falciparum*, inhibit parasite clearance of sulphadoxine–pyrimethamine-treated malaria, and increase subsequent recrudescence. The WHO recommends home fortification with micronutrient powders (MNPs) containing at least iron, vitamin A, and zinc to control childhood anaemia in resource-poor settings, and current MNP formulations generally include 88 μg folic acid. The safety and benefits of low-dose folic acid in MNPs in such settings using placebo-controlled, randomized trial designs have been called for (Kupka 2015).

While the evidence linking folate to the occurrence of NTDs is clear, research linking maternal folate status during pregnancy to later cognitive ability in the offspring is less conclusive. Studies in rodents have shown links between maternal folate deficiency and structural brain abnormalities in the offspring (Craciunescu et al. 2004). In humans, poor mental development has been reported in children of genetically susceptible mothers with low dietary folate intakes (del Río Garcia et al. 2009). A study examining associations between maternal intake of folate, vitamin B_{12}, and choline during the first and second trimesters of pregnancy, with tests of cognitive performance in children using data from 1210 participants in the U.S. Project Viva cohort study, reported that higher intake of folate in early pregnancy was associated with higher scores on a test of receptive language that predicts overall intelligence at 3 years of age. Vitamin B_{12} was only weakly associated with cognitive outcomes, and choline demonstrated no relationship (Villamor et al. 2012). A cohort study of 536 children aged 9–10 years from the Mysore Parthenon birth cohort in India reported a 0.1–0.2 SD increase in cognitive scores on the Kaufman Assessment Battery per SD increase in the maternal folate concentration. The associations with learning ability and long-term storage/retrieval, visuospatial ability, attention, and concentration were independent of several potential confounding factors such as body mass index and parity (Veena et al. 2010). In contrast, Tamura et al. (2005) reported that the folate status of mothers in the second half of pregnancy, as assessed by plasma and erythrocyte folate and plasma tHcy concentrations, had little impact on the neurodevelopment of their children at 5 years of age. This study was carried out among socially disadvantaged families in the United States, with 14% of mothers exhibiting 'poor folate' status (plasma folate concentrations $\leq$11.0 nmol/L), and the authors concluded that the severity of socio-economic factors may have superseded any effect of the maternal folate status in the first 5 years of life.

There is emerging evidence that maternal folic acid supplementation during pregnancy may be associated with reduced risk of neurodevelopmental disorders in children. In a follow-up study of an RCT, aspects of intellectual functioning including working memory, inhibitory control, and fine motor functioning in children aged 7–9 years have been reported to be positively associated with maternal prenatal iron/folic acid supplementation in an area where iron deficiency is prevalent (Christian et al. 2010). Children born to mothers in the folic acid–only supplementation group were not included in this follow-up study, however, so it is unclear whether folic acid alone would have had any effect on study outcomes. The large Norwegian Mother and Child Cohort Study (MoBa) of nearly 39,000 children found that maternal intake of folic acid supplements from 4 weeks before to 8 weeks after the start of pregnancy was associated with lower risk of severe language delay at 3 years of age (Roth et al. 2011) and a lower risk of autistic disorder (Suren et al. 2013). The authors acknowledge that, as the use of folic acid supplements was also associated with higher socio-economic status and more health-conscious maternal behaviour patterns, residual unmeasured confounding factors cannot be ruled out. Their findings, however, were consistent with a case–control study of autism spectrum disorder (ASD) which reported that the maternal intake of folic acid and prenatal vitamins during 3 months prior to pregnancy and the first month of pregnancy was associated with a lower risk of ASD in children. Complementary genetic analyses indicated that the association was modified by gene variants which determine the ability to utilize available folate, indicating genetic susceptibility for the condition in some mothers and their children (Schmidt et al. 2011, 2012).

5.9 VITAMIN B_{12} (COBALAMIN)

Vitamin B_{12}, also called cobalamin, plays a key role in the normal functioning of the brain and nervous system. It is not only involved in the metabolism of every cell in the body, particularly affecting DNA synthesis and regulation, but also in fatty acid synthesis and energy production. Vitamin B_{12} plays a crucial role in methionine and homocysteine metabolism in most cell types. Malabsorption of vitamin B_{12} can

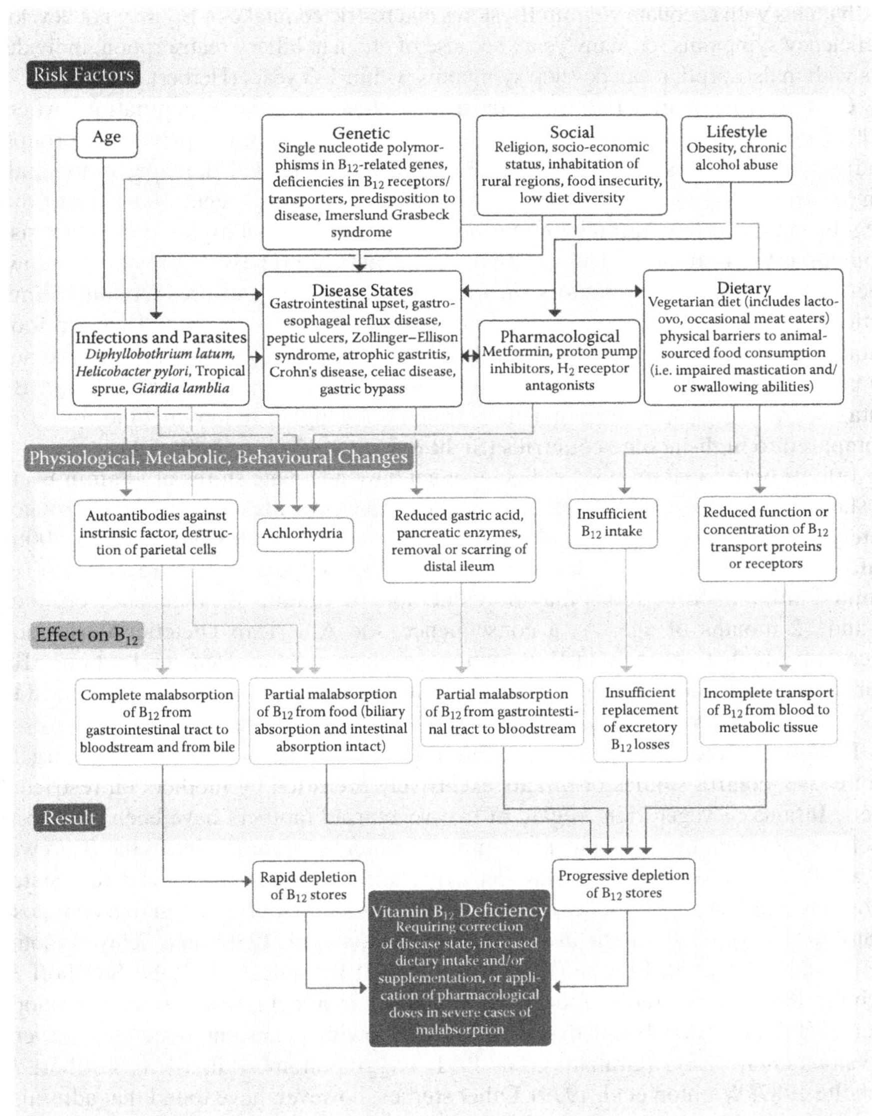

FIGURE 5.3 Factors which contribute to vitamin B deficiency. (From Sight & Life, Food Fortification with Vitamin B_{12}, 2012, available at: http://www.sightandlife.org/fileadmin/data/Magazine/2012/26_2_2012/sightandlife_magazine_26_2_2012.pdf, accessed May 24, 2016.)

result in the development of pernicious anaemia, which can lead to nerve damage if vitamin B_{12} supplements are not taken.

Vitamin B_{12} inadequacy is common worldwide. It is most frequently caused by low dietary intake and impaired absorption, which can in turn be influenced by a range of complex socio-demographic, cultural, and behavioural factors (Figure 5.3). While healthy individuals with adequate vitamin B_{12} stores and restricted intake of B_{12} may not develop deficiency symptoms for many years because of efficient biliary reabsorption, individuals with malabsorption can develop symptoms within 1–3 years (Herbert 1994).

Groups at particular risk of vitamin B_{12} deficiency include populations where nutritional deficiencies are common such as economically underprivileged groups; individuals with gastric and intestinal conditions and renal damage; individuals on special diets; and the elderly (Bender 2005). Vegans, vegetarians, lacto-ovo vegetarians, and low-animal source food consumers have a higher deficiency risk compared to omnivores (Antony 2003). Such diets are relatively prevalent in low-income countries, due to factors such as religious beliefs, culture, economic limitations, and physical access which may affect the access to animal source food intake. As a consequence, the prevalence of vitamin B_{12} inadequacy in women of childbearing age, infants (who depend primarily on their mothers' vitamin B_{12} intake), and children have been demonstrated to be higher in low-income countries compared to high-income countries (Sight & Life 2012) (see Table 5.1).

Infants born to vitamin B_{12} replete women have adequate stores of vitamin B_{12} to sustain them for several months post-partum, consequently, vitamin B_{12} deficiency rarely occurs before around 4 months of age in infants of such women (Black 2008). Infants born to vitamin B_{12}–deficient breastfeeding mothers or those receiving no or limited animal source foods may be vulnerable to vitamin B_{12} deficiency between 6 and 12 months of age. As a consequence, the American Dietetic Association recommends that vegans and lacto-ovo vegetarians take supplemental vitamin B_{12} during pregnancy and lactation to ensure that sufficient vitamin B_{12} is transferred to the fetus and infant (Kaiser & Allen 2008).

Evidence of the consequence of vitamin B_{12} deficiency in humans comes largely from case–control studies of infants exclusively breastfed by mothers on restricted diets. Infants of vegetarian, vegan, or ovo-vegetarian mothers have been described to have developmental delay and 'infant tremor syndrome' in India (Garewal et al. 1988); developmental delay, lethargy, and irritability in the United States (Higginbottom et al. 1978); neurological deterioration that progressed to a comatose state by the age of 9 months in Australia (Wighton et al. 1979); and delayed motor skills and lethargy in Europe (Kuhne et al. 1991; Renault et al. 1999; Stollhoff & Schulte 1987). Most studies found that, following treatment, restoration of developmental skills was variable, with some children showing persistent moderate or severe developmental delays (Graham et al. 1991; Higginbottom et al. 1978; Stollhoff & Schulte 1987; Wighton et al. 1979). Other studies, however, have found that administration of vitamin B_{12} to children who are deficient in the vitamin can lead to major improvements in functioning (Sklar 1986).

There is little consensus among studies investigating the association between maternal vitamin B_{12} intake and B_{12} status and cognitive development in their offspring. A large well-nourished population in a UK birth cohort study (ALSPAC) found no relationship between maternal vitamin B_{12} intakes in the third trimester and offspring IQ at 8 years of age (Bonilla et al. 2012). In contrast, a study of 253 mother–infant pairs in Mexico found that low maternal vitamin B_{12} intake (<2 μg/day) in the first trimester was significantly associated with lower Mental Development Index (MDI) on Bayley's Scale of Infant Development in their offspring (Del Rio Garcia et al. 2009).

TABLE 5.1
Prevalence of Vitamin B_{12} Deficiency in Infants, Children, and Women of Childbearing Age

Population Group	Country	Participants (Age, n)	% Deficient (Serum or Plasma B_{12})[a]	Cutoff Used (pmol/L)[b]	References
Infants and children	Mexico	Children (<6 years, n = 2099)	7.7	150	Cuevas-Nasu et al. (2012)
	Venezuela (nationwide)	Children (0–7 years, n = 1792)	11	150	García-Casal et al. (2005)
	Venezuela (Vargas State)	Children (0–15 years, n = 2720)	21	150	García-Casal et al. (2005)
	Guatemala (El Mezquital, Guatemala City)	Children (n = 553)	11	162	Rogers et al. (2003)
	Norway (Oslo)	Newborns (n = 4874)	3.3	100	Refsum et al. (2004)
	Kenya (Embu District, Eastern Province)	Schoolchildren (n = 512)	40	148	Siekmann et al. (2003)
	Colombia (Bogota)	Children (n = 2812)	1.6	148	Arsenault et al. (2009)
	India (Dakshinpuri)	Children (6–30 months, n = 2296)	28	150	Taneja et al. (2007)
Women of childbearing age	Germany	Women (18–40, n = 1266)	15	148	Thamm et al. (1999)
	Canada (Ontario)	Women of childbearing age (n = 6888)	6.9	125	Ray et al. (2008)
	Vietnam	Women of childbearing age (n = 1526)	12	148	Laillou et al. (2012)
	Denmark (Copenhagen Capital Region formerly Copenhagen Country)	Women (n = 3173)	8.4	148	Thuesen et al. (2010)
Pregnant women	Canada (Newfoundland)	Pregnant women (n = 1424)	25	130	House et al. (2000)
	Nepal (District of Sarlahi)	Pregnant women (n = 1158)	28	150	Jiang et al. (2005)
	Venezuela (Gran Caracas)	Pregnant women, 14–26 years (n = 1283)	61	150	García-Casal et al. (2005)
	Canada (Ontario)	Pregnant women <28 days (n = 1244)	5.2	125	Ray et al. (2008)
		Pregnant women >28 days (n = 2490)	10		

Source: Adapted from Sight & Life, Food fortification with vitamin B_{12}, Available at: http://www.sightandlife.org/fileadmin/data/Magazine/2012/26_2_2012/sightandlife_magazine_26_2_2012.pdf, 2012.

[a] Where data available.

[b] Conversions made for consistency where appropriate (1.35 pg/mL = 1 pmol/L).

A study conducted in rural India with a 70% prevalence of maternal vitamin B_{12} deficiency suggested that children of mothers with plasma vitamin B_{12} concentrations in the lowest decile (n = 49, <77 pmol/L) performed poorly on tests of attention and short-term memory at 9 years of age, compared to children of mothers in the highest decile of vitamin B_{12} concentrations (n = 59, >224 pmol/L) (Bhate et al. 2008). In contrast, studies of women in urban India (Veena et al. 2010) and in well-nourished women in Canada (Wu et al. 2012) reported that maternal vitamin B_{12} status was not related to cognitive performance in childhood. The absence of randomized controlled trials makes it difficult to draw a causal inference between maternal vitamin B_{12} intake and status and its effect on child cognitive abilities.

Studies of vitamin B_{12} status and cognitive outcomes in children are limited, particularly in early childhood. A study of infants of macrobiotic mothers in the Netherlands showed that infants had delayed motor and language development compared with infants of omnivores (Schneede et al. 1994). A follow-up study when the children were aged 12 years revealed that they still scored lower than the omnivores on cognitive tests (Louwman et al. 2000). Guatemalan school-aged children with vitamin B_{12} deficiency had poorer cognitive and neuromotor performance and lower academic performance, lower teacher ratings, and more attentional problems compared to those without deficiency (Allen et al. 1999). More recently, plasma concentrations of cobalamin (and folate) showed a significant positive relationship with cognitive performance in North Indian children aged 12–18 months (Strand et al. 2013). As with all observational studies which identify associations rather than causality, the influence of residual or unmeasured confounding such as the quality of mother and child interaction in early childhood and breastfeeding behaviours cannot be ruled out.

Several possible mechanisms to explain the link between vitamin B_{12} deficiency and developmental delay have been proposed. These include delayed myelination or demyelination of nerves, alteration in the SAM/SAH ratio, imbalance of neurotrophic and neurotoxic cytokines, and accumulation of lactate in brain cells. Rather than being one mechanism that is solely responsible, it is likely that multiple mechanisms contribute simultaneously to the outcome (Dror & Allen 2008).

5.10 CHOLINE

Choline is a vitamin-like essential nutrient, related to the B vitamins. As a methyl donor, it is involved in many physiological processes, including the metabolism and transport of lipids, methylation reactions, and neurotransmitter synthesis. Choline is present in many foods, with egg yolk, liver, and meat being the best sources.

Due to the importance of DNA methylation in normal brain development, neuronal functions, and cognitive processes, choline is essential for both optimal brain functioning and fetal brain development. Studies of rat pups exposed to supplemental choline before birth have been shown to have lifelong enhancement of memory and attention (for a review, see Zeisel 2004). The underlying physiology and biochemical basis for these changes are starting to be understood. Specific anatomical regions of the hippocampus play critical roles in learning and the acquisition of memory. In rats, prenatal choline supplementation increases the sensitivity of the CA1 hippocampal neurons to stimulation of long-term potentiation and increase working spatial memory (Zeisel 2004).

The limited studies investigating the relationship between maternal dietary choline and cognitive development in human offspring are inconclusive. The Seychelles Child Development Nutrition Cohort study failed to find an association between the cognitive abilities of 256 children aged 5 years and their plasma choline concentrations (Strain et al. 2013). Conversely, significant positive associations were found between 18-month-old infant cognitive test scores and maternal plasma free choline at 16 weeks of gestation in 154 mother–infant pairs (Wu et al. 2012). A prospective study of daily methyl donor nutrient intake of 1210 women during pregnancy reported that choline intake during the first and/or second trimester of pregnancy was not correlated with measures of cognitive performance in children aged 3 years (Villamor et al. 2012). The researchers did, however, find that higher visual memory scores were associated with higher maternal choline intakes during the second trimester of pregnancy in children aged 7 years (median intakes, 392 vs. 260 mg/day) (Boeke et al. 2013). A small randomized, double-blind, placebo-controlled trial of 99 pregnant women who consumed diets containing moderate amounts of choline found that maternal choline supplementation (750 mg/day of choline in the form of phosphatidylcholine) from 18 weeks of gestation to 3 months' post-partum did not result in significant benefit in short-term visuospatial memory, long-term episodic memory, language development, or global development in infants aged 10–12 months (Cheatham et al. 2012). As no follow-up was conducted, the study may have missed late-emerging effects, and future studies could focus on women with low chlorine diets, which is common in several low-income countries.

In adults, the Framingham Offspring Cohort study revealed a positive association between dietary choline intake and specific cognitive functions, such as verbal memory and visual memory in men and women aged 36–83 years (Poly et al. 2011). Significant associations were also found in the Hordaland Health cross-sectional study of men and women aged 70–74 years between high plasma concentrations of free choline (>8.36 mcmol/L) and a greater performance on cognitive tests assessing sensory motor speed, perceptual speed, executive function, and global cognition (Nurk et al. 2013). Such studies provide promising evidence for a possible protective role of choline in memory loss or dementia in older people, suggesting that intakes above the current recommended amounts may be warranted.

As choline is a methyl donor, it has been suggested that pregnant women with a low blood level or intake of choline are at higher risk for having children with neural tube defects (NTDs), but presently, the evidence is conflicting. A case–control study of 424 NTD cases and 440 controls reported that women in the highest (>498.46 mg/day) versus lowest (≤290.41 mg/day) quartile of periconceptual choline intake had a 51% lower risk of an NTD-affected pregnancy (Shaw et al. 2004b). Another study of 80 NTD-affected pregnancies and 409 controls found that women with the lowest concentrations of serum choline (<2.49 mmol/L) during mid-pregnancy had a 2.4-fold higher risk of NTDs (Shaw et al. 2009). However, more recent studies have found no evidence of a relationship between maternal choline intake and risk of NTDs (Carmichael et al. 2010; Chandler et al. 2012). Similarly, no association was found between maternal serum choline concentrations during pregnancy and risk of NTDs among women who either had NTD-affected pregnancies, pregnancies with non-NTD malformations, normal pregnancies with prior NTD-affected pregnancies, or normal pregnancies (Mills et al. 2014). However, it is important to note that dietary intake of choline is not accurately reflected by circulating choline concentrations. Whether supplemental choline could add to the protective effect currently being achieved by periconceptual folic acid supplementation requires further research.

5.11 CONCLUSION

The B vitamins and choline are essential nutrients in cell proliferation, myelination, neurotransmitter synthesis and functioning, and brain energy metabolism, and as a consequence are likely to have a number of influences on the development of the brain. There is increasing evidence that folate, thiamin, and vitamin B_{12} in particular influence cognitive development through two related neurochemical mechanisms involving hypomethylation and their influence on homocysteine metabolism. Several vitamin B deficiency disorders are typically characterized by neurological symptoms. While most vitamin B deficiencies have become rare in high-income countries where food has been enriched with several B vitamins, in some low-income countries recent evidence suggests that the prevalence of deficiencies in B vitamins such a thiamin and vitamin B_{12} may be common. Fortification of foodstuffs with B vitamins, in addition to other key nutrients, has shown promising results for preventing deficiencies and subsequent developmental delays, but further robust research in low- and middle-income countries which evaluates the long-term impact is needed.

REFERENCES

Allen, L.H. (2008). Causes of vitamin B_{12} and folate deficiency. *Food and Nutrition Bulletin* 29, S20–S34.

Allen, L.H. (2012). B vitamins in breast milk: Relative importance of maternal status and intake, and effects on infant status and function. *Advances in Nutrition: An International Review Journal* 3(3), 362–369.

Allen, L., de Benoist, B., Dary, O., & Hurrell, R. (eds). (2006). *Guidelines on Food Fortification with Micronutrients.* Geneva, Switzerland: World Health Organization and Food and Agricultural Organization of the United Nations.

Allen, L.H., Penland, J.G., Boy, E., DeBaessa, Y., & Rogers, L.M. (1999). Cognitive and neuromotor performance of Guatemalan schoolers with deficient, marginal and normal plasma B-12. *FASEB Journal* 13, A544.

Antony, A.C. (July 1, 2003). Vegetarianism and vitamin B_{12} (cobalamin) deficiency. *American Journal of Clinical Nutrition* 78(1), 3–6.

Anderson, O.S., Sant, K.E., & Dolinoy, D.C. (2012). Nutrition and epigenetics: an interplay of dietary methyl donors, one-carbon metabolism and DNA methylation. *Journal of Nutritional Biochemistry* 23(8), 853–859.

Arsenault, J.E., Mora-Plazas, M., Forero, Y., Lopez-Arana, S., Baylin, A., & Villamor, E. (2009). Hemoglobin concentration is inversely associated with erythrocyte folate concentrations in Colombian school-age children, especially among children with low vitamin B_{12} status. *European Journal of Clinical Nutrition* 63(7), 842–849.

Bailey, L.B. & Caudill, M.A. (2012). Folate. In: *Present Knowledge in Nutrition*, 10th edn., Erdman, J.W., Macdonald, I.A., & Zeisel, S.H. (eds.). Ames, IA: International Life Sciences Institute, pp. 321–342.

Bates, B., Lennox, A., Prentice, A., Bates, C., Page, P., Nicholson, S., & Swan, G. (2014). *National Diet and Nutrition Survey: Results from Years 1–4 (Combined) of the Rolling Programme (2008/2009–2011/12): Executive Summary*. London: Public Health England and Food Standards Agency.

Bates, C.J. (2006). Thiamin. In: *Present Knowledge in Nutrition*, 9th edn., Bowman, B.A. & Russell, R.M. (eds.). Washington, DC: International Life Sciences Institute, pp. 242–249.

Bates, C.J., Lui, D.-S., Fuller, N.J., & Lucas, A. (1985). Susceptibility of riboflavin and vitamin A in banked breast milk to photodegradation and its implications for the use of banked breast milk in infant feeding. *Acta Paediatrica Scandinavica* 74, 40–44.

Battaglia, A., Bruni, G., Ardia, A. et al. (1989). Nicergoline in mild to moderate dementia. A multicenter, double-blind, placebo-controlled study. *Journal of the American Geriatrics Society* 37, 295–302.

Bender, D.A. (2005). Water-soluble vitamins. In: *Human Nutrition*, 11th edn., Geissler, C. and Powers, H. (eds.). Elsevier, Edinburgh.

Bener, A., Al Maadid, M.G., Al-Bast, D.A., & Al-Marri, S. (2006). Maternal knowledge, attitude and practice on folic acid intake among Arabian Qatari women. *Reproductive Toxicology* 21(1), 21–25.

Bestwick, J.P., Huttly, W.J., Morris, J.K., & Wald, N.J. (2014). Prevention of neural tube defects: A cross-sectional study of the uptake of folic acid supplementation in nearly half a million women. *PLoS One* 9(2), e89354.

Bettendorff, L. (2012). Thiamin. In: *Present Knowledge in Nutrition*, 10th edn., Erdman, J.W., Macdonald, I.A., Zeisel, S.H. (eds.). Ames, IA: International Life Sciences Institute, pp. 261–279.

Bhate, V., Deshpande, S., Bhat, D. et al. (2008). Vitamin B_{12} status of pregnant women and cognitive function in their 9-yr-old children. *Food and Nutrition Bulletin* 29, 249–254.

Bitzer, J., von Stenglin, A., & Bannemerschult, R. (2013). Women's awareness and periconceptional use of folic acid: Data from a large European survey. *International Journal of Women's Health* 5, 201.

Black, M.M. (2008). Effects of vitamin B_{12} and folate deficiency on brain development in children. *Food and Nutrition Bulletin*, 29(2 Suppl), S126–S131.

Boeke, C.E., Gillman, M.W., Hughes, M.D., Rifas-Shiman, S.L., Villamor, E., & Oken, E. (2013). Choline intake during pregnancy and child cognition at age 7 years. *American Journal of Epidemiology* 177(12), 1338–1347.

Bonilla, C., Lawlor, D.A., Taylor, A.E. et al. (2012). Vitamin B_{12} status during pregnancy and child's IQ at age 8: A Medelian randomization study in the Avon longitudinal study of parents and children. *PLoS One* 7, e51084.

Bosch, A.M., Stroek, K., Abeling, N.G., Waterham, H.R., Ijlst, L., & Wanders, R.J. (2012). The Brown–Vialetto–Van Laere and Fazio Londe syndrome revisited: Natural history, genetics, treatment and future perspectives. *Orphanet Journal of Rare Diseases* 7(1), 83–83.

Boylan, L.M., Hart, S., Porter, K.B., & Driskell, J.A. (2002). Vitamin B-6 content of breast milk and neonatal behavioral functioning. *Journal of the American Dietetic Association* 102(10), 1433–1438.

British Dietetic Association (BDA). (2013). Folic acid. Available at: https://www.bda.uk.com/foodfacts/FolicAcid.pdf. Accessed on April 11, 2016.

Bryan, J., Osendarp, S., Hughes, D., Calvaresi, E., Baghurst, K., & van Klinken, J.W. (2004). Nutrients for cognitive development in school-aged children. *Nutrition Reviews* 62, 295–306.

Busby, A., Abramsky, L., Dolk, H., & Armstrong, B., Eurocat Folic Acid Working Group. (March 12, 2005). Preventing neural tube defects in Europe: Population based study. *BMJ* 330(7491), 574–575.

Butterworth, R.F. (2003). Thiamin deficiency and brain disorders. *Nutrition Research Reviews* 16(2), 277–284.

Calvaresi, E. & Bryan, J. (2001). B vitamins, cognition, and aging: A review. *Journals of Gerontology Series B: Psychological Sciences and Social Sciences* 56(6), P327–P339.

Carmichael, S.L., Yang, W., & Shaw, G.M. (2010). Periconceptional nutrient intakes and risks of neural tube defects in California. *Birth Defects Research, Part A, Clinical and Molecular Teratology* 88(8), 670–678.

Centers for Disease Control and Prevention (CDC). (May 7, 2004). Spina bifida and anencephaly before and after folic acid mandate – United States, 1995–1996 and 1999–2000. *MMWR Morbidity and Mortality Weekly Report* 53(17), 362–365.

Cervantes-Laurean, D., McElvaney, N.G., & Moss, J. (1999). Niacin. In: *Modern Nutrition in Health and Disease*, 9th edn., Shils, M., Olson, J.A., Shike, M., & Ross, A.C. (eds.). Baltimore, MD: Williams & Wilkins, pp. 401–411.

Chandler, A.L., Hobbs, C.A., Mosley, B.S. et al. (2012). Neural tube defects and maternal intake of micronutrients related to one-carbon metabolism or antioxidant activity. *Birth Defects Research, Part A, Clinical and Molecular Teratology* 94(11), 864–874.

Charles, D.H.M., Ness, A.R., Campbell, D., Smith, G.D., Whitley, E., & Hall, M.H. (2005). Folic acid supplements in pregnancy and birth outcome: Re-analysis of a large randomised controlled trial and update of Cochrane review. *Paediatric and Perinatal Epidemiology* 19, 112–124.

Cheatham, C.L., Goldman, B.D., Fischer, L.M., da Costa, K.A., Reznick, J.S., & Zeisel, S.H. (2012). Phosphatidylcholine supplementation in pregnant women consuming moderate-choline diets does not enhance infant cognitive function: A randomized, double-blind, placebo-controlled trial. *American Journal of Clinical Nutrition* 96(6), 1465–1472.

Christian, P., Murray-Kolb, L.E., Khatry, S.K. et al. (2010). Prenatal micronutrient supplementation and intellectual and motor function in early school-aged children in Nepal. *Journal of the American Medical Association* 304(24), 2716–2723.

Craciunescu, C.N., Brown, E.C., Mar, M.H., Albright, C.D., Nadeau, M.R., & Zeisel, S.H. (January 2004). Folic acid deficiency during late gestation decreases progenitor cell proliferation and increases apoptosis in fetal mouse brain. *Journal of Nutrition* 134(1), 162–166.

Cuevas-Nasu, L., Mundo-Rosas, V., Shamah-Levy, T., Méndez-Gómez Humaran, I., Ávila-Arcos, M.A., Rebollar-Campos, M., & Villalpando, S. (2012). Prevalence of folate and vitamin B_{12} deficiency in Mexican children aged 1 to 6 years in a population-based survey. *Salud Pública de México* 54(2), 116–124.

Cui, X., Chopp, M., Zacharek, A., Roberts, C., Buller, B., Ion, M., & Chen, J. (2010). Niacin treatment of stroke increases synaptic plasticity and axon growth in rats. *Stroke* 41(9), 2044–2049.

Cuskelly, G.J., Mooney, K.M., & Young, I.S. (2007). Folate and vitamin B_{12}: Friendly or enemy nutrients for the elderly. *Proceedings of the Nutrition Society* 66, 548–558.

Czeizel, A.E. & Dudás, I. (1992). Prevention of the first occurrence of neural-tube defects by periconceptional vitamin supplementation. *New England Journal of Medicine* 327, 1832–1835.

Da Silva, V.R., Russell, K.A., & Gregory, J.F. (2012). Vitamin B_6. In: *Present Knowledge in Nutrition*, 10th edn., Erdman, J.W., Macdonald, I.A., & Zeisel, S.H. (eds.). Ames, IA: International Life Sciences Institute, pp. 307–320.

De-Regil, L.M., Fernández-Gaxiola, A.C., Dowswell, T., & Peña-Rosas, J.P. (2010). Effects and safety of periconceptional folate supplementation for preventing birth defects. *Cochrane Database of Systematic Reviews* (10), Art. No.: CD007950. doi: 10.1002/14651858.CD007950.pub2.

Del Rio Garcia, C., Torres-Sanchez, L., Chen, J. et al. (2009). Maternal MTHFR 677C>T genotype and dietary intake of folate and vitamin (B_{12}): Their impact on child neurodevelopment. *Nutritional Neuroscience* 12, 13–20.

Dror, D.K. & Allen, L.H. (2008). Effect of vitamin B_{12} deficiency on neurodevelopment in infants: Current knowledge and possible mechanisms. *Nutrition Reviews* 66(5), 250–255.

European Surveillance of Congenital Abnormalities. (2009). Prevention of neural tube defects by periconceptional folic acid supplementation in Europe. Newtownabbey, Ireland: European Surveillance of Congenital Abnormalities.

Fattal-Valevski, A., Azouri-Fattal, I., Greenstein, Y.J., Guindy, M., Blau, A., & Zelnik, N. (2009). Delayed language development due to infantile thiamine deficiency. *Developmental Medicine and Child Neurology* 51(8), 629–634.

Fattal-Valevski, A., Kesler, A., Sela, B.-A. et al. (2005). Outbreak of life-threatening thiamine deficiency in infants in Israel caused by a defective soy-based formula. *Pediatrics* 115(2), e233–e238.

Fekete, K., Berti, C., Cetin, I., Hermoso, M., Koletzko, B.V., & Decsi, T. (2010). Perinatal folate supply: Relevance in health outcome parameters. *Maternal & Child Nutrition* 6, 23–38.

Figueiredo, J.C., Grau, M.V., Haile, R.W. et al. (2009). Folic acid and risk of prostate cancer: Results from a randomized clinical trial. *Journal of the National Cancer Institute* 101, 432–435.

Finch, S., Doyle, W., & Lowe, C. (1998). *The National Diet and Nutrition Survey: People Aged 65 Years and Older.* London, UK: TSO.

Foley, A.R., Menezes, M.P., Pandraud, A. et al. (2014). Treatable childhood neuronopathy caused by mutations in riboflavin transporter RFVT2. *Brain* 137(Pt 1): 44–56.

Food Fortification Initiative. (2014). New Grain, New Name: 2014 Year in Review. Available at: http://www.ffinetwork.org/about/stay_informed/publications/documents/FFI2014YearInReview.pdf#Annual Report. Accessed on April 11, 2016.

García-Casal, M.N., Osorio, C., Landaeta, M., Leets, I., Matus, P., Fazzino, F., & Marcos, E. (2005). High prevalence of folic acid and vitamin B_{12} deficiencies in infants, children, adolescents and pregnant women in Venezuela. *European Journal of Clinical Nutrition* 59(9), 1064–1070.

Garewal, G., Narang, A., & Das, K.C. (1988). Infantile tremor syndrome: A vitamin B_{12} deficiency syndrome in infants. *Journal of Tropical Pediatrics* 34, 174–178.

Gibson, G.E. & Blass, J.P. (1999). Nutrition and brain function. In: *Basic Neurochemistry: Molecular, Cellular and Medical Aspects*, Siegel, G.J. (ed.). Philadelphia, PA: Lippincott Williams & Wilkins, pp. 692–709.

Graham, S.M., Arvela, O.M., & Wise, G.A. (1991). Long-term neurologic consequences of nutritional vitamin B_{12} deficiency in infants. *Journal of Pediatrics* 121, 710–714.

Gregory, J. & Lowe, S. (2000). *National Diet and Nutrition Survey of Young People Aged 4–18 Years.* London, UK: The Stationary Office.

Haller, J. (2005). Vitamins and brain function. In: *Nutritional Neuroscience*, Lieberman, H.R., Kanarek, R.B., & Prasad, C. (eds.). Boca Raton, FL: CRC Press, pp. 207–234.

Hegyi, J., Schwartz, R.A., & Hegyi, V. (2004). Pellagra: Dermatitis, dementia, and diarrhea. *International Journal of Dermatology* 43(1), 1–5.

Herbert, V. (1994). Staging vitamin B-12 (cobalamin) status in vegetarians. *American Journal of Clinical Nutrition* 59(5), 1213S–1222S.

Herrmann, W. & Obeid, R. (2011). The mandatory fortification of staple foods with folic acid: A current controversy in Germany. *Deutsches Ärzteblatt International* 108(15), 249.

Herrmann, W.M., Stephan, K., Gaede, K. et al. (1997). A multicenter randomized double-blind study on the efficacy and safety of nicergoline in patients with multi-infarct dementia. *Dementia and Geriatric Cognitive Disorders* 8, 9–17.

Higdon, J. (2003). Biotin. In: *An Evidence-Based Approach to Vitamins and Minerals.* New York: Thieme, pp. 1–5.

Higginbottom, M.C., Sweetma, L., & Nyhan, W.L. (1978). A syndrome of methylmalonic aciduria, homocystinuria, megaloblastic anemia and neurologic abnormalities in a vitamin B_{12}-deficient breast-fed infant of a strict vegetarian. *New England Journal of Medicine* 299, 317–323.

Hisam, A., Rahman, M.U., & Mashhadi, S.F. (2014). Knowledge, attitude and practice regarding folic acid deficiency: A hidden hunger. *Pakistan Journal of Medical Sciences* 30(3), 583.

House, J.D., March, S.B., Ratnam, S., Ives, E., Brosnan, J.T., & Friel, J.K. 2000. Folate and vitamin B_{12} status of women in Newfoundland at their first prenatal visit. *Canadian Medical Association Journal* 162(11), 1557–1559.

Iesofsky-Vig, N. (1999). Pantothenic acid. In: *Modern Nutrition in Health and Disease*, Shils, M.E., Olson, J.A., Shike, M., & Ross, A.C. (eds.). Philadelphia, PA: Lippincott Williams & Wilkins, pp. 423–432.

IOM. (1998). *Dietary Reference Intakes for Thiamin, Riboflavin, Niacin, Vitamin B_6, Folate, Vitamin B_{12}, Pantothenic Acid, Biotin and Choline.* Available at: http://www.nap.edu/catalog/6015/dietary-reference-intakes-for-thiamin-riboflavin-niacin-vitamin-b6-folate-vitamin-b12-pantothenic-acid-biotin-and-choline (accessed November 21, 2015).

Ishii, N. & Nishihara, Y. (1981). Pellagra among chronic alcoholics: Clinical and pathological study of 20 necropsy cases. *Journal of Neurology, Neurosurgery and Psychiatry* 44(3), 209–215.

Jiang, T., Christian, P., Khatry, S.K., Wu, L., & West, K.P. 2005. Micronutrient deficiencies in early pregnancy are common, concurrent, and vary by season among rural Nepali pregnant women. *Journal of Nutrition* 135(5), 1106–1112.

Kaiser, L. & Allen, L.H. (2008). Position of the American Dietetic Association: Nutrition and lifestyle for a healthy pregnancy outcome. *Journal of the American Dietetic Association* 108, 553–561.

Kauffman, G., Coats, D., Seab, S., Topazian, M.D., & Fischer, P.R. (2011). Thiamine deficiency in ill children. *American Journal of Clinical Nutrition* 94(2), 616–617.

Kornreich, L., Bron-Harlev, E., Hoffmann, C. et al. (2005). Thiamine deficiency in infants: MR findings in the brain. *American Journal of Neuroradiology* 26(7), 1668–1674.

Kuhne, T., Bubl, R., & Baumgartner, R. (1991). Maternal vegan diet causing a serious infantile neurological disorder due to vitamin B_{12} deficiency. *European Journal of Pediatrics* 150, 205–208.

Kupka, R. (2015). The role of folate in malaria–implications for home fortification programmes among children aged 6–59 months. *Maternal and Child Nutrition* 11(S4), 1–15.

Laillou, A., Pham, T.V., Tran, N.T. et al. (2012). Micronutrient deficits are still public health issues among women and young children in Vietnam. *PLoS One* 7(4), e34906.

Langlais, P.J. & Savage, L.M. (1995). Thiamine deficiency in rats produces cognitive and memory deficits on spatial tasks that correlate with tissue loss in diencephalon, cortex and white matter. *Behavioural Brain Research* 68(1), 75–89.

Lima, L.F., Leite, H.P., & Taddei, J.A. (2011). Low blood thiamine concentrations in children upon admission to the intensive care unit: Risk factors and prognostic significance. *American Journal of Clinical Nutrition* 93, 57–61.

Lonn, E., Yusuf, S., Arnold, M.J. et al. (2006). Homocysteine lowering with folic acid and B vitamins in vascular disease. *New England Journal of Medicine* 354, 1567–1577.

Loriaux, S.M., Deijen, J.B., Orlebeke, J.F., & De Swart, J.H. (1985). The effects of nicotinic acid and xanthinol nicotinate on human memory in different categories of age. *Psychopharmacology* 87(4), 390–395.

Louwman, M.W., van Dusseldorp, M., van de Vijver, F.J., Thomas, C.M., Schneede, J., Ueland, P.M., Refsum, H., & van Staveren, W.A. (2000). Signs of impaired cognitive function in adolescents with marginal cobalamin status. *American Journal of Clinical Nutrition* 72, 762–769.

Mackey, A.D., Davis, S.R., & Gregory, J.F. (2006). Vitamin B_6. In: *Modern Nutrition in Health and Disease*, Shils, M.E., Shike, M., Ross, A.C., Caballero, B., & Cousins, R.J. (eds.). Philadelphia, PA: Lippincott Williams & Wilkins, pp. 452–461.

Maher, M. & Keriakos, R. (2014). Women's awareness of periconceptional use of folic acid before and after their antenatal visits. *Clinical Medicine Insights. Women's Health* 7, 9.

McCormick, D.B. (2012). Riboflavin. In: *Present Knowledge in Nutrition*, 10th edn., Erdman, J.W., Macdonald, I.A., & Zeisel, S.H. (eds.). Ames, IA: International Life Sciences Institute, pp. 280–292.

McCullough, A.L., Kirksey, A., Wachs, T.D., McCabe, G.P., Bassily, N.S., Bishry, Z., Galal, O.M., Harrison, G.G., & Jerome, N.W. (1990). Vitamin B-6 status of Egyptian mothers: Relation to infant behavior and maternal–infant interactions. *American Journal of Clinical Nutrition* 51, 1067–1074.

Miller, J.W. & Ruckner, R.B. (2012). Pantothenic acid. In: *Present Knowledge in Nutrition*, 10th edn., Erdman, J.W., Macdonald, I.A., & Zeisel, S.H. (eds.). Ames, IA: International Life Sciences Institute, pp. 375–390.

Mills, J.L., Fan, R., Brody, L.C. et al. (2014). Maternal choline concentrations during pregnancy and choline-related genetic variants as risk factors for neural tube defects. *American Journal of Clinical Nutrition* 100(4), 1069–1074.

Ministry of Health. (2006). *Food and Nutrition Guidelines for Healthy Pregnant and Breastfeeding Women: A Background Paper.* Wellington, New Zealand: Ministry of Health.

Morris, M.C., Evans, D.A., Bienias, J.L., Scherr, P.A., Tangney, C.C., Hebert, L.E., Bennett, D.A., Wilson, R.S., & Aggarwal, N. (2004). Dietary niacin and the risk of incident Alzheimer's disease and of cognitive decline. *Journal of Neurology, Neurosurgery and Psychiatry* 75(8), 1093–1099.

Morrison, L.A. & Driskell, J.A. (1985). Quantities of B_6 vitamers in human milk by high-performance liquid chromatography. Influence of maternal vitamin B_6 status. *Journal of Chromatography* 337, 249–258.

Morse, N.L. (2012). Benefits of docosahexaenoic acid, folic acid, vitamin D and iodine on foetal and infant brain development and function following maternal supplementation during pregnancy and lactation. *Nutrients* 4(7), 799–840.

MRC Vitamin Study Research Group. (1991). Prevention of neural tube defects: Results of the Medical Research Council Vitamin Study. *Lancet* 338, 131–137.

Nawapun, K. & Phupong, V. (2007). Awareness of the benefits of folic acid and prevalence of the use of folic acid supplements to prevent neural tube defects among Thai women. *Archives of Gynecology and Obstetrics* 276(1), 53–57.

New Zealand Ministry of Health. (2006). Folate/folic acid. Available at: http://www.health.govt.nz/our-work/preventative-health-wellness/nutrition/folate-folic-acid#how_much. Accessed on April 11, 2016.

Nurk, E., Refsum, H., Bjelland, I. et al. (2013). Plasma free choline, betaine and cognitive performance: The Hordaland Health Study. *British Journal of Nutrition* 109(3), 511–519.

Ogunleye, A.J. & Odutuga, A.A. (1989). The effect of riboflavin deficiency on cerebrum and cerebellum of developing rat brain. *Journal of Nutritional Science and Vitaminology* 35(3), 193–197.

Park, Y.K., Sempos, C.T., Barton, C.N., Vanderveen, J.E., & Yetley, E.A. (2000). Effectiveness of food fortification in the United States: The case of pellagra. *American Journal of Public Health* 90(5), 727–738.

Poly, C., Massaro, J.M., Seshadri, S. et al. (2011). The relation of dietary choline to cognitive performance and white-matter hyperintensity in the Framingham Offspring Cohort. *American Journal of Clinical Nutrition* 94(6), 1584–1591.

Powers, H.J., Hill, M.H., Mushtaq, S., Dainty, J.R., Majsak-Newman, G., & Williams, E.A. (2011). Correcting a marginal riboflavin deficiency improves hematologic status in young women in the United Kingdom (RIBOFEM). *American Journal of Clinical Nutrition* 93(6), 1274–1284.

Rabiu, T.B., Tiamiyu, L.O., & Awoyinka, B.S. (2012). Awareness of spina bifida and periconceptional use of folic acid among pregnant women in a developing economy. *Child's Nervous System* 28(12), 2115–2119.

Rahmanifar, A., Kirksey, A., Wachs, T.D., McCabe, G.P., Bishry, Z., Galal, O.M., Harrison, G.G., & Jerome, N.W. (1993). Diet during lactation associated with infant behavior and caregiver–infant interaction in a semirural Egyptian village. *Journal of Nutrition* 123, 164–175.

Ramakrishna, T. (1999). Vitamins and brain development. *Physiological Research* 48, 175–187.

Ray, J.G., Goodman, J., O'Mahoney, P.R.A., Mamdani, M.M., & Jiang, D. (2008). High rate of maternal vitamin B_{12} deficiency nearly a decade after Canadian folic acid flour fortification. *QJM* 101(6), 475–477.

Ray, J.G., Singh, G., & Burrows, R.F. (2004). Evidence for suboptimal use of periconceptional folic acid supplements globally. *BJOG: An International Journal of Obstetrics and Gynaecology* 111(5), 399–408.

Refsum, H., Grindflek, A.W., Ueland, P.M., Fredriksen, Å., Meyer, K., Ulvik, A., Guttormsen, A.B., Iversen, O.E., Schneede, J., & Kase, B.F. (2004). Screening for serum total homocysteine in newborn children. *Clinical Chemistry* 50(10), 1769–1784.

Ren, A., Zhang, L., Li, Z., Hao, L., Tian, Y., & Li, Z. (2006). Awareness and use of folic acid, and blood folate concentrations among pregnant women in northern China – An area with a high prevalence of neural tube defects. *Reproductive Toxicology* 22(3), 431–436.

Renault, F., Verstichel, P., Ploussard, J.P., & Costil, J. (1999). Neuropathy in two cobalamin-deficient breast-fed infants of vegetarian mothers. *Muscle Nerve* 22, 252–254.

Rogers, L.M., Boy, E., Miller, J.W., Green, R., Rodriguez, M., Chew, F., & Allen, L.H. (2003). Predictors of cobalamin deficiency in Guatemalan school children: Diet, *Helicobacter pylori*, or bacterial overgrowth? *Journal of Pediatric Gastroenterology and Nutrition* 36(1), 27–36.

Roth, C., Magnus, P., Schjølberg, S., Stoltenberg, C., Surén, P., McKeague, I.W., Davey Smith, G., Reichborn-Kjennerud, T., & Susser, E. (October 12, 2011). Folic acid supplements in pregnancy and severe language delay in children. *Journal of the American Medical Association* 306(14), 1566–1573.

Ruston, D., Hoare, J., Henderson, L., & Gregory, J. (2004). *The National Diet and Nutrition Survey: Adults Aged 19–64. Nutritional Status.* London, UK: The Stationary Office.

Schmidt, R.J., Hansen, R.L., Hartiala, J., Allayee, H., Schmidt, L.C., Tancredi, D.J., Tassone, F., & Hertz-Picciotto, I. (July 2011). Prenatal vitamins, one-carbon metabolism gene variants, and risk for autism. *Epidemiology* 22(4), 476–485.

Schmidt, R.J., Tancredi, D.J., Ozonoff, S., Hansen, R.L., Hartiala, J., Allayee, H., Schmidt, L.C., Tassone, F., & Hertz-Picciotto, I. (July 2012). Maternal periconceptional folic acid intake and risk of autism spectrum disorders and developmental delay in the CHARGE (CHildhood Autism Risks from Genetics and Environment) case–control study. *American Journal of Clinical Nutrition* 96(1), 80–89.

Schneede, J., Dagnelie, P.C., van Staveren, W.A., Vollset, S.E., Refsum, H., & Ueland, P.M. (1994). Methylmalonic acid and homocysteine in plasma as indicators of functional cobalamin deficiency in infants on macrobiotic diets. *Pediatric Research* 36, 194–201.

Setiawan, B., Giraud, D.W., & Driskell, J.A. (2000). Vitamin B-6 inadequacy is prevalent in rural and urban Indonesian children. *Journal of Nutrition* 130(3), 553–558.

Shaw, G.M., Carmichael, S.L., Nelson, V., Selvin, S., & Schaffer, D.M. (2004a). Occurrence of low birthweight and preterm delivery among California infants before and after compulsory food fortification with folic acid. *Public Health Reports* 119(2), 170.

Shaw, G.M., Carmichael, S.L., Yang, W., Selvin, S., & Schaffer, D.M. (2004b). Periconceptional dietary intake of choline and betaine and neural tube defects in offspring. *American Journal of Epidemiology* 160(2), 102–109.

Shaw, G.M., Finnell, R.H., Blom, H.J. et al. (2009). Choline and risk of neural tube defects in a folate-fortified population. *Epidemiology* 20(5), 714–719.

Siekmann, J.H., Allen, L.H., Bwibo, N.O., Demment, M.W., Murphy, S.P., & Neumann, C.G. (2003). Kenyan school children have multiple micronutrient deficiencies, but increased plasma vitamin B_{12} is the only detectable micronutrient response to meat or milk supplementation. *Journal of Nutrition* 133(11), 3972S–3980S.

Sight & Life. (2012). Food fortification with vitamin B_{12}. Available at: http://www.sightandlife.org/fileadmin/data/Magazine/2012/26_2_2012/sightandlife_magazine_26_2_2012.pdf. Accessed on May 24, 2016.

Singleton, C.K. & Martin, P.R. (2001). Molecular mechanism of thiamine utilization. *Current Molecular Medicine* 1, 197–207.

Sklar, R. (1986). Nutritional vitamin B_{12} deficiency in a breastfed infant of a vegan-diet mother. *Clinical Pediatrics (Philadelphia)* 25, 219–221.

Song, W.O., Chan, G.M., Wyse, B.W., & Hansen, R.G. (1984). Effect of pantothenic acid status on the content of the vitamin in human milk. *American Journal of Clinical Nutrition* 40(2), 317–324.

Stollhoff, K. & Schulte, F.J. (1987). Vitamin B_{12} and brain development. *European Journal of Pediatrics* 146, 201.

Strain, J.J., McSorley, E.M., van Wijngaarden, E. et al. (2013). Choline status and neurodevelopmental outcomes at 5 years of age in the Seychelles Child Development Nutrition Study. *British Journal of Nutrition* 110(2), 330–333.

Strand, T.A., Taneja, S., Ueland, P.M. et al. (2013). Cobalamin and folate status predicts mental development scores in North Indian children 12–18 mo of age. *American Journal of Clinical Nutrition* 97(2), 310–317.

Surén, P., Roth, C., Bresnahan, M. et al. (2013). Association between maternal use of folic acid supplements and risk of autism spectrum disorders in children. *Journal of the American Medical Association* 309(6), 570–577.

Tamura, T., Goldenberg, R.L., Chapman, V.R., Johnston, K.E., Ramey, S.L., & Nelson, K.G. (2005). Folate status of mothers during pregnancy and mental and psychomotor development of their children at 5 years of age. *Pediatrics* 116, 703–708.

Taneja, S., Bhandari, N., Strand, T.A., Sommerfelt, H., Refsum, H., Ueland, P.M., Schneede, J., Bahl, R., & Bhan, M.K. (2007). Cobalamin and folate status in infants and young children in a low-to-middle income com-munity in India. *American Journal of Clinical Nutrition* 86(5), 1302–1309.

Thamm, M., Mensink, G.B., & Thierfelder, W. (1999). Folic acid intake of women in childbearing age. *Gesundheitswesen (Bundesverband der Arzte des Offentlichen Gesundheitsdienstes* (Germany) 61, S207–S212.

Thuesen, B.H., Husemoen, L.L.N., Ovesen, L., Jørgensen, T., Fenger, M., & Linneberg, A. (2010). Lifestyle and genetic determinants of folate and vitamin B_{12} levels in a general adult population. *British Journal of Nutrition* 103(08), 1195–1204.

Vasconcelos, M.M., Silva, K.P., Vidal, G. et al. (1999). Early diagnosis of pediatric Wernicke's encephalopathy. *Pediatric Neurology* 20, 289–294.

Veena, S.R., Krishnaveni, G.V., Srinivasan, K. et al. (2010). Higher maternal plasma folate but not vitamin-B_{12} concentrations during pregnancy are associated with better cognitive function scores in 9–10 year old children in South India. *Journal of Nutrition* 140, 1014–1022.

Villamor, E., Rifas-Shiman, S.L., Gillman, M.W., & Oken, E. (2012). Maternal intake of methyl – Donor nutrients and child cognition at 3 years of age. *Paediatric and Perinatal Epidemiology* 26(4), 328–335.

Wellings, K., Jones, K.G., Mercer, C.H. et al. (2013). The prevalence of unplanned pregnancy and associated factors in Britain: Findings from the Third National Survey of Sexual Attitudes and Lifestyles (NATSAL-3). *Lancet* 382(9907), 1807–1816.

WHO. (2009). Recommendations on wheat and maize flour fortification meeting report: Interim Consensus Statement [Internet]. World Health Organization, Geneva. Available at: http://www.who.int/nutrition/publications/micronutrients/wheat_maize_fortification/en/. Accessed on April 11, 2016.

Wighton, M.C., Manson, J.I., Speed, I., Robertson, E., & Chapman, E. (1979). Brain damage in infancy and dietary vitamin B_{12} deficiency. *Medical Journal of Australia* 2, 1–3.

Wilson, R.D. & Genetics Committee. (2015). Pre-conception folic acid and multivitamin supplementation for the primary and secondary prevention of neural tube defects and other folic acid-sensitive congenital anomalies. *Journal of Obstetrics and Gynaecology Canada* 37(6), 534–549.

Wolff, T., Witkop, C.T., Miller, T., & Syed, S.B. (2009). U.S. Preventive Services Task Force. Folic acid supplementation for the prevention of neural tube defects: An update of the evidence for the US Preventive Services Task Force. *Annals of Internal Medicine* 150, 632–639.

Wu, B.T., Dyer, R.A., King, D.J., Richardson, K.J., & Innis, S.M. (2012). Early second trimester maternal plasma choline and betaine are related to measures of early cognitive development in term infants. *PLoS One* 7, e43448.

Wyalt, D.T., Michael, J.N., & Hillman, R.E. (1987). Infantile beriberi presenting as subacute necrotizing ncephalomyelopathy. *Journal of Pediatrics* 110, 888–891.

Zeisel, S.H. (2004). Nutritional importance of choline for brain development. *Journal of the American College of Nutrition* 23(Suppl. 6), 621S–626S.

Zempleni, J. & Mock, D.M. (1999). Biotin biochemistry and human requirements. *Journal of Nutritional Biochemistry* 10(3), 128–138.

6 Iron and the Developing Brain

Harry J. McArdle, Michael K. Georgieff, and William D. Rees

CONTENTS

6.1 INTRODUCTION

Iron is an essential element and its best-known function, accounting for about two-thirds of the iron in the body, is a component of the haemoglobin molecules which transport oxygen. Iron is also essential for mitochondria, with a key role in the electron transfer reactions which generate ATP during aerobic metabolism. The brain is the most metabolically active organ in the body, so its internal concentration of iron is exceptionally high and comparable to other active tissues such as the liver. Iron concentrations in several structures, including the globus pallidus, caudate nucleus, putamen, and substantia nigra, increase rapidly during development, reaching a plateau after the first decade (Höck et al. 1975). In addition to metabolism, iron is essential for brain-specific functions, which include the synthesis of fatty acids required for myelination and synthesis of neurotransmitters (serotonin, dopamine adrenalin, and noradrenalin). Iron is also found in cytochrome P450, which detoxifies a range of natural and xenobiotic compounds. Because of this role in a diverse spectrum of cellular functions, iron is indispensable for normal neural development and physiology.

Despite the essential role of protein bound iron, free iron is harmful as Fe^{3+} ions in solution enhance the production of peroxide free radicals. These cause oxidative damage to a range of biological molecules including polyunsaturated fatty acids which are key components of membrane structure. As free iron cannot be excreted, there are elaborate controls to regulate the uptake of iron and to ensure that almost all of the 4–5 g of elemental iron found in the adult human is tightly complexed to proteins. In considering the role of iron in the development of the brain, it is necessary to take into account all of the processes regulating its uptake and delivery as well as its actual role in neurogenesis.

6.2 IRON AS A NUTRIENT

Iron in food is present in two forms: in haem, with a porphyrin ring structure surrounding the Fe atom, and non-haem iron, usually complexed either to amino acids or in iron–sulphur clusters. Meat is the richest source of iron; however, other foods, which include fish, cereals, beans, nuts, and dark green vegetables, also contain relatively high levels. The main food groups contributing to iron in the Western diet are grains and grain products, followed by meat and then dark vegetables. Average iron intakes in the United Kingdom (from Dietary Reference Values given by the UK Scientific Advisory Committee for Nutrition [Scientific Advisory Committee on Nutrition (SACN) 2011], outlined in Table 6.1) are between 2.6 and 6 mg/day in infants, rising to 9.4 and 17.9 mg/day in adults.

6.2.1 Prevalence of Iron Deficiency

There are three levels of iron deficiency (ID): the mildest is a depletion of iron stores, followed by iron deficiency without anaemia, and finally iron deficiency anaemia (IDA). Changes in erythropoiesis which result in an abnormally low concentration of haemoglobin or haematocrit (the diagnostic criteria for IDA) are only observed once

TABLE 6.1
Dietary Reference Values for Iron, mg/Day (μmol/Day)[a]

Age	Lower Reference Nutrient Intake (LRNI)	Estimated Average Requirement (EAR)	Reference Nutrient Intake (RNI)
0–3 months	0.9 (15)	1.3 (20)	1.7 (30)
4–6 months	2.3 (40)	3.3 (60)	4.3 (80)
7–9 months	4.2 (75)	6.0 (110)	7.8 (140)
10–12 months	4.2 (75)	6.0 (110)	7.8 (140)
1–3 years	3.7 (65)	5.3 (95)	6.9 (120)
4–6 years	3.3 (60)	4.7 (80)	6.1 (110)
7–10 years	4.7 (80)	6.7 (120)	8.7 (160)
11–14 years (males)	6.1 (110)	8.7 (160)	11.3 (200)
11–14 years (females)	8.0 (140)	11.4 (200)	14.8 (260)
15–18 years (males)	6.1 (110)	8.7 (160)	11.3 (200)
15–18 years (females)	8.0 (140)	11.4 (200)	14.8 (260)
19–50 years (males)	4.7 (80)	6.7 (120)	8.7 (160)
19–50 years (females)	8.0 (140)	11.4 (200)	14.8 (260)
50+ years	4.7 (80)	6.7 (120)	8.7 (160)

Source: Department of Health, Dietary Reference Values for Food, Energy and Nutrients in the United Kingdom, Report on Health and Social Subjects No. 41, HMSO, London, UK, 1991.

[a] The conversion factor 1 μmol = 55.9 μg of iron is based on the molecular weight of iron.

whole-body iron status has fallen substantially. However, the clinical diagnosis of IDA during pregnancy is complicated by the natural changes in blood volume which reduce the haematocrit and mask effects associated with iron deficiency (Scholl 2005). Currently, there are no global figures for iron deficiency, but estimates using anaemia as an indirect indicator suggest that one in four people are affected and that pregnant women and preschool-age children are at the greatest risk (WHO Global Database on Iron Deficiency and Anaemia). Many women of childbearing age have a dietary intake of absorbable iron that is insufficient to compensate for the losses from menstruation, leaving them in negative iron balance. Data from the WHO suggest that up to 70% of women worldwide may be classed as either iron deficient or suffering from IDA.

Prior to the introduction of complementary foods, the developing fetus and infant is dependent on iron from the mother, via the placenta before birth and from milk after birth. As human breast milk is low in iron, stores of iron acquired *in utero* are important for the first 4–6 months after birth. If the stores are exhausted, additional iron must be obtained from the diet. Unfortunately, several important elements in the diet of infants and toddlers, such as cow's milk, fruits, and vegetables, are all low in iron. Furthermore, there is evidence to suggest that the consumption of cow's milk actually worsens infants iron status by interfering with intestinal uptake (Ziegler 2011). The prevalence of iron deficiency in neonates reflects the distribution of maternal iron deficiency and in exclusively breastfed infants at 6 months of age varies from 6% in developed countries to in excess of 35% in developing nations (Yang et al. 2009).

In predominantly agrarian populations such as the rural poor in India, IDA prevalence is 49.5% in 6 to 23-month-old and 39.9% in 24 to 58-month-old children (Plessow et al. 2015). Although IDA is less common in infants and toddlers in developed countries such as the United States, mothers and infants still present with ID and IDA (Eden & Sandoval 2012). Risk factors include socio-economic status, immigrant status, low birthweight (LBW), high cow's milk intake, and a low intake of iron-rich complementary foods.

6.2.2 Iron Status and Effects on Pregnancy Outcome and Fetal and Neonatal Growth

Anaemia and iron deficiency during pregnancy are associated with an increase in placental weight and a higher ratio of placental to fetal weight (Godfrey et al. 1991). There is a decrease in fetal growth reflected in an association between maternal haemoglobin concentration, birthweight, and risk of preterm birth in iron-deficient pregnancies. There are clear benefits of pre-pregnancy supplementation with daily iron in reducing the risk of maternal anaemia in pregnancy (Pena-Rosas et al. 2015); however, supplementation of anaemic or non-anaemic pregnant women with iron, folic acid, or both does not appear to increase either birthweight or the duration of gestation (Haider et al. 2013; Rasmussen 2001). The benefits also have to be balanced against the disadvantage that iron supplements during pregnancy consistently increase the risk of adverse outcomes in mothers with high maternal haemoglobin and high levels of the iron storage protein ferritin (Scholl 2011). In addition, prenatal stress has also been shown to reduce neonatal iron stores in primate models. The post-partum effect was most pronounced when the disturbance occurred early in pregnancy, suggesting that changes which perturbed iron storage preceded the increased placental transfer of iron occurring later in gestation (Coe et al. 2007).

Most (>66%) of the infant's total body iron is acquired during the final trimester of pregnancy, and as a result, healthy, normal birthweight infants born at term are self-sufficient for iron during the first 6 months of life. There is little evidence that iron supplements are beneficial for growth in the first few months of life as iron-replete infants redistribute iron from haemoglobin to iron stores (Ziegler et al. 2009). In contrast, babies born to mothers with poor iron status or low birthweight (LBW, <2500 g) or preterm have reduced iron stores and are more likely to experience ID during the first 6 months of life. Trials show that giving these babies iron supplements results in a slightly higher haemoglobin level and a lower risk of developing IDA when compared with those who have not received supplements; however, there is no conclusive evidence for long-term benefits in terms of growth (Mills & Davies 2012).

As it is common for formula milk and milk substitutes to be fortified with iron, often to levels well in excess of those found in breast milk, many infants in the developed world actually receive an excess of iron. Since the accumulation of iron in neural tissues is associated with degenerative diseases in adults (Piñero & Connor 2000), it has been suggested that this excess may have long-term adverse effects in the offspring. While there is good evidence that iron supplementation causes no adverse effects on short-term health (Singhal et al. 2000), there is some evidence from animal studies to suggest that the infant brain is not as well protected against systemic iron overload compared to the adult (Fredriksson et al. 1999). It has been suggested that excess iron in infancy may alter the trajectory of brain iron uptake and amplify the risk of iron-associated neurodegeneration in later life (Hare et al. 2015).

In rats fed iron-deficient rations throughout pregnancy, neonatal size is reduced; however, supplementation from the beginning of the first, second, or third week all reduced the effect (Gambling et al. 2004). Although gestational and neonatal iron deficiency in rodents does not affect overall brain size, there is evidence for a decrease in the size of specific regions including the hippocampus (Rao et al. 2011). In addition to poor growth, physiological systems are compromised in the iron-deficient offspring. Babies born to mothers with poorer iron status have an increased risk of compromised lung function, which is still significant at age 11 (Nwaru et al. 2014). Furthermore, it has been suggested that iron deficiency, whether induced genetically or by dietary means, can increase the damage caused by inflammation (Kim et al. 2011). In rat models, iron deficiency during pregnancy results in hypertension in the offspring (Gambling et al. 2003) as a result of a reduction in nephron number, although to date, the evidence does not support a similar change in blood pressure in humans (Belfort et al. 2008; Brion et al. 2008).

6.2.3 Iron Deficiency and Early Life: Development of Cognitive Deficits

Observational studies of the acute and long-term effects of early life iron deficiency in humans show a clear association between prenatal and early postnatal iron deficiency and long-term disruptions in cognitive, social, and behavioural developments. The impact depends on the precise time period when the deficiency was encountered and its extent. The most severe cases of ID leading to IDA in pregnancy and early life predispose the offspring to a range of social problems such as increased anxiety, increased likelihood of depression, and poor attention (Lozoff et al. 1998, 2000; Wachs et al. 2005). Educational outcomes such as arithmetic achievement, written expression, and some specific cognitive processes such as spatial memory and selective recall are all affected (Lozoff et al. 2000). Unfortunately, many of these studies are carried out in developing or low-income countries where iron is just one of several micronutrient deficiencies. Poor social conditions further confound the interpretation of these studies, making it difficult to conclusively describe the effects of specific micronutrient deficiencies on neurodevelopment.

The acute effects of ID in pregnancy on the term or preterm new-born include poorer discrimination memory (Siddappa et al. 2004), altered temperament and interactions with the caregiver (Wachs et al. 2005), slower speed of neural processing (Amin et al. 2010), and a greater number of abnormal neurological reflexes (Armony-Sivan et al. 2004). Children with the lowest concentrations of ferritin in cord blood at birth were most acutely affected, demonstrating significantly lower IQ and poorer language ability, tractability, and fine motor skills at 5 years (Tamura et al. 2002). There are also reports that the offspring of women who had IDA with a haemoglobin concentration <100 g/L during pregnancy have a 3.7-fold greater risk of schizophrenia as adults (Insel et al. 2008).

Acute postnatal ID has been reported to result in slower neural conduction velocities in 6-month-olds with ID (Roncagliolo et al. 1998), which has been attributed to disruptions in myelination. Toddlers with ID have a lower developmental quotient than iron-sufficient toddlers, and the gap in cognitive functioning between these groups widens with age (Lozoff et al. 2000). Toddlers currently suffering from ID also have socio-emotional alterations, including increased hesitancy and wariness in novel situations (Lozoff et al. 1998). These are thought to relate to alterations in monoamine neurotransmission (Lozoff et al. 2006). Infants with ID anaemia demonstrate poorer performance for both gross and fine motor skills at 9 months of age (Angulo-Barroso et al. 2011) and abnormal sleep patterns (Peirano et al. 2010).

Crucially, the deleterious effects of iron deficiency are persistent and are not resolved by iron supplementation later in life. Children diagnosed anaemic before they reach 2 years of age, but normal thereafter, are still showing deficits in cognition and school achievement when tested at 4, 19 (Lozoff et al. 2006), and 25 years of age (Lozoff et al. 2013). Four-year-olds, who were iron deficient early in their postnatal lives, have long-lasting effects on both auditory and visual systems when compared to controls who were never anaemic. Early postnatal iron deficiency causes poorer visual processing and myelination, as well as longer visual evoked potential latencies (Algarin et al. 2003). Changes in higher functions, which manifest as features such as abnormal sleep patterns (Peirano et al. 2010), an increased risk of anxiety and depression (Lukowski et al. 2010), and poorer inhibitory control (Algarin et al. 2013), have all been described in formerly ID children, adolescents, and adults.

6.2.4 Intervention Studies in Humans

Intervention studies, usually in the form of iron supplementation either alone or in combination with other micronutrients, provide one means of resolving the role of iron in fetal and neonatal neurodevelopment in humans; however, these are still subject to many of the confounding factors which complicate observational studies. The majority of studies are carried out on populations in the developing world and have concentrated either on children who are already iron deficient (treatment) or have provided supplemental iron to mothers and/or children who are at risk (prevention). A meta-analysis of 10 treatment studies in former iron-deficient anaemic or chronically iron-deficient individuals found that iron therapy that corrected their anaemia in infancy produced some improvement in cognitive outcomes; however, when compared with their non-anaemic peers, there were still long-term effects on IQ, socialization, and attention span (Walker et al. 2013). There is also evidence that prenatal iron supplementation may be beneficial; however, the results are contradictory (Prado & Dewey 2014). The variability of prevention studies probably reflects uncertainty in the measurement of iron status (whether iron sufficient or extremely deficient), coupled with confounding factors due to the presence of multiple micronutrient deficiencies. Despite these drawbacks, comparisons demonstrate that treatment is better than no treatment, although there are often residual effects in the treated children not seen in the iron-sufficient controls (Wachs et al. 2014). Supplementation studies of infants in low- and middle-income countries are more encouraging, consistently showing that iron supplements improve outcomes at the end of the intervention period (Black et al. 2011).

These treatment or supplementation studies highlight the importance of starting iron supplementation at the earliest possible stage. For example, prenatal iron and folic acid supplementation in pregnant women from rural Nepal who had a high risk of ID resulted in positive effects on neurodevelopmental outcomes when the offspring were subsequently studied at 7–9 years of age (Christian et al. 2010), whereas providing supplements to infants between ages 12 and 36 months did not provide additional benefits (Christian et al. 2011). These results indicate that adverse effects can be prevented and/or reversed, at least to some extent, with iron early in development or before iron deficiency becomes severe or chronic (Lozoff 2007) and demonstrate that the timing of supplementation is critical. Ideally, early iron supplementation during the prenatal period is better for the developing brain (Cusick & Georgieff 2012; Wachs et al. 2014).

Another group of babies at risk of ID are preterm and low-birthweight (LBW) infants who, because iron is accreted in the last trimester, are often born with inadequate iron stores. Studies suggest that iron supplementation in LBW infants during the first 6 months of life may reduce clinical symptoms in early childhood. For example, early iron supplementation of marginally LBW infants did not affect cognitive functions at 3.5 years of age but significantly reduced the prevalence of behavioural problems (Berglund et al. 2013). Another study of very low-birthweight infants (<1301 g) indicated a trend towards better neurocognitive and motor development when iron supplementation was initiated at the earliest opportunity (Steinmacher et al. 2007).

Despite the clear benefits of early interventions, several studies report marked improvements in cognitive and motor skills following interventions in the postnatal period. The majority of studies report neurological improvements, suggesting that iron-dependent processes continue during the postnatal development of the brain (Lozoff et al. 2006). Studies where ID infants are given supplements (Lozoff et al. 2003), as well as those aimed at preventing ID in infancy, all demonstrate positive changes in neurological development as well as improved iron status (Black et al. 2004; Stoltzfus et al. 2001), despite the fact that children who were anaemic in infancy often fail to achieve the same level of cognitive development as non-anaemic infants (Grantham-McGregor & Ani 2001). In one study, 5-year-olds who received iron supplementation in infancy to correct IDA still showed lower physical activity levels, less positive affect, and less verbalization (Corapci et al. 2006), again emphasizing the long-term risk when ID occurs early in life. Another study showed no effect of iron supplementation and this was attributed to the supplementation being given in the period of 12–36 months, missing the early period of rapid brain development (Murray-Kolb et al. 2012). In general, neurological domains that are affected by acute ID in toddlerhood show persistent negative effects over time even after correction of ID (Georgieff 2011; Lozoff et al. 2006). Cognitive abilities such as literacy and numeracy are often poorer in formerly iron-deficient children, consistent with abnormalities in hippocampal and prefrontal cortical development (Lukowski et al. 2010).

Unfortunately, the analysis of the behavioural and cognitive outcomes gives no information on the underlying changes in brain development. Pharmacological and neuroimaging techniques have been employed to test hypotheses derived from animal models (reviewed in Lozoff 2011). Dopamine is a neurotransmitter important in regulating cognition and emotion, reward and pleasure, movement, and hormone release (Seamans & Yang 2004). Iron is a cofactor for tyrosine hydroxylase, a critical enzyme in dopamine production, and animal studies have shown that impaired emotional behaviours are associated with iron deficiency through altered dopamine metabolism (Li et al. 2011). The analysis suggests that there are changes in the frontal-striatal circuits and the mesocortical dopamine pathway and the mesolimbic pathway in ID infants, which may help explain changes in social-emotional behaviour. Other neurotransmitters including serotonin, noradrenaline (Kaladhar & Narasinga Rao 1983), gamma amino-butyric acid, and glutamine (Kim & Wessling-Resnick 2014) are also implicated in animal studies. Unfortunately, ethical considerations, the complexity of the problem, and technical limitations limit the ability to conduct mechanistic studies in humans. Much of what is known about the role of iron in brain development is drawn from the studies of experimental animals. While there is a need to exercise caution in interpreting the results, as brain development differs greatly across species, the fundamental mechanisms are probably similar and many of the findings in rodents have been subsequently supported by studies in primates (Golub 2010; Golub & Hogrefe 2015).

6.2.5 Physiology of Iron Homeostasis

With a large amount of iron associated with red blood cells, the natural turnover of erythrocytes results in substantial quantities of iron (~20 mg/day) cycling into and out of haemoglobin. This is much less than the amounts of iron absorbed from the diet (~1 mg/day in adults). There is no specific mechanism to excrete excess iron in humans and, although there is some evidence for loss through excretion across the gut, overall iron status is maintained by regulating absorption.

Iron is largely absorbed in the duodenum and jejunum. Very little iron is absorbed in the lower intestine or colon, and iron in the colon may, in fact, be harmful, since it has the capacity to go through redox cycling, with risk of damage to colon cells. Haem iron is more bioavailable than non-haem iron, but in normal diets, non-haem iron is present in much higher amounts (up to about 90%). Additionally, there are components in the diet that can increase or decrease bioavailability. Phytate, for example, can bind iron and reduce its absorption, while vitamin C will increase absorption by reducing Fe^{3+} to Fe^{2+}, which is the form taken up by the enterocyte. Additionally, meat contains factors that stimulate absorption, possibly by increasing the solubility of the iron.

The liver is the major regulator of whole-body iron status, coordinating an elaborate system to store surplus iron to make it available when it is needed and also to regulate uptake from the gut (Linder 2013). The liver stores iron safely in ferritin. The ferritin apo-protein consists of approximately 20 monomers which combine to form a hollow shell, within which the iron is stored. Some of the ferritin finds its way into serum and circulating levels can be used to estimate liver iron stores with a reasonable degree of accuracy. When ferritin stores are adequate, the liver produces a small peptide, hepcidin, which enters the circulation and binds to ferroportin, the protein regulating iron efflux from the gut. The ferroportin becomes ubiquitinated and is degraded by the proteasome in the gut, reducing iron efflux from the cell as shown in Figure 6.1. Hepcidin also acts on macrophages to reduce the production of iron from the destruction of outdated erythrocytes. Hepcidin itself is regulated by many different factors (Figure 6.2) which unfortunately means that it cannot be used as a biomarker of iron status.

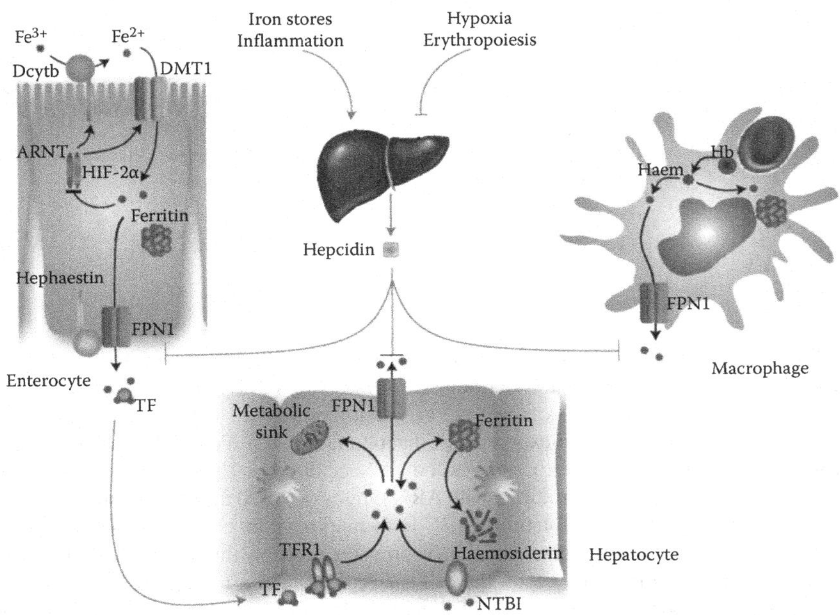

FIGURE 6.1 Systemic regulation of whole-body iron homeostasis. (From Darshan, D. et al., *Expert Rev. Mol. Med.*, 12, e36. Copyright Cambridge University Press 2010.) Iron is reduced at the brush-border membrane of duodenal enterocytes (Dcytb is a candidate ferric reductase) and transported across the membrane by DMT1. Excess iron is stored in ferritin and the remainder is transported across the basolateral membrane and into the circulation by the iron exporter FPN1. Excess iron can also suppress the ARNT–HIF-2α complex, which normally induces DMT1 and Dcytb expression. Iron which enters the bloodstream is bound to circulating plasma TF. TF delivers iron to various tissues, including hepatocytes where it is either stored in ferritin or utilized for cellular metabolism. Iron which is not bound to TF (NTBI) can also enter hepatocytes and contributes to the labile iron pool. Excess iron is stored in ferritin and its degradation product, haemosiderin. When required, iron can be removed from ferritin and exported from hepatocytes. Senescent red blood cells are engulfed by reticuloendothelial macrophages. Hb is broken down, and iron is either released into the circulation or stored in ferritin. The liver-derived peptide hepcidin blocks cellular iron release by binding to FPN and facilitating its removal from the membrane, thereby regulating iron entry into the plasma. Iron stores and inflammation positively regulate hepcidin levels, whereas hypoxia and increased erythropoiesis down-regulate it. (Abbreviations: ARNT, aryl hydrocarbon receptor nuclear translocator; DMT1, divalent-metalion transporter 1; FPN1, ferroportin; Hb, haemoglobin; HIF-2α, hypoxia-inducible factor 2α; NTBI, non-transferrin-bound iron; TF, transferrin; TFR1, transferrin receptor 1.)

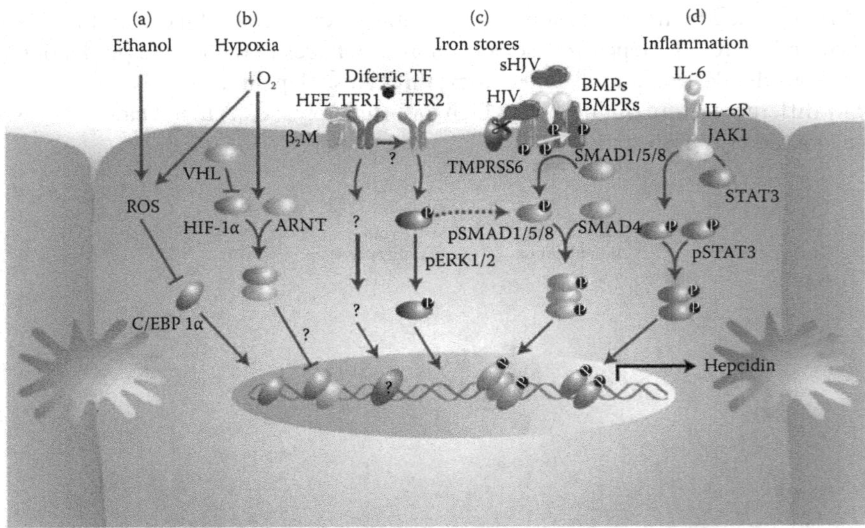

FIGURE 6.2 Molecular regulation of hepcidin expression. (From Darshan, D. et al., *Expert Rev. Mol. Med.*, 12, e36. Copyright Cambridge University Press 2010.) In hepatocytes, hepcidin can be regulated by ethanol, hypoxia, iron stores, and inflammation. (a, b) C/EBPα binds to the promoter and stimulates hepcidin expression. Ethanol and hypoxia induce ROS, down-regulate C/EBPα binding, and thus lead to suppression of hepcidin. (b) Under hypoxic conditions, HIF-1α is stabilized, forms a heterodimer with ARNT, translocates to the nucleus, and downregulates hepcidin expression. VHL destabilizes HIF-1α by marking it for ubiquitination and degradation. (c) Diferric transferrin stimulates hepcidin expression, probably through its interactions with TFR2 and the HFE–TFR1 complex on the cell surface. Signalling through the ERK pathway appears to be involved. BMPs, notably BMP6, bind to BMPRs and the co-receptor HJV to induce signalling through the SMAD pathway to modulate hepcidin expression. TMPRSS6 down-regulates hepcidin expression by cleaving HJV. (d) Inflammatory cytokines, such as IL-6, bind to their receptors (IL-6R) and stimulate STAT3 to induce hepcidin expression. (Abbreviations: ARNT, aryl hydrocarbon receptor nuclear translocator; BMPRs, BMP receptors; BMPs, bone morphogenetic proteins; C/EBPα, CCAAT/enhancer-binding protein alpha; pERK1/2, phosphorylated extracellular signal–regulated kinase 1/2; HIF-1α, hypoxia-inducible factor 1α; HJV, haemojuvelin; IL-6, interleukin-6; JAK1, Janus kinase 1; β2M, β2-microglobulin; ROS, reactive oxygen species; SMAD, small mothers against decapentaplegic homologue; STAT, signal transducer and activator of transcription; TF, transferrin; TFR, transferrin receptor; TMPRSS6, transmembrane protease, serine 6; VHL, von Hippel–Lindau.)

6.2.6 Iron Absorption and Excretion

As described in the previous section, iron from food in the intestinal lumen consists of haem iron and non-haem iron. Non-haem iron is reduced from Fe^{3+} to Fe^{2+} by a reductase (duodenal cytochrome B, DcytB) in the enterocyte membrane or by components in the diet itself, such as vitamin C, and the reduced iron is transported across the apical membrane by the divalent metal transporter-1 (DMT1). Inside the cell, the iron is incorporated into ferritin, held for excretion, or transferred to the basolateral side through ferroportin, and re-oxidized by hephaestin prior to incorporation into transferrin (Figure 6.1).

The mechanism for haem iron uptake and transfer is not so well delineated. Some time ago, a possible haem transporter was identified in the enterocyte membrane (Shayeghi et al. 2005) but closer examination determined that it was, in fact, a folate transporter. Other potential haem transporters have been proposed, but to date, it is not clear whether or how they are involved in metabolism in the gut. Following uptake into the enterocyte, haem is broken down by haem oxygenase, and the iron is incorporated into the same pool as non-haem iron and thereafter treated in the same manner. A similar mechanism for haem absorption may exist in placenta (see the following).

6.2.7 Regulation of Iron Status in the Cell

Within the cell, the iron status is regulated by two iron-binding proteins, IRP1 and IRP2 (Anderson et al. 2012). If the IRP does not have its full complement of iron, it binds to an iron regulatory element (IRE) on the mRNAs coding for proteins involved in iron regulation such as transferrin receptor (TfR) or ferritin. Depending on whether the IRE is located on the 3′ or 5′ end of the mRNA, the message is degraded or stabilized, resulting in increased levels of the protein (Figure 6.3). So, in the case of adequate iron status, transferrin receptor expression

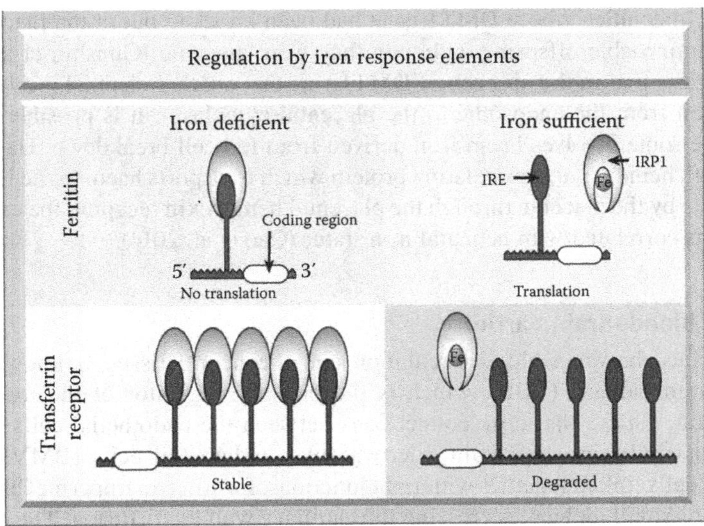

FIGURE 6.3 Regulation of translation and mRNA stability by iron response elements. (Modified from Anderson, C.P. et al., *Biochim. Biophys. Acta*, 1823, 1468, 2012.) IRPs bind to IREs located in either the 5′ or 3′ untranslated regions of specific mRNAs. When iron is limited, IRPs bind with high affinity to 5′ IRE mRNAs and repress translation. IRPs also bind to the five 3′ IREs in TfR1mRNA, stabilizing the mRNAs. When iron is abundant, IRPs do not bind IREs, resulting in the translation of 5′ IRE-containing mRNAs and degradation of TfR1 mRNA.

is reduced and ferritin is increased. In iron deficiency, the reverse occurs. This is a very elegant and efficient system and one which results in very tight control of intracellular iron status.

6.2.7.1 Iron Uptake in the Placenta

Iron is transferred from the maternal liver on transferrin, a serum protein with two iron-binding sites. Protein without iron is called apo-transferrin, while the term for protein carrying iron is holo-transferrin. In pregnancy, approximately 30% or so of the iron-binding sites are occupied. Holo-transferrin binds to the transferrin receptor (TfR) on the apical surface of the trophoblast. The complex is internalized into vesicles, which become acidified by the action of an H^+-ATPase. The pH inside the vesicles drops to about 6.0 and at this pH, the affinity of the transferrin receptor for transferrin drops. Additionally, the iron is released from the protein and moves out of the vesicle through the DMT1 transporter. The iron crosses the cell, through unknown mechanisms, but given the potential toxicity of Fe^{2+} in solution and the insolubility of Fe^{3+} at neutral pH, this is unlikely to be a simple diffusion. The iron effluxes into the fetal circulation through ferroportin and is oxidized from Fe^{2+} to Fe^{3+} by a copper oxidase, zyklopen, following which it binds to fetal transferrin and is carried to the fetal liver and erythron (McArdle et al. 2013) (Figure 6.4).

There is however evidence to suggest that there is an alternative to DMT1-mediated transport since mice whose DMT1 gene had been knocked out in the placenta still gave birth to viable offspring, although they were anaemic (Gunshin et al. 2005). This suggests that in the absence of DMT1 was that another channel is available to deliver iron from the endosome to the placental cytoplasm. It is possible that this alternative route involves haem iron derived from red cell breakdown. Haem complexed with hemopexin, a circulating protein which transports haem to the liver, may be taken up by the placenta through the placental hemopexin receptor, the expression of which is correlated with neonatal iron status (Cao et al. 2014).

6.2.7.2 Blood–Brain Barrier

The interface between blood circulation and the neural tissue is known as the 'blood–brain barrier' (BBB), which is the primary regulator of the iron supply to the brain. Unlike the loose connections between the endothelial cells found in peripheral capillaries, the brain microvascular endothelial cells (BMVECs) are polarized cells linked together with tight junctions, forming an impermeable barrier which stops small molecules crossing the capillary wall by diffusion. The only way for nutrients, including iron, to cross this barrier and enter the brain is by transcellular transport through the BMVEC. Specific proteins in the apical membranes of the BMVEC transport iron and other nutrients from the circulation into the cytoplasm of the cell, from where it is subsequently released through the basolateral membranes into the interstitial spaces between the cells of the brain. This process is highly regulated and protects the neurons from variations in the iron content of

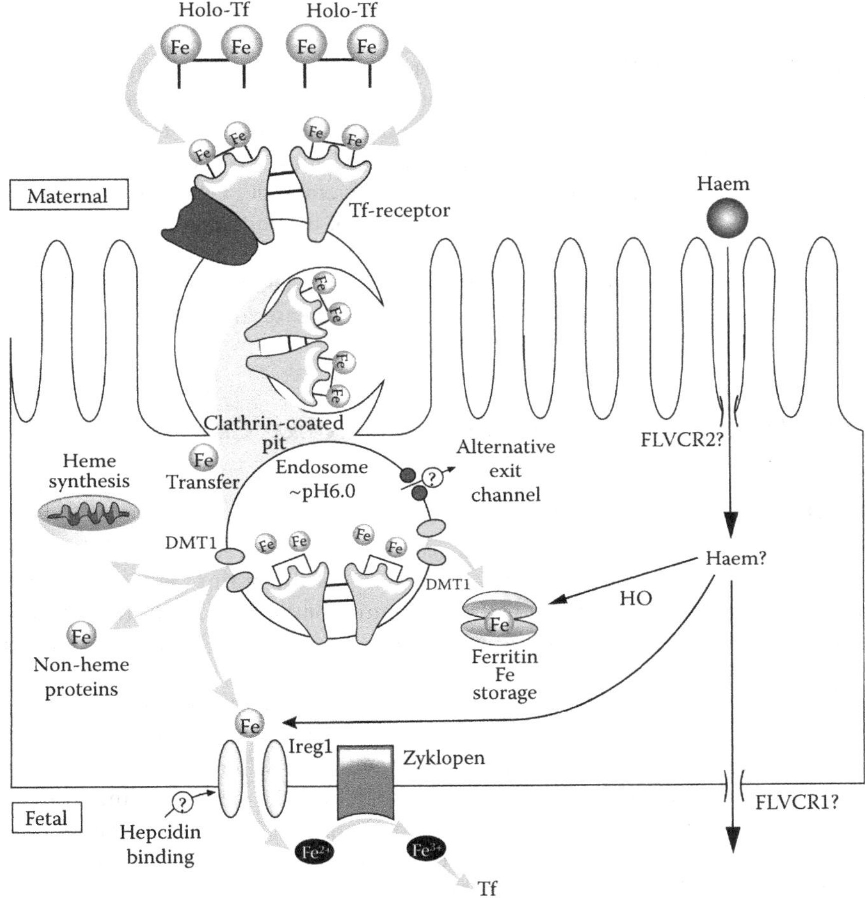

FIGURE 6.4 Iron transport by the placenta. (From Mcardle, H.J. et al., *Nutr. Rev.*, 69(Suppl 1), S17, 2011.) The steps involved are described in the text.

the peripheral circulation (Obermeier et al. 2013). The exact timing of the development of the BBB is unclear, but since the genes specific for the tight junctions characteristic of BMVEC are expressed at a very early stage of embryonic development (between e10 and e12 in the mouse), it is possible that the free flow of small molecules is restricted from an early stage, although the full barrier may not be fully functional until later in gestation (Hagan & Ben-Zvi 2015). Once the BBB has formed, there is evidence that both free iron and iron–transferrin complexes are taken up by the BMVEC. Although the divalent iron transporter DMT1 is present at the apical surface of BMVEC, there is very little free iron in serum, suggesting that this route is of minor importance (McCarthy & Kosman 2012).

As most of the iron in the circulation is complexed to transferrin, it is likely that the binding of iron–transferrin to the transferrin receptor-1 expressed on the apical membrane of the BMVEC accounts for the bulk of iron uptake into the brain. Once bound, the iron–transferrin–receptor complex is taken into the cell by endocytosis. Acidification of the internalized endosome releases Fe^{3+} from transferrin, and following reduction to Fe^{2+} by endosomal reductases is then transported into the cytosol by DMT1 present in the endosomal membrane. Ferroportin present in the basolateral membrane allows iron to pass out of the cell and into the interstitial space (McCarthy & Kosman 2014a). However, this simple model fails to account for several aspects of iron transport (Simpson et al. 2015) and the role of apo-transferrin and hepcidin secreted on the basolateral side to increase and decrease the rate of iron release is discussed further in the following.

6.2.8 Direct Effects of Iron Deficiency on Neural Growth and Differentiation

6.2.8.1 Brain Development

The brain develops from the anterior end of the neural tube where a series of swellings form and give rise to the various parts of the brain: the forebrain containing the cerebral hemispheres, the midbrain containing important pathways to and from the forebrain, and the hindbrain containing the brainstem and cerebellum. While the process of neural development is underway, the stem cells destined to become glia form the supportive tissue that surrounds the nerve cells. Neurogenesis precedes gliogenesis; in the case of the newborn rat, >90% of the cells in the brain are neurons and glial cell growth and differentiation takes place during the postnatal period of development. While the general principles and mechanisms underlying neurogenesis have been identified, much remains to be elucidated about the subtle differences in molecular mechanisms which mediate the formation of the different neuronal subtypes found in distinct brain regions (Paridaen & Huttner 2014).

6.2.8.2 Stem Cell Proliferation

Iron is essential for the proliferation of neural progenitor cells which like all cells progress through the well-recognized stages of the cell cycle (Fu & Richardson 2007; Nurtjahja-Tjendraputra et al. 2006; Renton & Jeitner 1996). Iron deficiency, induced *in vitro* by adding chelators such as desferoxamine (DFO) to the culture medium (Blatt & Stitely 1987; Lederman et al. 1984), halts progress at both the G1 and S phases of the cell cycle (Yu & Richardson 2011, Siriwardana & Seligman 2013). Quiescent cells stimulated to grow in media containing DFO arrest in late G1 due to elevated levels of the cyclin-dependent kinase inhibitor p27(Kip1), CDK4 (Kulp et al. 1996), p53 (Liang & Richardson 2003), p21 (Fu & Richardson 2007) and inhibition of CDK2 activity (Wang et al. 2004). However, cells which have already passed the G1 checkpoint continue until they enter the S phase of the cell cycle when they arrest with incompletely replicated DNA. This is because the synthesis of all four deoxyribonucleotides found in DNA is dependent on the Fe-containing enzyme, ribonucleotide reductase (Nyholm et al. 1993). Since iron-limited cells entering the S phase cannot maintain the supply of deoxynucleotides, DNA synthesis is halted. Growth arrest in both G1 and S phases leads to downregulation of the anti-apoptotic gene Bcl-2 and upregulation of the pro-apoptotic protein Bax along with increases in caspase-3, caspase-8, and caspase-9 and the induction of apoptosis and cell death (Greene et al. 2002). The analysis of gene expression in iron-deficient rats during embryonic development demonstrates the upregulation of pro-apoptotic genes in the kidney (Swali et al. 2011).

The source of iron for the neural stem cells is not clear but is likely to be transferrin-bound iron from the fetal circulation; however, as the BBB becomes established during development, the source is likely to change to transferrin produced by oligodendrocytes and choroid plexus epithelial cells (Espinosa de los et al. 1999).

6.2.8.3 Neuronal Cell Commitment and Differentiation

The innermost cells within the neural tube are the precursors of nerve cells (neurons) and the supportive tissue components (glia). The differentiation of neuronal progenitor cells is highly dependent on the pattern of growth factors to which the cells are exposed during their proliferation/expansion phase and cannot be significantly altered during differentiation phase (Sanalkumar et al. 2010). The availability of nutrients influences the production of growth factors: for example, IGF-I stimulates neuron progenitor proliferation and promotes neuron survival, outgrowth, and synaptogenesis. IGF-I also stimulates oligodendrocyte progenitor proliferation despite inhibiting apoptosis in oligodendrocyte lineage cells and stimulating myelin production (D'Ercole & Ye 2008). Gestational iron deficiency suppresses hippocampal IGF signalling in rats, an effect which is reversed by iron supplementation. The rapid increase in the expression of neuron-specific synaptogenesis markers suggests that there is a greater response following supplementation in the IGF-I-dependent neurons compared to the slower response of the IGF-II-dependent glia-specific myelination markers (Tran et al. 2012). Transferrin is an important source of iron for the developing neurons, since genetic ablation of the transferrin receptor in neural cells impaired spatial memory and disorganized the structure of the apical dendrites (Fretham et al. 2012). Transferrin-bound iron is also important in regeneration following hypoxia/ischaemia as an intraventricular injection of transferrin is able to promote cell proliferation (Clausi et al. 2010).

6.2.8.4 Gliogenesis

During the first 3 weeks of postnatal development, there is a sixfold increase in the mass of the rodent brain due to a corresponding increase in the population of glial cells (Bandeira et al. 2009). Glial proliferation also coincides (around P15 in the rat) with a rapid increase in dendritic arborization and an overproduction of synapses. Astrocytes which make up the largest glial population are crucial to the regulation of synaptic connectivity and play an important role in stabilizing synaptic structures (Ge et al. 2012). Synapses which are unused are subsequently lost during a period of maturation and pruning, forming the neural networks responsible for higher brain activity.

Iron is present in every cell type of the mature brain; oligodendrocytes are the predominant iron-containing cells, but iron is also found in neurons, astrocytes, and microglia (Zecca et al. 2004). Both astrocytes and oligodendrocytes have foot-like processes reaching out to and surrounding the BMVEC (Abbott 2013). A glycophosphosinositide-linked ceruloplasmin found in the foot processes oxidizes Fe^{2+} released by the BMVEC. Two molecules of Fe^{3+} are then bound to apotransferrin secreted by the oligodendrocytes and possibly neurons (McCarthy & Kosman 2014a). The transferrin receptor (TfR1) present on the surface of neurons binds the diferric transferrin and internalizes it, supplying the cells with iron. Studies *in vitro* suggest that transferrin may also have an important role as a trophic factor, promoting the differentiation of stem cells into neurons and astrocytes. The availability of iron-transferrin also promotes the differentiation of distinct population of glial precursor cells into oligodendrocytes (Morath & Mayer-Pröschel 2001).

Astrocytes are the most abundant cells in the brain and although they do not store large amounts of iron, they do have a central role in the regulation of iron. Astrocytes do not express detectable levels of TfR1 protein or mRNA, instead their main source of iron appears to be non-transferrin-bound iron (NTBI) taken up from the BMVEC through DMT1 expressed where the end-feet contact with the capillaries (Lane et al. 2010; Pelizzoni et al. 2013). The astrocyte end-feet also express ferroxidase activity and produces hepcidin which modulates the expression of ferroportin in the basal membranes of the BMVEC (McCarthy & Kosman 2014b). This creates a feedback loop which increases the supply of iron to the brain in response to deficiency or suppresses transport when iron is in excess. Although astrocytes do not appear to have a high metabolic requirement for iron, they do contain ferritin. This is an efficient intracellular store of iron which can be exported from the astrocyte via ferroportin and ceruloplasmin when iron is required elsewhere in the brain (Dringen et al. 2007). In addition to the BMVEC, astrocytes also clear iron from the synaptic environment, protecting the synapse from iron overload (Pelizzoni et al. 2013). This tight regulation is important to protect the cells of the brain from the oxidative stress and membrane damage caused by free iron. A failure in this system has been implicated in the pathology of a number of neurodegenerative diseases (Ward et al. 2014).

6.2.8.5 Myelination

Oligodendrocytes are the myelin-forming cells of the central nervous system (Baumann & Pham-Dinh 2001). Myelin accounts for ~30% of the dry weight of the adult human brain and is a lipid-rich multilamellar structure which encloses segments of axons insulating the nerves and stabilizing synapses (Schmitt et al. 2015). The active phase of myelination is an energetically demanding process, membrane precursors have to be synthesized rapidly as large quantities of myelin membrane are produced in a relatively short period of time. Iron has a number of critical roles in this process, it is essential for ATP production by mitochondria as well as for the enzymes which synthesize cholesterol and fatty acids (Au & Schilling 1986;

Bailey-Wood et al. 1975). Especially important are the iron-dependent lipid saturase and desaturase enzymes, which are involved in increasing and decreasing number of double bonds in fatty acids (Rao et al. 1983).

It is therefore not surprising that iron deficiency for as little as 10 days during the peak period of myelination in the postnatal period can significantly alter the function of oligodendrocytes and the production of myelin (Beard 2003; Beard et al. 2003). Infants with a history of IDA have increased latency in auditory brainstem and evoked visual potentials which are consistent with changes in myelination affecting transmission through the nerves of the auditory and visual systems (Algarin et al. 2003). Because these changes in myelination occur during critical windows of development, they cannot be reversed by subsequent iron supplementation.

During the differentiation of oligodendrocytes, the expression of both transferrin receptor-1 and ferritin heavy chain is up-regulated (Connor & Menzies 1996), implying an increased requirement for iron (Li et al. 2013). Microglia found in close proximity to the oligodendrocyte precursors are the first brain cells to accumulate substantial quantities of iron (Cheepsunthorn et al. 1998; Connor et al. 1995), storing it as a ferritin complex (Jorgenson et al. 2005; Rao et al. 2003). When it is required to support the developing oligodendrocyte precursor cells, the ferritin is released from the microglia and taken up as H-ferritin via receptor-mediated endocytosis (Todorich et al. 2008, 2011). Microglia also release cytokines or other factors regulating oligodendrocyte development (Zhang et al. 2006). Transferrin is also able to increase myelin content during early postnatal development in the rat (Escobar Cabrera et al. 1994, 1997; Marta et al. 2000) although it is not clear if this is by direct uptake of transferrin via its receptor or through the microglia acting as intermediates (Todorich et al. 2009).

6.2.8.6 Neurotransmitter Synthesis

The sending and receiving of messages between the cells of the nervous system rely on chemical messengers. By supporting signalling between nerves, neurotransmitters are intimately involved in the growth, development, and neural plasticity. An accumulating body of evidence has demonstrated that iron deficiency is closely associated with altered neurotransmission, especially monoamine metabolism (Beard & Connor 2003). Iron is a cofactor for tyrosine hydroxylase, tryptophan hydroxylase, and enzymes involved in the formation of catecholamines and 5-hydroxytryptamine (5-HT), respectively (Youdim & Green 1978). There is evidence that levels of dopamine, serotonin, norepinephrine, glutamate, and GABA are influenced by iron deficiency (Kim & Wessling-Resnick 2014). The analysis of the metabolomic profile of the developing hippocampus of the rat shows that iron deficiency induces changes in a number of different neurochemicals, including phosphocreatine, phosphoethanolamine glutamate, N-acetylaspartate, aspartate, γ-aminobutyric acid, and taurine (Rao et al. 2003). While some of these changes are related to altered myelination (see the earlier texts), they are also indicative of altered neurotransmitter synthesis. A similar set of observations have been made in the CSF of iron-deficient primates (Rao et al. 2013)

Changes in brain iron metabolism are known to occur in Parkinson's disease, and the relationship between iron and dopamine has been extensively studied in the adult and may be related to defects in mitochondrial function (de Vries &

Przedborski 2013). Although iron deficiency perturbs dopamine concentrations in the post-weaning rat brain, there is no evidence for changes in the activity of tyrosine hydroxylase or tryptophan hydroxylase, or for changes in the serotonin, adrenergic, or gabaminergic receptor populations (Youdim et al. 1989). Rather than affecting synthesis, iron deficiency elevates extracellular dopamine in the caudate putamen and nucleus accumbens by decreasing the abundance of dopamine transporters (Nelson et al. 1997). The analysis of brains subjected to iron efficiency post-weaning found changes in the expression of genes associated with not only dopaminergic neurons but also with metabolic and energy metabolism (Jellen et al. 2013).

6.2.9 Indirect Effects of Iron Deficiency on Cellular Growth and Differentiation

In addition to the direct requirement of the cells in the developing brain for iron, there are also systemic effects of iron deficiency, such as reduced oxygen transport to the fetus and brain. Gene knockout studies in which the DMT-1 gene is deleted mimic the most severe effects of iron deficiency, suggesting that the requirement for iron within the hippocampus itself is critical (Pisansky et al. 2013). Iron is also essential for brain metabolism and studies in primates show that citrate/pyruvate, citrate/lactate, and pyruvate/glutamine ratios differed significantly in the CSF of iron-deficient infants, suggesting that iron deficiency reduces oxidative metabolism in the brain (Rao et al. 2013), even though the fetus is to some extent protected from maternal iron deficiency by the increased transport of iron via the placenta (Gambling et al. 2011).

Iron is also essential for lipid metabolism in both maternal and fetal compartments, especially the production of polyunsaturated fatty acids and eicosanoids via the fatty acid desaturases (LeBlanc et al. 2009). The polyunsaturated fatty acids docosahexaenoic acid (DHA) and arachidonic acid (AA) are important structural fatty acids in the brain and are essential for brain growth and myelination. An interruption in the supply of these critical precursors for membrane synthesis from the maternal plasma or later from milk has the potential for indirectly reducing rates of neurite proliferation. Studies in both humans and animals have demonstrated that combined supplementation with iron and DHA/EPA is superior to supplementation with each component alone (Baumgartner et al. 2012).

6.2.9.1 Windows of Susceptibility

Iron-dependent events during brain development are age dependent (e.g. myelination) and specific for particular regions (e.g. dopamine synthesis). The most profound effect of iron on brain development appears to be during the period of myelination, during weaning in the rat. Intracranial injection of apo-transferrin at 3 days of age into the brain of iron-deficient neonatal rats completely reversed the effects of iron deficiency, both changing the migration pattern and increasing the number of mature cells and myelin formation (Rosato-Siri et al. 2010). In humans, brain development takes place over a much longer period (Figure 6.5) so that susceptibility to changes in nutrition extends over a considerable time.

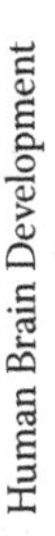

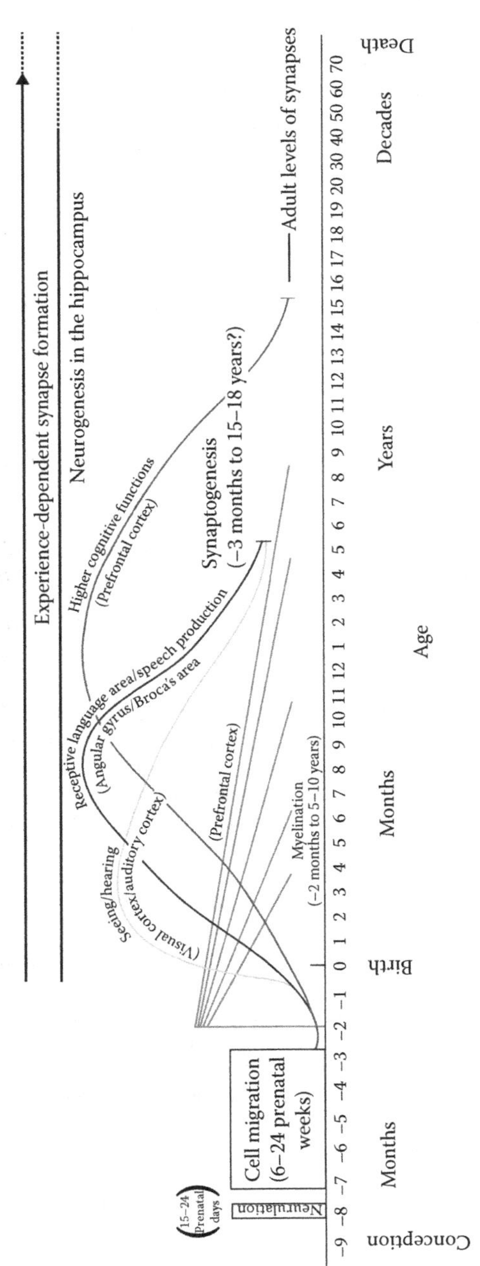

FIGURE 6.5 Time course of development of the human brain, illustrating the windows of susceptibility to suboptimal nutrition. (From Georgieff, M.K. & Innis, S.M., *Pediatr. Res.*, 57, 99R, 2005.)

6.3 CONCLUSION

In this chapter, we have examined how iron plays a role in brain development and that the general metabolism of iron is central to its function in the CNS. In doing so, we have clarified how important it is that a woman enters pregnancy with an adequate reserve of iron, and shown how, if these are not sufficient, her developing baby is at risk of not achieving its genetic potential for brain development and function.

REFERENCES

Abbott, N. J. 2013. Blood–brain barrier structure and function and the challenges for CNS drug delivery. *J Inherit Metab Dis*, 36, 437–449.

Algarin, C., Nelson, C. A., Peirano, P., Westerlund, A., Reyes, S., & Lozoff, B. 2013. Iron-deficiency anemia in infancy and poorer cognitive inhibitory control at age 10 years. *Dev Med Child Neurol*, 55, 453–458.

Algarin, C., Peirano, P., Garrido, M., Pizarro, F., & Lozoff, B. 2003. Iron deficiency anemia in infancy: Long-lasting effects on auditory and visual system functioning. *Pediatr Res*, 53, 217–223.

Amin, S. B., Orlando, M., Eddins, A., Macdonald, M., Monczynski, C., & Wang, H. 2010. In utero iron status and auditory neural maturation in premature infants as evaluated by auditory brainstem response. *J Pediatr*, 156, 377–381.

Anderson, C. P., Shen, M., Eisenstein, R. S., & Leibold, E. A. 2012. Mammalian iron metabolism and its control by iron regulatory proteins. *Biochim Biophys Acta*, 1823, 1468–1483.

Angulo-Barroso, R. M., Schapiro, L., Liang, W., Rodrigues, O., Shafir, T., Kaciroti, N., Jacobson, S. W., & Lozoff, B. 2011. Motor development in 9-month-old infants in relation to cultural differences and iron status. *Dev Psychobiol*, 53, 196–210.

Armony-Sivan, R., Eidelman, A. I., Lanir, A., Sredni, D., & Yehuda, S. 2004. Iron status and neurobehavioral development of premature infants. *J Perinatol*, 24, 757–762.

Au, Y. P. & Schilling, R. F. 1986. Relationship between anemia and cholesterol metabolism in sex-linked anemic (gene symbol, sla) mouse. *Biochim Biophys Acta*, 883, 242–246.

Bailey-Wood, R., Blayney, L. M., Muir, J. R., & Jacobs, A. 1975. The effects of iron deficiency on rat liver enzymes. *Br J Exp Pathol*, 56, 193–198.

Bandeira, F., Lent, R., & Herculano-Houzel, S. 2009. Changing numbers of neuronal and non-neuronal cells underlie postnatal brain growth in the rat. *Proc Natl Acad Sci*, 106, 14108–14113.

Baumann, N. & Pham-Dinh, D. 2001. Biology of oligodendrocyte and myelin in the mammalian central nervous system. *Physiol Rev*, 81, 871–927.

Baumgartner, J., Smuts, C. M., Malan, L., Kvalsvig, J., Van Stuijvenberg, M. E., Hurrell, R. F., & Zimmermann, M. B. 2012. Effects of iron and n–3 fatty acid supplementation, alone and in combination, on cognition in school children: A randomized, double-blind, placebo-controlled intervention in South Africa. *Am J Clin Nutr*, 96, 1327–1338.

Beard, J. 2003. Iron deficiency alters brain development and functioning. *J Nutr*, 133, 1468S–1472S.

Beard, J. L. & Connor, J. R. 2003. Iron status and neural functioning. *Annu Rev Nutr*, 23, 41–58.

Beard, J. L., Wiesinger, J. A., & Connor, J. R. 2003. Pre- and postweaning iron deficiency alters myelination in Sprague–Dawley rats. *Dev Neurosci*, 25, 308–315.

Belfort, M. B., Rifas-Shiman, S. L., Rich-Edwards, J. W., Kleinman, K. P., Oken, E., & Gillman, M. W. 2008. Maternal iron intake and iron status during pregnancy and child blood pressure at age 3 years. *Int J Epidemiol*, 37, 301–308.

Berglund, S. K., Westrup, B., Hagglof, B., Hernell, O., & Domellof, M. 2013. Effects of iron supplementation of LBW infants on cognition and behavior at 3 years. *Pediatrics*, 131, 47–55.

Black, M. M., Baqui, A. H., Zaman, K., Ake Persson, L., El Arifeen, S., Le, K., Mcnary, S. W., Parveen, M., Hamadani, J. D., & Black, R. E. 2004. Iron and zinc supplementation promote motor development and exploratory behavior among Bangladeshi infants. *Am J Clin Nutr*, 80, 903–910.

Black, M. M., Quigg, A. M., Hurley, K. M., & Pepper, M. R. 2011. Iron deficiency and iron-deficiency anemia in the first two years of life: Strategies to prevent loss of developmental potential. *Nutr Rev*, 69, S64–S70.

Blatt, J. & Stitely, S. 1987. Antineuroblastoma activity of desferoxamine in human cell lines. *Cancer Res*, 47, 1749–1750.

Brion, M. J., Leary, S. D., Smith, G. D., Mcardle, H. J., & Ness, A. R. 2008. Maternal anemia, iron intake in pregnancy, and offspring blood pressure in the Avon Longitudinal Study of Parents and Children. *Am J Clin Nutr*, 88, 1126–1133.

Cao, C., Pressman, E. K., Cooper, E. M., Guillet, R., Westerman, M., & O'Brien, K. O. 2014. Placental heme receptor LRP1 correlates with the heme exporter FLVCR1 and neonatal iron status. *Reproduction*, 148, 295–302.

Cheepsunthorn, P., Palmer, C., & Connor, J. R. 1998. Cellular distribution of ferritin subunits in postnatal rat brain. *J Comp Neurol*, 400, 73–86.

Christian, P., Morgan, M. E., Murray-Kolb, L., Leclerq, S. C., Khatry, S. K., Schaefer, B., Cole, P. M., Katz, J., & Tielsch, J. M. 2011. Preschool iron-folic acid and zinc supplementation in children exposed to iron-folic acid in utero confers no added cognitive benefit in early school-age. *J Nutr*, 141, 2042–2048.

Christian, P., Murray-Kolb, L. E., Khatry, S. K. et al. 2010. Prenatal micronutrient supplementation and intellectual and motor function in early school-aged children in Nepal. *JAMA*, 304, 2716–2723.

Clausi, M. G., Pasquini, L. A., Soto, E. F., & Pasquini, J. M. 2010. Apotransferrin-induced recovery after hypoxic/ischaemic injury on myelination. *ASN Neuro*, 2, e00048.

Coe, C. L., Lubach, G. R., & Shirtcliff, E. A. 2007. Maternal stress during pregnancy predisposes for iron deficiency in infant monkeys impacting innate immunity. *Pediatr Res*, 61, 520–524.

Connor, J. R. & Menzies, S. L. 1996. Relationship of iron to oligodendrocytes and myelination. *GLIA*, 17, 83–93.

Connor, J. R., Pavlick, G., Karli, D., Menzies, S. L., & Palmer, C. 1995. A histochemical study of iron-positive cells in the developing rat brain. *J Comp Neurol*, 355, 111–123.

Corapci, F., Radan, A. E., & Lozoff, B. 2006. Iron deficiency in infancy and mother-child interaction at 5 years. *J Dev Behav Pediatr*, 27, 371–378.

Cusick, S. E. & Georgieff, M. K. 2012. Nutrient supplementation and neurodevelopment: Timing is the key. *Arch Pediatr Adolesc Med*, 166, 481–482.

Darshan, D., Frazer, D. M., & Anderson, G. J. 2010. Molecular basis of iron-loading disorders. *Expert Rev Mol Med*, 12, e36.

Department of Health. 1991. Dietary Reference Values for Food Energy and Nutrients in the United Kingdom. (Report on Health and Social Subjects, No 41). London HMSO.

De Vries, R. L. A. & Przedborski, S. 2013. Mitophagy and Parkinson's disease: Be eaten to stay healthy. *Mol Cell Neurosci*, 55, 37–43.

D'ercole, J. A. & Ye, P. 2008. Expanding the mind: Insulin-like growth factor I and brain development. *Endocrinology*, 149, 5958–5962.

Dringen, R., Bishop, G. M., Koeppe, M., Dang, T. N., & Robinson, S. R. 2007. The pivotal role of astrocytes in the metabolism of iron in the brain. *Neurochem Res*, 32, 1884–1890.

Eden, A. N. & Sandoval, C. 2012. Iron deficiency in infants and toddlers in the United States. *Pediatr Hematol Oncol*, 29, 704–709.

Escobar Cabrera, O. E., Bongarzone, E. R., Soto, E. F., & Pasquini, J. M. 1994. Single intracerebral injection of apotransferrin in young rats induces increased myelination. *Dev Neurosci*, 16, 248–254.

Escobar Cabrera, O. E., Zakin, M. M., Soto, E. F., & Pasquini, J. M. 1997. Single intracranial injection of apotransferrin in young rats increases the expression of specific myelin protein mRNA. *J Neurosci Res*, 47, 603–608.

Espinosa De Los, M. A., Kumar, S., Zhao, P., Huang, C. J., Nazarian, R., Pan, T., Scully, S., Chang, R., & De, V. J. 1999. Transferrin is an essential factor for myelination. *Neurochem Res*, 24, 235–248.

Fredriksson, A., Schröder, N., Eriksson, P., Izquierdo, I., & Archer, T. 1999. Neonatal iron exposure induces neurobehavioural dysfunctions in adult mice. *Toxicol Appl Pharmacol*, 159, 25–30.

Fretham, S. J. B., Carlson, E. S., Wobken, J., Tran, P. V., Petryk, A., & Georgieff, M. K. 2012. Temporal manipulation of transferrin-receptor-1-dependent iron uptake identifies a sensitive period in mouse hippocampal neurodevelopment. *Hippocampus*, 22, 1691–1702.

Fu, D. & Richardson, D. R. 2007. Iron chelation and regulation of the cell cycle: 2 mechanisms of posttranscriptional regulation of the universal cyclin-dependent kinase inhibitor p21CIP1/WAF1 by iron depletion. *Blood*, 110, 752–761.

Gambling, L., Andersen, H. S., Czopek, A., Wojciak, R., Krejpcio, Z., & McArdle, H. J. 2004. Effect of timing of iron supplementation on maternal and neonatal growth and iron status of iron-deficient pregnant rats. *J Physiol*, 561, 195–203.

Gambling, L., Dunford, S., Wallace, D. I., Zuur, G., Solanky, N., Srai, S. K., & Mcardle, H. J. 2003. Iron deficiency during pregnancy affects postnatal blood pressure in the rat. *J Physiol*, 552, 603–610.

Gambling, L., Lang, C., & McArdle, H. J. 2011. Fetal regulation of iron transport during pregnancy. *Am J Clin Nutr*, 94, 1903S–1907S.

Ge, W. P., Miyawaki, A., Gage, F. H., Jan, Y. N., & Jan, L. Y. 2012. Local generation of glia is a major astrocyte source in postnatal cortex. *Nature*, 484, 376–380.

Georgieff, M. K. 2011. Long-term brain and behavioral consequences of early iron deficiency. *Nutr Rev*, 69(Suppl 1), S43–S48.

Georgieff, M. K. & Innis, S. M. 2005. Controversial nutrients that potentially affect preterm neurodevelopment: Essential fatty acids and iron. *Pediatr Res*, 57, 99R–103R.

Godfrey, K. M., Redman, C. W., Barker, D. J., & Osmond, C. 1991. The effect of maternal anaemia and iron deficiency on the ratio of fetal weight to placental weight. *Br J Obstet Gynaecol*, 98, 886–891.

Golub, M. S. 2010. Recent studies of iron deficiency during brain development in nonhuman primates. *BioFactors*, 36, 111–116.

Golub, M. S. & Hogrefe, C. E. 2015. Fetal iron deficiency and genotype influence emotionality in infant rhesus monkeys. *J Nutr*, 145, 647–653.

Grantham-Mcgregor, S. & Ani, C. 2001. A review of studies on the effect of iron deficiency on cognitive development in children. *J Nutr*, 131, 649S–666S.

Greene, B. T., Thorburn, J., Willingham, M. C., Thorburn, A., Planalp, R. P., Brechbiel, M. W., Jennings-Gee, J., Wilkinson, J., Torti, F. M., & Torti, S. V. 2002. Activation of caspase pathways during iron chelator-mediated apoptosis. *J Biol Chem*, 277, 25568–25575.

Gunshin, H., Fujiwara, Y., Custodio, A. O., Direnzo, C., Robine, S., & Andrews, N. C. 2005. Slc11a2 is required for intestinal iron absorption and erythropoiesis but dispensable in placenta and liver. *J Clin Invest*, 115, 1258–1266.

Hagan, N. & Ben-Zvi, A. 2015. The molecular, cellular, and morphological components of blood–brain barrier development during embryogenesis. *Semin Cell Dev Biol* 8, 7–15.

Haider, B. A., Olofin, I., Wang, M., Spiegelman, D., Ezzati, M., & Fawzi, W. W. 2013. Anaemia, prenatal iron use, and risk of adverse pregnancy outcomes: Systematic review and meta-analysis. *BMJ*, 346, f3443.

Hare, D. J., Arora, M., Jenkins, N. L., Finkelstein, D. I., Doble, P. A., & Bush, A. I. 2015. Is early-life iron exposure critical in neurodegeneration? *Nat Rev Neurol* 11, 536–544.

Höck, A., Demmel, U., Schicha, H., Kasperek, K., & Feinendegen, L. E. 1975. Trace element concentration in human brain. *Brain*, 98, 49–64.

Insel, B. J., Schaefer, C. A., McKeague, I. W., Susser, E. S., & Brown, A. S. 2008. Maternal iron deficiency and the risk of schizophrenia in offspring. *Arch Gen Psychiatry*, 65, 1136–1144.

Jellen, L. C., Lu, L., Wang, X., Unger, E. L., Earley, C. J., Allen, R. P., Williams, R. W., & Jones, B. C. 2013. Iron deficiency alters expression of dopamine-related genes in the ventral midbrain in mice. *Neuroscience*, 252, 13–23.

Jorgenson, L. A., Sun, M., O'Connor, M., & Georgieff, M. K. 2005. Fetal iron deficiency disrupts the maturation of synaptic function and efficacy in area CA1 of the developing rat hippocampus. *Hippocampus*, 15, 1094–1102.

Kaladhar, M. & Narasinga Rao, B. S. 1983. Effect of maternal iron deficiency in rat on serotonin uptake in vitro by brain synaptic vesicles in the offspring. *J Neurochem*, 40, 1768–1770.

Kim, J., Molina, R. M., Donaghey, T. C., Buckett, P. D., Brain, J. D., & Wessling-Resnick, M. 2011. Influence of DMT1 and iron status on inflammatory responses in the lung. *Am J Physiol Lung Cell Mol Physiol*, 300, L659–L665.

Kim, J. & Wessling-Resnick, M. 2014. Iron and mechanisms of emotional behavior. *J Nutr Biochem*, 25, 1101–1107.

Kulp, K. S., Green, S. L., & Vulliet, P. R. 1996. Iron deprivation inhibits cyclin-dependent kinase activity and decreases cyclin D/CDK4 protein levels in asynchronous MDA-MB-453 human breast cancer cells. *Exp Cell Res*, 229, 60–68.

Lane, D. J., Robinson, S. R., Czerwinska, H., Bishop, G. M., & Lawen, A. 2010. Two routes of iron accumulation in astrocytes: Ascorbate-dependent ferrous iron uptake via the divalent metal transporter (DMT1) plus an independent route for ferric iron. *Biochem J*, 432, 123–132.

LeBlanc, C. P., Fiset, S., Surette, M. E., Turgeon O'Brien, H., & Rioux, F. M. 2009. Maternal iron deficiency alters essential fatty acid and eicosanoid metabolism and increases locomotion in adult guinea pig offspring. *J Nutr*, 139, 1653–1659.

Lederman, H. M., Cohen, A., Lee, J. W., Freedman, M. H., & Gelfand, E. W. 1984. Deferoxamine: A reversible S-phase inhibitor of human lymphocyte proliferation. *Blood*, 64, 748–753.

Li, Y., Guan, Q., Chen, Y., Han, H., Liu, W., & Nie, Z. 2013. Transferrin receptor and ferritin-H are developmentally regulated in oligodendrocyte lineage cells. *Neural Regen Res*, 8, 6–12.

Li, Y., Kim, J., Buckett, P. D., Böhlke, M., Maher, T. J., & Wessling-Resnick, M. 2011. Severe postnatal iron deficiency alters emotional behavior and dopamine levels in the prefrontal cortex of young male rats. *J Nutr*, 141, 2133–2138.

Liang, S. X. & Richardson, D. R. 2003. The effect of potent iron chelators on the regulation of p53: Examination of the expression, localization and DNA-binding activity of p53 and the transactivation of WAF1. *Carcinogenesis*, 24, 1601–1614.

Linder, M. C. 2013. Mobilization of stored iron in mammals: A review. *Nutrients*, 5, 4022–4050.

Lozoff, B. 2007. Iron deficiency and child development. *Food Nutr Bull*, 28, S560–S571.

Lozoff, B. 2011. Early iron deficiency has brain and behavior effects consistent with dopaminergic dysfunction. *J Nutr*, 141, 740S–746S.

Lozoff, B., Beard, J., Connor, J., Barbara, F., Georgieff, M., & Schallert, T. 2006. Long-lasting neural and behavioral effects of iron deficiency in infancy. *Nutr Rev*, 64, S34–S43.

Lozoff, B., De Andraca, I., Castillo, M., Smith, J. B., Walter, T., & Pino, P. 2003. Behavioral and developmental effects of preventing iron-deficiency anemia in healthy full-term infants. *Pediatrics*, 112, 846–854.

Lozoff, B., Jimenez, F., Hagen, J., Mollen, E., & Wolf, A. W. 2000. Poorer behavioral and developmental outcome more than 10 years after treatment for iron deficiency in infancy. *Pediatrics*, 105, E51.

Lozoff, B., Klein, N. K., Nelson, E. C., McClish, D. K., Manuel, M., & Chacon, M. E. 1998. Behavior of infants with iron-deficiency anemia. *Child Dev*, 69, 24–36.

Lozoff, B., Smith, J. B., Kaciroti, N., Clark, K. M., Guevara, S., & Jimenez, E. 2013. Functional significance of early-life iron deficiency: Outcomes at 25 years. *J Pediatr*, 163, 1260–1266.

Lukowski, A. F., Koss, M., Burden, M. J., Jonides, J., Nelson, C. A., Kaciroti, N., Jimenez, E., & Lozoff, B. 2010. Iron deficiency in infancy and neurocognitive functioning at 19 years: Evidence of long-term deficits in executive function and recognition memory. *Nutr Neurosci*, 13, 54–70.

Marta, C. B., Escobar Cabrera, O. E., Garcia, C. I., Villar, M. J., Pasquini, J. M., & Soto, E. F. 2000. Oligodendroglial cell differentiation in rat brain is accelerated by the intracranial injection of apotransferrin. *Cellular and molecular biology (Noisy-le-Grand, France)*, 46, 529–539.

McArdle, H. J., Gambling, L., & Kennedy, C. 2013. Iron deficiency during pregnancy: The consequences for placental function and fetal outcome. *Proc Nutr Soc*, 73, 9–15.

McArdle, H. J., Lang, C., Hayes, H., & Gambling, L. 2011. Role of the placenta in regulation of fetal iron status. *Nutr Rev*, 69(Suppl 1), S17–S22.

McCarthy, R. & Kosman, D. 2014a. Iron transport across the blood–brain barrier: Development, neurovascular regulation and cerebral amyloid angiopathy. *Cell Mol Life Sci*, 72, 709–727.

McCarthy, R. C. & Kosman, D. J. 2012. Mechanistic analysis of iron accumulation by endothelial cells of the BBB. *BioMetals*, 25, 665–675.

McCarthy, R. C. & Kosman, D. J. 2014b. Glial cell ceruloplasmin and hepcidin differentially regulate iron efflux from brain microvascular endothelial cells. *PLoS ONE*, 9, e89003.

Mills, R. J. & Davies, M. W. 2012. Enteral iron supplementation in preterm and low birth weight infants. *Cochrane Database Syst Rev*, 3, CD005095.

Morath, D. J. & Mayer-Pröschel, M. 2001. Iron modulates the differentiation of a distinct population of glial precursor cells into oligodendrocytes. *Dev Biol*, 237, 232–243.

Murray-Kolb, L. E., Khatry, S. K., Katz, J. et al. 2012. Preschool micronutrient supplementation effects on intellectual and motor function in school-aged nepalese children. *Arch Pediatr Adolesc Med*, 166, 404–410.

Nelson, C., Erikson, K., Piñero, D. J., & Beard, J. L. 1997. In vivo dopamine metabolism is altered in iron-deficient anemic rats. *J Nutr*, 127, 2282–2288.

Nurtjahja-Tjendraputra, E., Fu, D., Phang, J. M., & Richardson, D. R. 2006. Iron chelation regulates cyclin D1 expression via the proteasome: A link to iron deficiency-mediated growth suppression. *Blood*, 109, 4045–4054.

Nwaru, B. I., Hayes, H., Gambling, L. et al. 2014. An exploratory study of the associations between maternal iron status in pregnancy and childhood wheeze and atopy. *Br J Nutr*, 112, 2018–2027.

Nyholm, S., Mann, G. J., Johansson, A. G., Bergeron, R. J., Grãslund, A., & Thelander, L. 1993. Role of ribonucleotide reductase in inhibition of mammalian cell growth by potent iron chelators. *J Biol Chem*, 268, 26200–26205.

Obermeier, B., Daneman, R., & Ransohoff, R. M. 2013. Development, maintenance and disruption of the blood-brain barrier. *Nat Med*, 19, 1584–1596.

Paridaen, J. T. & Huttner, W. B. 2014. Neurogenesis during development of the vertebrate central nervous system. *EMBO Rep*, 15, 351–364.

Peirano, P. D., Algarín, C. R., Chamorro, R. A., Reyes, S. C., Durán, S. A., Garrido, M. I., & Lozoff, B. 2010. Sleep alterations and iron deficiency anemia in infancy. *Sleep Med*, 11, 637–642.

Pelizzoni, I., Zacchetti, D., Campanella, A., Grohovaz, F., & Codazzi, F. 2013. Iron uptake in quiescent and inflammation-activated astrocytes: A potentially neuroprotective control of iron burden. *Biochim Biophys Acta*, 1832, 1326–1333.

Pena-Rosas, J. P., De-Regil, L. M., Garcia-Casal, M. N., & Dowswell, T. 2015. Daily oral iron supplementation during pregnancy. *Cochrane Database Syst Rev*, 7, CD004736.

Piñero, D. J. & Connor, J. R. 2000. Iron in the brain: An important contributor in normal and diseased states. *Neuroscientist*, 6, 435–453.

Pisansky, M. T., Wickham, R. J., Su, J., Fretham, S., Yuan, L. L., Sun, M., Gewirtz, J. C., & Georgieff, M. K. 2013. Iron deficiency with or without anemia impairs prepulse inhibition of the startle reflex. *Hippocampus*, 23, 952–962.

Plessow, R., Arora, N. K., Brunner, B., Tzogiou, C., Eichler, K., Brügger, U., & Wieser, S. 2015. Social costs of iron deficiency anemia in 6–59-month-old children in India. *PLoS ONE*, 10, e0136581.

Prado, E. L. & Dewey, K. G. 2014. Nutrition and brain development in early life. *Nutr Rev*, 72, 267–284.

Rao, G. A., Crane, R. T., & Larkin, E. C. 1983. Reduction of hepatic stearoyl-CoA desaturase activity in rats fed iron-deficient diets. *Lipids*, 18, 573–575.

Rao, R., Ennis, K., Oz, G., Lubach, G., Georgieff, M., & Coe, C. 2013. Metabolomic analysis of cerebrospinal fluid indicates iron deficiency compromises cerebral energy metabolism in the infant monkey. *Neurochem Res*, 38, 573–580.

Rao, R., Tkac, I., Schmidt, A. T., & Georgieff, M. K. 2011. Fetal and neonatal iron deficiency causes volume loss and alters the neurochemical profile of the adult rat hippocampus. *Nutr Neurosci*, 14, 59–65.

Rao, R., Tkac, I., Townsend, E. L., Gruetter, R., & Georgieff, M. K. 2003. Perinatal iron deficiency alters the neurochemical profile of the developing rat hippocampus. *J Nutr*, 133, 3215–3221.

Rasmussen, K. M. 2001. Is there a causal relationship between iron deficiency or iron-deficiency anemia and weight at birth, length of gestation and perinatal mortality? *J Nutr*, 131, 590S–603S.

Renton, F. J. & Jeitner, T. M. 1996. Cell cycle-dependent inhibition of the proliferation of human neural tumor cell lines by iron chelators. *Biochem Pharm*, 51, 1553–1561.

Roncagliolo, M., Garrido, M., Walter, T., Peirano, P., & Lozoff, B. 1998. Evidence of altered central nervous system development in infants with iron deficiency anemia at 6 mo: Delayed maturation of auditory brainstem responses. *Am J Clin Nutr*, 68, 683–690.

Rosato-Siri, M. V., Badaracco, M. E., Ortiz, E. H., Belforte, N., Clausi, M. G., Soto, E. F., Bernabeu, R., & Pasquini, J. M. 2010. Oligodendrogenesis in iron-deficient rats: Effect of apotransferrin. *J Neurosci Res*, 88, 1695–1707.

Sanalkumar, R., Vidyanand, S., Lalitha Indulekha, C., & James, J. 2010. Neuronal vs. glial fate of embryonic stem cell-derived neural progenitors (ES-NPs) is determined by FGF2/EGF during proliferation. *J Mol Neurosci*, 42, 17–27.

Schmitt, S., Castelvetri, L. C., & Simons, M. 2015. Metabolism and functions of lipids in myelin. *Biochim Biophys Acta*, 1851, 999–1005.

Scholl, T. O. 2005. Iron status during pregnancy: Setting the stage for mother and infant. *Am J Clin Nutr*, 81, 1218S–1222S.

Scholl, T. O. 2011. Maternal iron status: Relation to fetal growth, length of gestation, and iron endowment of the neonate. *Nutr Rev*, 69, S23–S29.

Scientific Advisory Committee on Nutrition (SACN). Iron and health, 2011. Available from: http://www.gov.uk/government/publications/sacn-iron-and-health-report (accessed October 5, 2015).

Seamans, J. K. & Yang, C. R. 2004. The principal features and mechanisms of dopamine modulation in the prefrontal cortex. *Progr Neurobiol*, 74, 1–58.

Shayeghi, M., Latunde-Dada, G. O., Oakhill, J. S. et al. 2005. Identification of an intestinal heme transporter. *Cell*, 122, 789–801.

Siddappa, A. M., Georgieff, M. K., Wewerka, S., Worwa, C., Nelson, C. A., & Deregnier, R.-A. 2004. Iron deficiency alters auditory recognition memory in newborn infants of diabetic mothers. *Pediatr Res*, 55, 1034–1041.

Simpson, I. A., Ponnuru, P., Klinger, M. E., Myers, R. L., Devraj, K., Coe, C. L., Lubach, G. R., Carruthers, A., & Connor, J. R. 2015. A novel model for brain iron uptake: Introducing the concept of regulation. *J Cereb Blood Flow Metab*, 35, 48–57.

Singhal, A., Morley, R., Abbott, R., Fairweather-Tait, S., Stephenson, T., & Lucas, A. 2000. Clinical safety of iron-fortified formulas. *Pediatrics*, 105, E38.

Siriwardana, G. & Seligman, P. A. 2013. Two cell cycle blocks caused by iron chelation of neuroblastoma cells: Separating cell cycle events associated with each block. *Physiol Rep*, 1, e00176.

Steinmacher, J., Pohlandt, F., Bode, H., Sander, S., Kron, M., & Franz, A. R. 2007. Randomized trial of early versus late enteral iron supplementation in infants with a birth weight of less than 1301 grams: Neurocognitive development at 5.3 years' corrected age. *Pediatrics*, 120, 538–546.

Stoltzfus, R. J., Kvalsvig, J. D., Chwaya, H. M., Montresor, A., Albonico, M., Tielsch, J. M., Savioli, L., & Pollitt, E. 2001. Effects of iron supplementation and anthelmintic treatment on motor and language development of preschool children in Zanzibar: Double blind, placebo controlled study. *BMJ*, 323, 1389–1393.

Swali, A., Mcmullen, S., Hayes, H., Gambling, L., McArdle, H. J., & Langley-Evans, S. C. 2011. Cell cycle regulation and cytoskeletal remodelling are critical processes in the nutritional programming of embryonic development. *PLoS ONE*, 6, e23189.

Tamura, T., Goldenberg, R. L., Hou, J., Johnston, K. E., Cliver, S. P., Ramey, S. L., & Nelson, K. G. 2002. Cord serum ferritin concentrations and mental and psychomotor development of children at five years of age. *J Pediatr*, 140, 165–170.

Todorich, B., Pasquini, J. M., Garcia, C. I., Paez, P. M., & Connor, J. R. 2009. Oligodendrocytes and myelination: The role of iron. *Glia*, 57, 467–478.

Todorich, B., Zhang, X., & Connor, J. R. 2011. H-ferritin is the major source of iron for oligodendrocytes. *GLIA*, 59, 927–935.

Todorich, B., Zhang, X., Slagle-Webb, B., Seaman, W. E., & Connor, J. R. 2008. Tim-2 is the receptor for H-ferritin on oligodendrocytes. *J Neurochem*, 107, 1495–1505.

Tran, P. V., Fretham, S. J. B., Wobken, J., Miller, B. S., & Georgieff, M. K. 2012. Gestational-neonatal iron deficiency suppresses and iron treatment reactivates IGF signaling in developing rat hippocampus. *Am J Physiol Endocrinol Metabol*, 302, E316–E324.

Wachs, T. D., Georgieff, M., Cusick, S., & McEwen, B. S. 2014. Issues in the timing of integrated early interventions: Contributions from nutrition, neuroscience, and psychological research. *Ann N Y Acad Sci*, 1308, 89–106.

Wachs, T. D., Pollitt, E., Cueto, S., Jacoby, E., & Creed-Kanashiro, H. 2005. Relation of neonatal iron status to individual variability in neonatal temperament. *Dev Psychobiol*, 46, 141–153.

Walker, S. P., Wachs, T. D., Meeks Gardner, J., Lozoff, B., Wasserman, G. A., Pollitt, E., & Carter, J. A. 2013. Child development: Risk factors for adverse outcomes in developing countries. *Lancet*, 369, 145–157.

Wang, G., Miskimins, R., & Miskimins, W. K. 2004. Regulation of p27(Kipl) by intracellular iron levels. *BioMetals*, 17, 15–24.

Ward, R. J., Zucca, F. A., Duyn, J. H., Crichton, R. R., & Zecca, L. 2014. The role of iron in brain ageing and neurodegenerative disorders. *Lancet Neurol*, 13, 1045–1060.

Yang, Z., Lönnerdal, B., Adu-Afarwuah, S., Brown, K. H., Chaparro, C. M., Cohen, R. J., Domellöf, M., Hernell, O., Lartey, A., & Dewey, K. G. 2009. Prevalence and predictors of iron deficiency in fully breastfed infants at 6 mo of age: Comparison of data from 6 studies. *Am J Clin Nutr*, 89, 1433–1440.

Youdim, M. B., Ben-Shachar, D., & Yehuda, S. 1989. Putative biological mechanisms of the effect of iron deficiency on brain biochemistry and behavior. *Am J Clin Nutr*, 50, 607–615.

Youdim, M. B. H. & Green, A. R. 1978. Iron deficiency and neurotransmitter synthesis and function. *Proc Nutr Soc*, 37, 173–179.

Yu, Y. & Richardson, D. R. 2011. Cellular iron depletion stimulates the JNK and p38 MAPK signaling transduction pathways, dissociation of ASK1-thioredoxin, and activation of ASK1. *J Biol Chem*, 286, 15413–15427.

Zecca, L., Youdim, M. B. H., Riederer, P., Connor, J. R., & Crichton, R. R. 2004. Iron, brain ageing and neurodegenerative disorders. *Nat Rev Neurosci*, 5, 863–873.

Zhang, X., Surguladze, N., Slagle-Webb, B., Cozzi, A., & Connor, J. R. 2006. Cellular iron status influences the functional relationship between microglia and oligodendrocytes. *GLIA*, 54, 795–804.

Ziegler, E. E. 2011. Consumption of cow's milk as a cause of iron deficiency in infants and toddlers. *Nutr Rev*, 69, S37–S42.

Ziegler, E. E., Nelson, S. E., & Jeter, J. M. 2009. Iron supplementation of breastfed infants from an early age. *Am J Clin Nutr*, 89, 525–532.

7 Zinc in the Developing Brain

Andreas M. Grabrucker

CONTENTS

7.1 INTRODUCTION

In 1933, zinc was reported for the first time to be essential for the growth of rats (Todd et al. 1933). Thirty years later, the first studies in human subjects from the Middle East showed that this was also true for humans (Prasad et al. 1961, 1963a,b). However, with the exception of mental lethargy, little was mentioned in these reports on possible neurological effects of zinc deficiency in these patients. Only in later studies was it found that zinc deficiency might compromise emotional and cognitive functioning (Bhatnagar & Taneja 2001; Black 1998). To date, many studies have been performed, investigating the influence of zinc deficiency and zinc supplementation on human well-being and mental performance. However, particularly in mechanistic and behavioural studies, the majority of data available to date regarding the effects of zinc deficiency on brain development and function later in life come from findings in animal models (Hagmeyer et al. 2014).

7.2 HUMAN ZINC HOMEOSTASIS

Zinc is an essential and ubiquitous ionic signal and structural component in a myriad of cells and tissues such as the brain. Within the body, two major pools of zinc can be found. A slow-exchange zinc pool which contains as much as 90% of the body's zinc is mainly located in muscle and bone and a rapid-exchange zinc pool in the plasma. The latter, which contains 10% of the body's zinc, is located, for example, in the GI tract, liver, and other viscera. The rapid-exchange zinc pool is also the one which is especially reactive to the amount of absorbed zinc and is the first to be depleted under conditions of zinc deficiency.

To maintain adequate zinc levels, endogenous losses and demands, for example, for tissue synthesis during pregnancy or milk secretion during lactation, must be provided by the absorption of zinc from dietary sources. This dietary requirement thus may vary over a wide range, depending on age and physiological state of an individual as well as factors influencing the bioavailability of zinc in the food. During pregnancy, the incremental daily need for zinc can be calculated from the rate of tissue weight gain and the concentration of zinc found in these tissues. Swanson & King (1987) calculated the mean rate of zinc accumulation for the four successive quarters of pregnancy to be 0.08, 0.24, 0.53, and 0.73 mg/day. To cover these requirements, recommended daily intakes of zinc range from 10 to 15 mg in adults (+5 – 10 mg for pregnant and lactating women).

However, zinc status also affects zinc absorption and excretion and thus, the requirements of an individual adjusted to low zinc intake might be different from someone not adapted to low zinc availability. In 1996, WHO therefore indicated the recommended daily zinc intake of an adult male (18–60 years of age) consuming a diet with high zinc bioavailability to be 5.6 mg, with a medium zinc bioavailability diet to be 9.4 mg, and a low zinc bioavailability diet to be 18.7 mg (female: 6, 10, 20 mg, respectively). The influence of dietary zinc bioavailability on the required daily zinc intake was also taken into account by several other countries for the calculation of recommended dietary intakes. For example, in the United States, a mixed diet with 20% zinc absorption was the basis for the estimation of Recommended Dietary Allowance (RDA) values, while in the United Kingdom, a 30% absorption rate was assumed. Dietary Reference Intakes for zinc in the United States are shown in Table 7.1.

A tolerable upper intake level (UL) for zinc has also been set (40 mg/day for adults), given that high intakes may be harmful. Although zinc is not considered to be very toxic, consumption of more than 1 g at once may cause nausea, vomiting, diarrhoea, and lethargy. Ingestion of high amounts of zinc (>75 mg/day) chronically might interfere with the absorption of other trace elements such as copper.

High levels of zinc can be found in food sources like lamb, beef, molluscs, and crustacean, while low levels are present in fruit, refined cereal products, and most vegetables. Thus, while a common diet consumed in Europe and North America might provide about 150% of the required daily amount of zinc, the prevalent diet in poorer countries may only reach 50%. Currently, an estimated 17.3% of the global population is at risk of developing zinc deficiency (Wessells & Brown 2012), although estimates vary between studies. The prevalence of inadequate zinc intake has been estimated to range from 7.5% in high-income regions to 30% in poorer

TABLE 7.1
Data from the U.S. Food and Nutrition Board

Life Stage/Group	RDA (mg/Day)		UL (mg/Day)	
Infants				
0–6 months	2		4	
7–12 months	3		5	
Children				
1–3 years	3		7	
4–8 years	5		12	
	Males	**Females**	**Males**	**Females**
Adolescents/Adults				
9–13 years	8	8	23	23
14–18 years	11	9	34	34
19 years	11	8	40	40
Pregnancy				
≤18 years		12		34
19 years		11		40
Lactation				
≤18 years		13		34
19 years		12		40

Source: National Academy of Sciences, Dietary Reference Intakes for vitamin A, vitamin K, arsenic, boron, chromium, copper, iodine, iron, manganese, molybdenum, nickel, silicon, vanadium, and zinc, National Academy Press, Washington, DC, 2001.

RDA, Recommended Dietary Allowance; UL, Tolerable Upper Intake Levels.

countries (Wessells & Brown 2012). This is not only based on less consumption of meat in poorer countries, but on the amount of dietary zinc absorbed. Absorption of zinc can be decreased in response to dietary fibre, phytic acid (inositol hexa- and penta-phosphate), folic acid, or copper (Vela et al. 2015). Conversely, several endogenous substances such as citric acid, picolinic acid, prostaglandins, and amino acids like histidine and cysteine may serve as ligands for zinc and enhance absorption (Gropper et al. 2009). Once absorbed, zinc passes into portal blood and is transported bound to proteins such as albumin, alpha-2 macroglobulin (Chesters 1981), or S100, and amino acids such as histidine.

7.3 ZINC ABSORPTION AND TRANSPORT

7.3.1 Zinc Absorption

Zinc is taken up from our dietary sources. To ensure uptake and delivery of zinc to the target tissue in the right concentration, the body is equipped with sophisticated mechanisms that ensure specificity and safe transport and prevent depletion or excess. The proximal small intestine, most likely the jejunum, is the main site of absorption of zinc. There, zinc is taken up by zinc transporters into enterocytes (Figure 7.1). There are at least 10 zinc transporters (ZnT/SLC30A) and 15 Zrt- and Irt-like protein (ZIP/SLC39A) transporters in human cells. Trans-membrane transporters mediate the uptake (mostly ZIP) and removal (mostly ZnT) of zinc and both the ZnT and ZIP transporter families exhibit unique tissue-specific expression (Roohani et al. 2013). For example, the ZIP4 (SLC39A4) gene is involved in zinc absorption in the small intestine (Cousins and McMahon 2000). ZIP4 is expressed along the entire gastrointestinal tract and localizes to the apical membrane of enterocytes (the side exposed to lumen of the intestine). There, Zip4 imports zinc into enterocytes. In mouse models, it was shown that in times of decreased dietary zinc intake, Zip4 is up-regulated and thus contributes to the homeostatic control of zinc levels. In humans, mutations in ZIP4 cause *acrodermatitis enteropathica*, a rare and, if left untreated, lethal autosomal recessive genetic disorder of zinc uptake (Andrews 2008). However, animal studies indicate that other ZIP family members such as ZIP1 and 2 are also able to contribute to zinc uptake into enterocytes. Within enterocytes, intracellular transporters, such as ZnT7 (SLC30A7), and zinc-buffering proteins, such as metallothioneins (MTs), influence the transport of zinc across the enterocyte. Studies on mice have shown that the release of zinc into the blood stream is mediated by ZnT1 (SLC30A1), a zinc transporter located at the basolateral membrane of enterocytes (Cousins 2010) (Figure 7.1).

7.3.2 Zinc Transport across the Placenta

Placental transport of zinc is determined by the number and size of fetuses present and can be a fast process. In rabbits, in the last trimester, half of an injected dose of zinc was taken up within 3 h (Terry et al. 1960). In the fetus, zinc is taken up from the blood by the liver but retrograde placental transport (transport of zinc from the blood of the fetus back into the maternal blood) was also observed. Consumption of alcohol leads to a reduction of placental zinc transport and it is hypothesized that the consequences of 'fetal alcohol syndrome' may unfold through both effects of ethanol and zinc deficiency (Keppen et al. 1985).

7.3.3 Zinc Uptake by the Brain

In 1955, it was discovered that zinc is highly enriched in the hippocampus and neocortical region of the mammalian brain (Maske 1955). However, interest in the role of zinc in the brain was not raised until the late 1960s by pioneering studies reporting the abnormal development of the central nervous system (CNS) in zinc-deficient rat embryos and behavioural abnormalities in zinc-deprived animals (Apgar 1968; Caldwell et al. 1970; Hurley and Swenerton 1966). Subsequent studies identified a growing number of effects of zinc deficiency and excess on the CNS, which have also been associated with neurological disorders. These effects can be caused either by teratological or by functional impairments acting on brain development, or functional impairments later in life.

Zinc is one of the most prevalent trace metals in the human and animal brain. Passive diffusion of zinc from the blood into the brain is prevented by the blood–brain barrier (BBB) and thus requires active transport. This transport may be mediated by L-histidine. Histidine may play a role in the transfer of zinc to plasma membrane transporters such as DMT1 (divalent metal [ion] transporter 1/SLC11A2) that import zinc into brain capillary endothelial cells. Alternatively, currently unidentified zinc transporters may be localized in the endothelial cells (Takeda 2000). The mechanism of export of zinc once within those cells into the brain's extracellular fluid is so far unknown. Zinc may also be taken up by choroidal epithelial cells and transported into the cerebrospinal fluid (CSF) across the blood–CSF barrier.

Active transport is also expected to occur within the brain, given that some brain regions such as the hippocampus accumulate zinc at high concentrations (100-fold higher) compared to cerebrospinal fluid (CSF) (Crawford 1983). Although the turnover of zinc in the CNS of adult animals seems rather slow and homeostatic mechanisms are able to maintain proper brain zinc levels for weeks in zinc-deficient animals (Kasarskis 1984), zinc deficiency in the embryo has a rapid onset and also affects brain development within few days (Dreosti et al. 1985). This most likely is due to the absence of an intact BBB in very early embryos (Pardridge 1986).

While most of the total brain zinc exists in a protein-bound state (>80%), 'free' zinc can be found predominantly within synaptic vesicles of nerve cells (Cole et al. 1999; Palmiter et al. 1996). The mechanisms which modulate the free zinc pool are key to health and performance given that excess of free zinc has been shown to be neurotoxic. In general, zinc can be bound firmly to high-affinity binding sites of proteins, thereby regulating protein structure. Weakly bound zinc can be released from proteins and similar to free zinc act as signaling ion. In particular, metallothioneins (MTs) are a group of proteins which can transiently bind up to seven zinc ions (Li & Maret 2008) and act as major zinc-buffering proteins. While MT-1 and MT-2 proteins are expressed ubiquitously including the brain, MT-3 and MT-4 are especially abundant in the CNS (Hidalgo et al. 2001). Under physiological conditions,

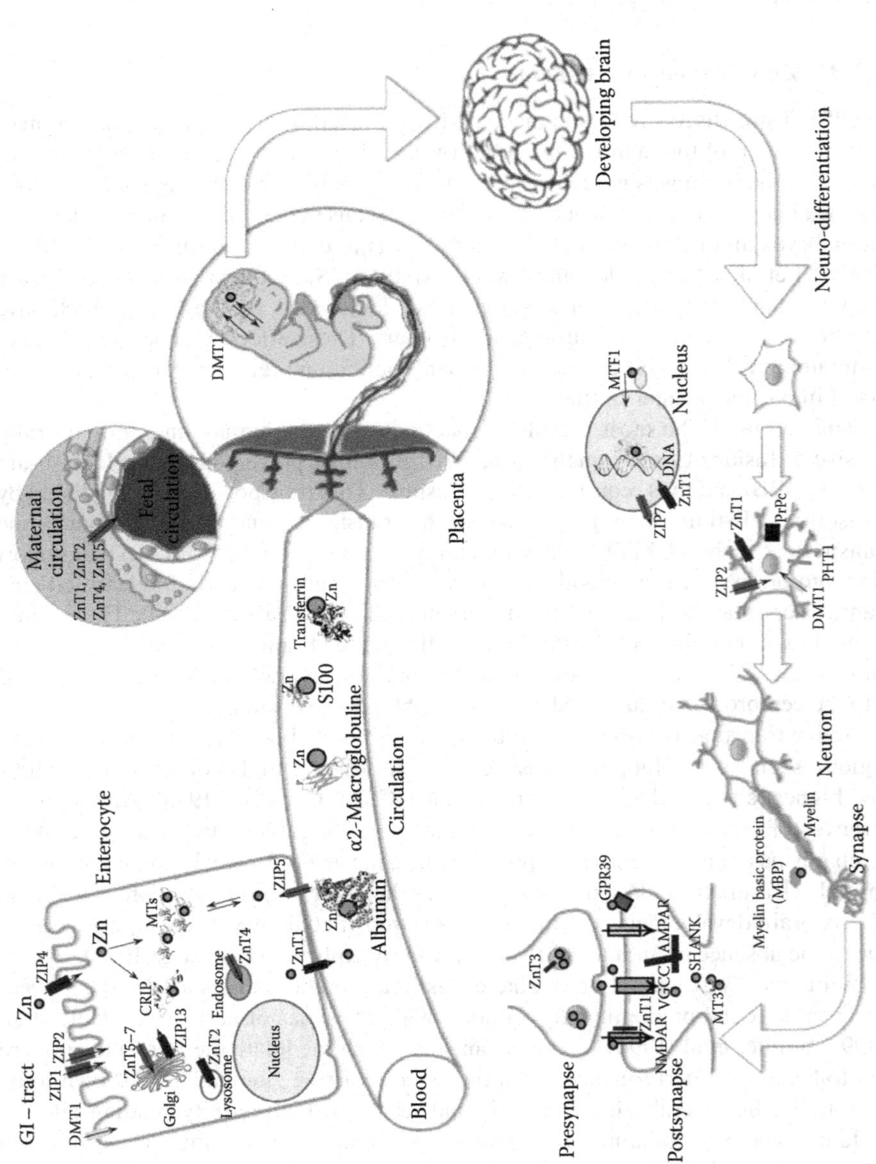
GI – tract
Zn
DMT1
ZIP1
ZIP2
ZIP4
Zn
Enterocyte
CRIP
MTs
ZnT5–7
ZIP13
Golgi
ZnT2
Lysosome
Endosome
ZnT4
Nucleus
ZnT1
ZIP5
Zn
Albumin
Blood
α2-Macroglobuline
Circulation
Zn
S100
Zn
Transferrin
Maternal circulation
Fetal circulation
ZnT1, ZnT2
ZnT4, ZnT5
Placenta
DMT1
Developing brain
Neuro-differentiation
MTF1
Nucleus
DNA
ZIP7
ZnT1
ZIP2
ZnT1
PrPc
DMT1
PHT1
Neuron
Myelin
Myelin basic protein (MBP)
Synapse
ZnT3
GPR39
AMPAR
SHANK
VGCC
ZnT1
NMDAR
MT3
Presynapse
Postsynapse

FIGURE 7.1 Zinc in brain development – from maternal uptake to the embryo's synapse. Zinc is taken up from the diet in the maternal gastrointestinal (GI) tract by zinc transporters. Import into enterocytes is mediated by ZIP4 and other ZIP family members such as ZIP1 and 2 but also unspecific divalent metal transporters such as DMT1. Within enterocytes, zinc can be transiently exported from the cytoplasm into the Golgi apparatus, that is, via ZnT7, and back via ZIP13. Additionally, zinc can be buffered by zinc-binding proteins such as metallothioneins (MTs) or CRIP. Zinc can also be imported into lysosomes (by ZnT2) and endosomes (by ZnT4). Release of zinc in the blood stream is mediated by ZnT1, located at the basolateral membrane of the enterocyte. Within the blood, zinc is transported bound to proteins such as albumin, α-2 macroglobulin, histidine, or to a lesser extent, S100, and transferrin. Through the maternal circulation, zinc reaches the placenta and is actively imported into the fetal circulation by ZnTs (most likely ZnT1, 2, 4, and 5). Once inside the embryo, zinc reaches the developing brain by passive diffusion in the very early stages of brain development, where a fully intact blood–brain barrier (BBB) is not yet established. Later, passive diffusion of zinc from the blood into the brain is prevented by the BBB and requires active transport, probably mediated by transporters such as DMT1. Within the embryo's brain, zinc is again actively transported from the extracellular fluid or CSF into neurons and glial cells. DMT1, ZIP2, PHT1, and the prion protein PrP^C appear to be involved in zinc uptake in neurons; ZnT1 is associated with zinc efflux. Within neurons, zinc is bound to proteins or found as 'free' zinc within presynaptic vesicles of specific 'zincergic' neurons. Zinc is imported into the nucleus by ZnT1 and shuttled back to the cytoplasm via ZIP7. Additionally, zinc may enter the nucleus bound to enzymes and transcription factors, in particular, MTF1 which translocates from the cytoplasm into the nucleus upon zinc binding. Zinc is also found in glial cells and might be released as gliotransmitter or contribute to the stabilization of the myelin sheath probably by binding to myelin basic protein (MBP). Within the mature neuron, zinc can be locally released from MT-3 after synaptic activity. Additionally, upon synaptic activity, zinc is released with glutamate from presynaptic terminals. There, zinc is enriched in synaptic vesicles via ZnT3. Zinc in the synaptic cleft can bind to several receptors and channels, such as GPR39, TrkB, NMDA, and kainate receptors or enter into the postsynaptic compartment through NMDARs, AMAPRs, and VGCCs. In the postsynapse, zinc can participate in structural changes via Shank2 and Shank3 proteins and influence various signalling pathways, ultimately modulating synaptic function and plasticity.

zinc is often the sole metallic constituent of MTs. However, under zinc deficiency or exposure to toxic metals, cadmium, mercury, platinum, lead, and bismuth might also be associated with MTs. However, in addition to the known functions in heavy metal detoxification and metal buffering, MTs such as MT-3 might also play a role in synaptic signalling given that zinc might be locally released from MT-3 due to activity-dependent nitrosylation or oxidation of the thiol ligands by nitric oxide (NO) (Grabrucker et al. 2014; Maret 2000). NO is generated through the process of synaptic activity. Additionally, upon synaptic activity, zinc is released with glutamate from glutamatergic (zincergic) presynaptic terminals (Frederickson & Bush 2001; Frederickson & Moncrieff 1994). Although zinc might act on several receptors and channels, such as GPR39 (G-protein-coupled receptor 39) (Chorin et al. 2011), TrkB (tropomyosin receptor kinase B) (Huang et al. 2008), and NMDA (*N*-methyl-D-aspartate) and kainate receptors (Mott et al. 2008; Veran et al. 2012; Vergnano et al. 2014) in the synaptic cleft, zinc might also enter into the postsynaptic compartment through NMDA and AMPA (α-amino-3-hydroxy-5-methyl-4-isoxazolepropionic acid) receptors, and calcium channels (Frederickson et al. 2005).

7.3.4 Zinc Interactions

Trace metals are in equilibrium with each other and thus do not operate independently (Pfaender & Grabrucker 2014). Copper and zinc interact at the intestinal mucosal level influencing each other's absorption and are found in balance in the blood, where the concentrations of both trace metals are inversely related. Additionally, exposure to lead decreases zinc levels in the brain and lead competes with zinc at binding sites of metalloproteins and enzymes, inhibiting their activity. Similarly, nickel and cadmium may compete with zinc. Thus, it is possible that some effects of the exposure to high levels of these metals are established through interfering with zinc-dependent processes during brain development and in the adult CNS.

7.3.5 Zinc as a Cofactor

Within the cell, zinc is a cofactor for a variety of enzymes and can have a catalytic, co-catalytic and structural role. It is therefore involved in many signalling and metabolic pathways in the CNS. Examples include DNA and RNA polymerases, histone deacetylases (Marks 2010), metalloproteinases, dehydrogenases (Tapiero & Tew 2003) such as glutamate dehydrogenase (Dreosti et al. 1981; Wolf & Schmidt 1983), and other important enzymes in the CNS like ERK (extracellular signal–regulated kinase) (Nutall & Oteiza 2012), dopamine-β-hydroxylase (Wenk & Stemmer 1982), and superoxide dismutase (SOD1) (Hayward et al. 2002). However, more than 300 enzymes were shown to bind zinc, most of them are also expressed within the CNS. Together with enzymes, the human genome encodes for ca. 2800 zinc-binding proteins corresponding to 10% of the human proteome (Andreini et al. 2006), many of them also expressed in the CNS. Additionally, zinc acts as structural component in zinc-finger proteins, a family of DNA-binding transcription factors (O'Halloran 1993). Furthermore, zinc ions may serve as link in between two proteins. Thus, given that excess or in particular deficiency of zinc might interfere with a great number of biological processes, the investigation of the underlying molecular mechanisms related to abnormal behaviour and functioning of deficient animals and humans is hampered. Nevertheless, some important insights have been gained over recent years.

7.4 FUNCTION OF ZINC IN THE BRAIN

7.4.1 Zinc in Neurogenesis and Differentiation, Neuronal Migration, and Myelination

Neurogenesis is an essential first step of CNS development. To that end, cells in the developing embryo must undergo asymmetric divisions to form the embryonic notochord, neural tube, and neural crest. Additionally, cells must migrate to their target destination. There, the process of cell differentiation into mature neurons must be completed, followed by synaptogenesis and synaptic pruning. Programmed cell death (apoptosis) is an important part along these steps in CNS development. On a cellular level, zinc is involved in processes such as DNA replication, transcriptional control, mRNA translation, apoptosis (Pang et al. 2013), and microtubule stabilization, thereby affecting cell differentiation, division, growth, and neural migration (Adamo & Oteiza 2010; Levenson & Morris 2011). Thus, it is not surprising that zinc plays a critical role in the control of CNS development given that these effects may be particularly important in a developing organism. Indeed, reduced food intake in rodents after dietary restriction of zinc most likely is a compensatory mechanism to decrease growth rates and thus the need for zinc. Zinc-deficient animals force-fed with a diet comparable to controls become unwell and die within short time.

7.4.1.1 Zinc in Neurogenesis and Differentiation

The formation of the CNS starts very early in embryonic development. In humans, the neural plate is established already during the third week following conception. Subsequently, neural folds rise up on each side of the plate to form the neural tube. In the fourth week, a complete closure of the tube should be achieved. A failure of closure at the lower end of the neural tube that normally forms the spinal cord results in a condition known as *spina bifida*. In contrast, a failure of closure of the top end that generates the cerebral hemispheres results in anencephaly, a lethal condition.

Pregnant women have increased demand for zinc and, thus, are at risk of zinc deficiency (King & Cousins 2006; Vela et al. 2015) that might affect the developing brain of the offspring. A role of zinc in neurogenesis became obvious in animals suffering from early prenatal zinc deficiency. Although all organ systems are affected by systemic zinc depletion, the development of the CNS seems particularly vulnerable resulting, among others, in neural tube defects. In humans, women suffering from *acrodermatitis enteropathica* show a high incidence of birth defects (Hambridge et al. 1975), underlining the importance of zinc in brain development. In general, the developing brain seems most vulnerable to zinc deficiency due to high rates of cell proliferation and differentiation.

Within the developing brain, regional growth takes place. Here, periods of rapid development occur referred to as the brain growth spurt. Within this critical period, adverse influences might have the greatest effect on brain growth. Fetuses of pregnant rats are at maximum risk to develop abnormalities during days 9–12 of pregnancy, coinciding with the period when tissue differentiation is maximal (Hurley et al. 1971). However, in different species, the growth spurt of the brain can vary in respect of the time after conception.

ZIP12 (SLC39A12) is a zinc uptake transporter, which is highly expressed in the human brain. Zinc depletion or knockdown of ZIP12 reduces cAMP response element–binding (CREB) protein activation, which acts as a key molecular switch in a pathway for neuronal differentiation. ZIP12 shows a conserved pattern of high expression in the human, mouse, and frog nervous systems (Chowanadisai et al. 2013a). Thus, zinc homeostasis and the regulation of zinc transporters such as ZIP12 are critical for neuronal differentiation, neurulation, and embryonic development (Chowanadisai et al. 2013b). In the frog (*Xenopus tropicalis*), ZIP12 knockdown impairs neural tube closure and arrests development during neurulation along with a decreased tubulin polymerization in the neural plate (Chowanadisai et al. 2013a). In line with these findings, previous studies have reported that zinc deficiency in rodents impairs neurite outgrowth in the brain (Dvergsten et al. 1984; Gao et al. 2009).

In the adult brain of rodents and most likely humans, neurogenesis, and in particular adult neurogenesis, occurs in the subgranular zone of the dentate gyrus. Within this region, high levels of presynaptic vesicular zinc can be found in synaptic terminals of neurons. Dietary zinc deprivation, zinc chelation (using 5-chloro-7-iodo-8-hydroxyquinoline [clioquinol]), and vesicular zinc depletion caused by genetic disruption of the ZnT3 gene all lead to a significant decrease in hippocampal progenitor cell proliferation in the normal brain or after hypoglycaemia (hypoglycaemia is known to transiently increase the number of proliferating progenitor cells) in mice (Suh et al. 2009). These data support the hypothesis of an essential role of zinc in modulating hippocampal neurogenesis.

In line with this, the microarray analysis of hippocampal gene expression revealed several genes involved in cellular proliferation to be regulated by zinc (Gower-Winter et al. 2013), including the nuclear retinoic acid receptor, retinoid X receptor (RXR), doublecortin, and transforming growth factor-beta (TGF-β). Moreover, suboptimal zinc nutrition during gestation might cause long-term effects through a deregulation of the transcription factors AP-1 (activating protein-1), NF-κB (nuclear factor 'kappa-light-chain-enhancer' of activated B cells), and NFAT (nuclear factor of activated T cells) (Aimo et al. 2010). Thus, zinc may play a role in the control of both developmental and adult neurogenesis mediated by proliferating stem cells (Gower-Winter et al. 2013). In line with this, Nestin expression, a marker for the proliferation of neural stem cells, is reduced in offspring that experienced maternal zinc deficiency (Wang et al. 2001).

7.4.1.2 Zinc in Proliferation and Neuronal Migration

In the CNS, both cell proliferation and apoptosis occur during the perinatal period and are critical for normal brain development. Zinc deficiency leads to the inhibition of cell proliferation through the arrest of the cell cycle and induces apoptosis in neuronal cells via modulating a number of pro-survival (ERK, Akt, and NF-κB) and pro-apoptotic (JNK and p53) pathways (Adamo et al. 2010).

Zinc deficiency in utero is also associated with decreased rates of DNA synthesis and decreased DNA polymerase and thymidine kinase activities in the fetus. Indeed, most DNA polymerases contain zinc. However, evidence shows that the mechanistic process of DNA synthesis is not severely affected in zinc-deficient animals. In fact, the general impairment of DNA synthesis is more likely to be a result of the inability of a cell to induce the expression of genes necessary to establish the competence to undergo DNA synthesis prior to the entry into the S phase of the cell cycle.

Zinc deficiency may also interfere with cell division through the cytoskeletal protein tubulin. Zinc is able to bind to tubulin with low affinity and stimulates the assembly of microtubules *in vitro*. Zinc deficiency in turn reduces the rate of tubulin aggregation *in vitro* and *in vivo* (Oteiza et al. 1988, 1990). Tubulin may play a role in the formation of the mitotic spindle during mitosis. However, tubulin might also play a role in cell migration. It was found that division and migration of cerebellar granular cells are delayed after severe zinc deficiency (Dvergsten et al. 1983). Also, ZIP12 knockdown was shown to reduce tubulin polymerization.

7.4.1.3 Zinc and Myelination

Fetal and neonatal malnutrition including zinc deficiency can also have global or circuit-specific effects. In the case of zinc deficiency, hippocampal connectivity in the developing brain might be most affected. However, detailed studies mapping brain connectivity of prenatally zinc-deficient animals and humans during development and later in life are currently missing. Recently, a putative zinc–metalloprotease–BDNF axis was suggested to play an important role in establishing proper brain connectivity (Koh et al. 2014). Induction of metalloproteases may activate BDNF/TrkB signalling. An impairment of this pathway was speculated to contribute to hyperconnectivity in young patients with autism spectrum disease (Koh et al. 2014).

During vertebrate brain development, the first period of rapid cell division and differentiation does not coincide with an increase in myelination that is established in a brain region–specific manner, sometimes even months or years after birth. Myelination is the process by which myelin, which is produced by different cell types such as oligodendrocytes, accumulates around neurons. Myelin might vary in chemical composition (70%–85% lipids such as cholesterol, 15%–30% protein) and enables neurons to transmit axon potentials (signals encoding information) faster due to an insulating function. Thus, an intact brain myelination is important for establishing a healthy CNS function. Offspring from marginal zinc-deficient rats and monkeys showed a delay in myelin maturation. In particular, myelin protein profiles were found altered although brain cortex weights were similar to control animals (Liu et al. 1992). Thus, myelination of the brain in the offspring might be vulnerable to maternal zinc deficiency during the perinatal period.

Taken together, zinc deficiency might impair CNS development by affecting neurogenesis via a decrease in neuronal precursor cell proliferation, neuronal migration, differentiation, and myelination.

7.4.2 Zinc in Neurophysiology

In the developing brain, zinc is selectively enriched in distinct regions and subcellular structures. For example, in rat striatum, only low levels of zinc can be detected at postnatal day 3, but zinc is found enriched in distinct patches at day 6 that disappear again at day 11. These patches correspond to areas innervated by dopaminergic neurons (Vincent & Semba 1989).

Apart from these zinc-rich areas, zinc appears to accumulate in synaptic vesicles in presynaptic terminals (Crawford & Connor 1972; Frederickson et al. 1983; Haug 1967). Transport of zinc into vesicles is mediated by the ZnT3 transporter (Cole et al. 1999; Palmiter et al. 1996) which shows expression in several brain regions during brain development and later concentrates in areas rich in vesicular zinc (Valente & Auladell 2002). Similarly, ZnT1 levels and distribution strongly correlate with the occurrence of zincergic terminals during development (Nitzan et al. 2002).

In most brain regions, zinc concentrations are maintained similar from birth into adulthood. However, zinc levels in the hippocampus increase significantly during the first 3 postnatal weeks (Szerdahelyi & Kasa 1983) with zinc ions shifting from perikarya into axon terminals (Wolf et al. 1984). Vesicular zinc is involved in synaptic signalling and neuromodulation (Gower-Winter & Levenson 2012). For example, zinc is able to influence synaptic transmission by modulating receptors and channels, cell adhesion proteins (Connor & Chavkin 1992; Davies et al. 1993; Heiliger et al. 2015; Huang et al. 1993; Xie & Smart 1993), as well as pre- and postsynaptic uptake of calcium (Browning & O'Dell 1994; O'Dell & Browning 2013). Moreover, zinc is an important factor regulating dynamic processes at the postsynaptic density (PSD) (Grabrucker 2014; Jan et al. 2002). Following synaptic activity, free zinc released into the synaptic cleft transiently elevates local concentrations from a low nM range to concentrations up to approximately 100–300 μM (Assaf & Chung 1984; Howell et al. 1984). Depletion of zinc attenuates the induction of hippocampal long-term potentiation (LTP) (Takeda et al. 2010). LTP is the molecular mechanism thought to underlie synaptic plasticity in learning and memory formation and manifests as a lasting increase of the response to repeated activation of a synapse.

Although the mossy fibre pathway in the hippocampus of mammals is famous for its strong accumulation of zinc in presynaptic vesicles, zinc-containing vesicles have also been found in various other brain areas. However, almost no zinc-containing neurons can be found in the brain stem and cerebellum.

Moreover, apart from zinc-loaded vesicles, all brain cells contain zinc that is mostly protein bound and that has many neurobiological functions. Zinc deficiency during gestation leads to a reduced cell number in both the mesoderm and the neuroepithelium of zinc-deficient rat embryos (Dreosti et al. 1985) along with a high incidence rate of malformations in 11.5-day-old zinc-deficient embryos. No evidence was found about impaired implantation of embryos in the zinc-deficient dams nor was an increased intrauterine death rate reported at that stage (Dreosti et al. 1985). However, even in non-teratogenic conditions, marginal zinc deficiency during gestation can have long-term effects on the offspring's nervous system. For example, impaired learning behaviour has been reported in zinc-deficient animal models such as rats with mild or moderate zinc deficiency from day 16 of gestation to postnatal day 15 even when tested with 70 days of age, where zinc deficiency was no longer present (Golub et al. 1983), hinting at an important role of zinc for cognitive development.

7.5 ZINC AND COGNITIVE DEVELOPMENT

Cognition is defined as mental process leading to a gain of knowledge and comprehension through processing information based on skills of perception, memory, learning, and attention.

In animals, suboptimal zinc levels or zinc deficiency during late prenatal or early postnatal life, which does not have severe teratogenic effects, was shown to lead to changes in behaviour (Hagmeyer et al. 2014). These changes can persist into adulthood even in the absence of further zinc deficiency (Golub et al. 1983; Grabrucker et al. 2014; Halas et al. 1983, 1986; Halas & Sandstead 1975; Lokken et al. 1973; Sandstead et al. 1978; Strobel & Sandstead 1984). Typically, zinc-deficient animals show a reduced memory and learning capacity, increased anxiety, decreased emotional control, less exploratory activity as part of other signs of depression-like behaviour and are more prone to seizures (Halas 1983; Młyniec et al. 2014; Strobel & Sanstead 1984; Takeda et al. 2003). However, clear differences are visible between animals exposed to a prenatal versus postnatal zinc deficiency. For example, prenatal zinc deficiency seems to have more impact on the social behaviour.

7.5.1 Prenatal Zinc Deficiency

Impoverished zinc levels in pregnancy have been shown to increase aggressiveness in zinc-depleted animals, with juveniles unable to retain previously learned tasks and exhibiting difficulties in learning new problems (Halas et al. 1977; Peters 1978; Strobel & Sandstead 1984). For example, mice with mild or moderate zinc deficiency from embryonic day 16 on until postnatal day 15 were tested as adults and displayed impaired learning and memory (Golub et al. 1983). In another study, the effects of severe zinc deprivation during pregnancy and lactation were investigated, again measuring adult rats. The results showed a severe learning deficit and some working memory deficit (Halas et al. 1983, 1986). Another study on rats that had been subjected to low zinc levels during the late nursing period investigated memory of conditionally learnt associations when the offspring were adults. Animals which were severely zinc deprived exhibited poorer memory as adults (Halas et al. 1979). Zinc deficiency during the last trimester of pregnancy and during lactation was also reported to impair spatial learning and memory in the offspring (Tahmasebi et al. 2009). Similarly, using the Morris water maze test, changes in the learning and memory ability of offspring of mildly zinc-deficient rats during pregnancy and lactation were reported to be consistent with changes in hippocampal neuron morphology (Yu et al. 2013). These learning and memory deficits were observed not only in rodent models but also in the offspring of rhesus monkeys with a severe zinc deficiency during the third trimester (Sandstead et al. 1978; Strobel & Sandstead 1984).

7.5.2 Postnatal Zinc Deficiency

In animal models, postnatal zinc deficiency in turn was shown to result in lethargy and altered activity levels. This phenotype was associated with increased depression-like behaviour in general. Some studies additionally report learning and memory deficits. However, it cannot always be concluded that the behavioural changes observed are a direct consequence of zinc deficiency, since in some studies, especially those with severe zinc depletion, the tested animals were too unwell to conclude on specific changes. In humans, prenatal and early postnatal zinc deficiency may affect cognitive development by alterations in attention, activity, and neuropsychological behaviour (Bhatnagar & Taneja 2001). However, data are very scarce on the cognitive development of prenatal zinc-deficient children and most insights are derived from supplementation studies.

7.5.3 Zinc Supplementation Studies

Zinc deficiency during pregnancy was suspected to influence survival rates, lead to congenital malformations, a reduced fetal and postnatal growth, altered neurobehavioural development, and an increased risk for infections based on animal studies. However, alterations observed in animal studies are produced by zinc deficiency in isolation from any other nutritional deprivation, which is in contrast to the human situation, where zinc deficiency in most cases is caused by undernutrition. Probably in part influenced by this, the findings in human studies show wide variation, with some of them reporting beneficial effects of zinc supplementation and some not (Shah & Sachdev 2006). This may be also based on differences in timing of sampling, laboratory methods and quality, sample size, and underlying zinc nutriture of the different populations observed. Most consistent to animal studies, maternal zinc supplementation has shown a benefit in infant immunity and decreased morbidity from infectious diseases (Shah & Sachdev 2006).

Studies on the cognitive performance of older zinc supplemented children are limited. Zinc deficiency among schoolchildren may increase infectious morbidity and reduce linear growth and cognitive function (Sandstead 2012). Some studies report that even in schoolchildren without marginal zinc deficiency, zinc supplementation improves specific cognitive abilities (de Moura et al. 2013). Recent meta-analyses of data from randomized controlled trials (RCTs) which gave supplemental zinc to infants (Nissensohn et al. 2013) and children (Warthon-Medina et al. 2015) revealed no significant impact of zinc supplementation on intelligence, executive function, and motor skills. These findings were consistent with an earlier Cochrane review and meta-analysis of eight studies which reported data on the Bayley Scales of Infant Development (BSID) in 2134 participants. No significant effect of zinc supplementation was found between supplementation and placebo groups on development as measured by the Mental Development Index (MDI) and Psychomotor Development Index (PDI) (Gogia & Sachdev 2012). All three meta-analyses however showed significant heterogeneity in included studies, which was not adequately explained by subgroup analyses.

Nevertheless, when studies were interrogated individually, some small indicators of improvement on aspects of cognition following zinc supplementation were identified, with 9 of the 18 studies included in a recent review reporting a positive association between zinc intake and status with one or more measure of cognitive function (Warthon-Medina et al. 2015). For example, a positive association between zinc intake or plasma zinc levels and measures of intelligence (Umamaheswari et al. 2011), memory (Gewa et al. 2009; Tupe & Chiplonkar 2009; Umamaheswari et al. 2011), and motor skills (Penland et al. 1997) has been reported in children. The existing inconsistencies among studies may be based on differences in study design and the type of cognitive test administered per cognitive domain, the lack of a reliable biomarker of zinc status in humans, the paucity of carefully controlled long-term trials, and the absence of standardization among studies. Furthermore, most trials involved only healthy children.

Undernourished children in turn are likely to benefit from normalized zinc levels. Better motor development in low-birthweight infants, increased functional activity in malnourished infants, and improved neuropsychological functions in school-age children have been reported in some studies (Bhatnagar & Taneja 2001). However, in one study (Sandstead et al. 1998), supplementation with zinc only improved performance when combined with multiple nutrients, again hinting at some limiting effects caused by other deficiencies due to general malnourishment. Studies which investigate the influence of zinc supplementation, intake, or status during pregnancy or early childhood on measures other than cognitive ability, such as the occurrence of neurodevelopmental disorders like autism, or other neuropsychiatric disorders later in life, are almost completely missing.

Various studies using animal models for zinc deficiency have reported an association of low zinc levels and thymic atrophy, abnormally low level of lymphocytes in the blood, and compromised cell- and antibody-mediated immune responses (Murakami & Hirano 2008). Maternal zinc deficiency might therefore also contribute to altered brain development in the offspring through increasing the likelihood of activation of the immune system during early development due to lowered immunocompetence which may have deleterious effect on the developing CNS. Via the NF-κB pathway, zinc is able to down-regulate the production of inflammatory cytokines and thus might act as an anti-inflammatory agent (Prasad et al. 2011). An increase in inflammation during pregnancy might have influence on CNS development of the embryo.

The underlying molecular mechanisms of how zinc deficiency might lead to impaired cognitive performance are currently not well understood. However, zinc deficiency is associated with a variety of other neuropathologies that in some cases can be caused, but also accompanied or modified, by altered zinc levels.

7.6 ZINC AND NEUROPATHOLOGIES

Zinc plays a role both in adult brain physiology and during brain development. It was shown that prenatal zinc deficiency impairs neurulation and the development of the neural tube. Moreover, severe zinc deficiency in rodents is associated with cleft lip and brain malformations. In humans, maternal zinc deficiency, resulting, for example, from diabetes, alcoholism, poor dietary intake, impaired absorption, increased excretion through the urinary and GI tract, or maternal stress, may cause growth retardation, impaired immunocompetence, and abnormal behaviour (Keen et al. 1993). Additionally, prenatal zinc deficiency is associated with a high incidence rate of spina bifida and exencephalus (Hurley 1981; Warkany & Petering 1972). It has been speculated that these effects are mediated by the role of zinc in the nucleus, given that nucleases, nucleotidases, nucleotidyl transferase, or DNA polymerase all contain zinc. In line with this, it was shown that zinc deficiency reduces the total amount of DNA and the incorporation of thymidine into the DNA and leads to impaired DNA–RNA protein synthesis (Yasui et al. 1997).

Apart from the striking teratogenic effects of severe early prenatal zinc deficiency, mild or late prenatal and early postnatal zinc deficiency result in much less defined clinical pictures. Here, zinc-related dysfunctions lead to behavioural abnormalities and impaired cognitive function in most cases. This might be attributed to the role of zinc in several neurochemical processes which are additionally influenced by the genetic background of an individual.

7.6.1 Zinc Deficiency and Neurodevelopmental Disorders

Autism spectrum disorders (ASDs) are neurodevelopmental disorders characterized by their core symptoms – delayed acquisition of speech, deficits in social interactions, and stereotypic behaviours. Multiple molecular genetic studies in the past have provided evidence that the pathogenesis of ASD has a strong genetic component (Delorme et al. 2013). However, although genetic factors might be largely responsible for the occurrence of ASD, they cannot fully account for all cases. It is thus likely that in addition to a combination of ASD-related genes, specific non-genetic factors act as risk factors triggering the development of ASD (Grabrucker 2012). One such 'environmental' factor might be the presence of imbalances in biometal homeostasis, such as maternal and perinatal zinc deficiency, given that a strong association of low zinc levels and ASD has been reported in recent studies using serum, hair, cerebrospinal fluid (CSF), and other tissues (Bjorklund 2013; Pfaender & Grabrucker 2014). Intriguingly, early studies conducted between 1970 and the early 1980s using prenatal zinc-deficient animals reported altered emotionality, altered states of anxiety, and aggression, as well as altered social behaviour in the offspring later in life. Furthermore, in 1976, it was noted that mood disturbances occurring in infant and young patients with *acrodermatitis enteropathica* can be described as 'schizoid' and that these children display some features similar to autistic children (Moynahan 1976). Nowadays, the incidence rate of zinc deficiency is found to be very high among children with autism, especially in young age, with some studies indicating rates as high as 50% in the age group below

3 years (Jen & Yan 2010; Yasuda et al. 2011) and zinc deficiency is highly discussed as non-genetic modifier of ASD (Grabrucker 2012; Vela et al. 2015). Additionally, some candidate genes for ASD are members of zinc-regulating pathways such as ZnT5 or regulated by zinc such as SHANK3. One unanswered question, however, is whether and how this zinc deficiency is generating, contributing, or modifying the phenotype seen in ASD.

7.6.2 Zinc and Epilepsy

Zinc deficiency may also render a developing brain more susceptible to the manifestation of epileptic seizures. Seizure susceptibility was shown to be decreased by zinc supplementation in an epilepsy mouse model and conversely increased by zinc deficiency (Barry-Sterman et al. 1986; Elsas et al. 2009; Fukahori & Itoh 1990; Takeda et al. 2003). These findings are consistent with studies showing that ZnT3 knockout mice, being depleted of vesicular synaptic zinc, were more susceptible to kainic acid–induced seizures (Cole et al. 2000). Several molecular mechanisms might underlie this phenomenon.

Zinc, for example, released from the presynapse upon synaptic activity is able to bind the GPR39 receptor. GPR39 is a G-protein-coupled receptor that after activation leads to an enhancement of K^+/Cl^- cotransporter 2 (KCC2) activity (Chorin et al. 2011). KCC2 is the major Cl^- exporter in neurons. Activation of KCC2 is absent in slices from ZnT3 knockout animals. KCC2 activity is closely associated with seizure activity. Knockdown of KCC2 in mice impairs synaptic inhibition by increasing neuronal excitability (Hübner et al. 2001) and variants of KCC2 increase the risk of epilepsy in men (Hübner 2014). This effect is achieved through the alteration of the electrochemical gradient for Cl^-. Inhibitory $GABA_A$ receptor channels establish their inhibitory action by Cl^- import. However, import depends critically on the magnitude of the Cl^- concentration gradient, which is mainly established by KCC2. Thus, decreased zinc levels at synapses may contribute to the development of seizures. In line with these findings, Zip1 and Zip3 knockout mice, which lack zinc influx, were shown to have reduced sensitivity to seizure-induced neuronal death (Qian et al. 2011) probably due to increased zinc signaling at synapses.

7.6.3 Zinc Deficiency and Mood Disorders

Zinc deficiency in adult animals and humans is associated with depression, neurosensory impairments of taste and smell, as well as deficits in learning and memory, and may lead to peripheral neuropathy (O'Dell 1993). Additionally, low serum zinc levels are often observed in clinical depression and a correlation between the severity of zinc deficiency and the severity of clinical depression has been demonstrated in both clinical studies and animal models (Amani et al. 2010; Cope & Levenson 2010; Levenson 2006; Maes et al. 1994). In line with this, zinc deficiency is able to cause depression- and anxiety-like behaviours in humans, whereas zinc supplementation has been used to treat depression in animal models and humans. For example, very low doses of zinc co-administered with otherwise ineffective doses of two antidepressant drugs enhanced the antidepressant effects of both drugs (Kroczka et al. 2001; Szewczyk et al. 2002). Intriguingly, zinc modulates drug binding to dopamine uptake complexes (Richfield 1993).

Induction of severe zinc deficiency in humans leads to a reproducible sequence of effects. In a study by Henkin et al. (1975), zinc deficiency was induced by large doses of histidine. The participants became anorexic after 2–3 days and developed a dysfunction of taste and smell. Thereafter, subjects became lethargic, depressed, irritable, and easy to anger, and an impairment of short-term memory was seen. Additionally, participants showed signs of cerebellar dysfunction, such as fine tremor, ataxia, and slurred speech. Supplementation with 50 mg zinc was found to reverse the symptoms (Henkin et al. 1975).

7.7 CONSEQUENCES OF ZINC DEFICIENCY AND EXCESS

The clinical diagnosis of marginal zinc deficiency in humans is difficult and zinc deficiency commonly overlooked. It is estimated that more than 20% of the worldwide population indeed is zinc deficient. However, the prevalence of mild zinc deficiency is currently not known due to the inconsistency of clinical symptoms (Willoughby & Bowen 2014). So far, blood plasma/serum (with 70–150 mg/dL [10.7–22.9 mmol/L] regarded normal in paediatric populations), hair zinc concentration, and dietary intake are frequently used indicators of zinc deficiency (Roohani et al. 2013; Willoughby & Bowen 2014). Apart from teratogenic effects and effects on mental functions as described earlier, the functional consequences of zinc deficiency can be best seen in the occurrence of skin lesions, anorexia, growth retardation, depressed wound healing, altered immune function, impaired night vision, and alterations in taste and smell acuity. In some cases, zinc-deficient babies were reported to cry excessively and to be irritable and inconsolable (Aggett et al. 1980; Sivasubramanian & Henkin 1978).

In contrast to zinc deficiency, excess zinc in the CNS might occur as a consequence of an inherited disorder, such as hyperzincaemia (Selimoglu et al. 2006; Smith et al. 1976) or environmental exposure. However, it is uncertain whether familial hyperzincaemia apart from plasma zinc levels also increases CNS zinc levels and patients do not present apparent phenotypes. So far, it is not well investigated whether excess of zinc during pregnancy has adverse effects on brain development of the offspring. Effects of excess zinc levels in the adult brain might be secondary through an antagonistic influence on copper, iron, and calcium metabolism. Some studies report an association of high zinc levels in the CNS with increased cell death after neuronal injury (Shuttleworth and Weiss 2011). However, zinc has been implicated to play a role after traumatic brain injury (TBI) in both, a neuroprotective and neurotoxic manner. Although there are preclinical and clinical findings for zinc to act as a neuroprotective agent following TBI, excessive zinc, released from neurons acutely after TBI, might contribute to neuronal death (Morris & Levenson 2013). This release of synaptic zinc after injury is mainly based on the release of vesicular zinc, but other pools of free zinc, such as zinc from mitochondria, may contribute, too. On a molecular level, zinc causes neuronal death via multiple different mechanisms including p38 and protein ubiquitination. Thus, despite the acute toxicity of zinc acting on neurons directly after a TBI, zinc supplementation in the recovery phase might be beneficial. The acute toxicity of excess zinc was also associated with ischaemia-induced neuronal death (Kawahara et al. 2014).

7.8 CONCLUSION

The turnover of zinc in the adult brain is slow. The half-time for the elimination of zinc from the rat brain, for example, is in the range of 16–43 days (Takeda 2000). Thus, only chronic zinc deficiency may influence brain zinc levels over time in adults. In contrast, the developing brain of an embryo is much more susceptible to changes in maternal zinc levels, and only few days of zinc deficiency might severely affect brain development. Therefore, adequate nutrition for pregnant mothers and infants is necessary, given that nutrients and growth factors regulate brain development during fetal and early postnatal life. During this time, the foundation for the development of cognitive, motor, and socio-emotional skills throughout childhood and adulthood is laid. Among the many nutrients, zinc availability certainly has a considerable effect on brain development. Animal models have shown that prenatal and perinatal zinc deficiency causes deficits in activity, social behaviour, attention, and learning and memory. Although data on benefits of zinc supplementation during pregnancy or infancy on child cognitive development in human show mixed results, in human studies, in contrast to animal studies, the detection and quantification of zinc deficiency is a difficult task, and specific impairments might be overlaid by the more general effects of under- or malnutrition. Nevertheless, enough data have accumulated over the years to prove the clinical relevance and public health importance of zinc deficiency. The observation that mild zinc deficiency may be widespread in human populations, including people who are adequately nourished (Skinner et al. 1997), raises pertinent questions on how in the future, the complexities of zinc metabolism can be better understood, biomarkers of zinc status identified to assess populations or individuals at special risk and to determine the prevalence of zinc deficiency, and how strategies such as zinc supplementation or fortification for the management and prevention of zinc deficiency can be implemented.

REFERENCES

Adamo AM, Oteiza PI. Zinc deficiency and neurodevelopment: The case of neurons. *Biofactors* 36(2) (2010): 117–124.

Adamo AM, Zago MP, Mackenzie GG et al. The role of zinc in the modulation of neuronal proliferation and apoptosis. *Neurotox Res* 17(1) (2010): 1–14.

Aggett PJ, Atherton DJ, More J, Davey J, Delves HT, Harries JT. Symptomatic zinc deficiency in a breast-fed preterm infant. *Arch Dis Child* 55(7) (1980): 547–550.

Aimo L, Mackenzie GG, Keenan AH, Oteiza PI. Gestational zinc deficiency affects the regulation of transcription factors AP-1, NF-κB and NFAT in fetal brain. *J Nutr Biochem* 21(11) (2010): 1069–1075.

Amani R, Saeidi S, Nazari Z, Nematpour S. Correlation between dietary zinc intakes and its serum levels with depression scales in young female students. *Biol Trace Elem Res* 137(2) (2010): 150–158.

Andreini C, Banci L, Bertini I, Rosato A. Counting the zinc-proteins encoded in the human genome. *J Proteome Res* 5(1) (2006): 196–201.

Andrews GK. Regulation and function of Zip4, the acrodermatitis enteropathica gene. *Biochem Soc Trans* 36(6) (2008): 1242–1246.

Apgar J. Comparison of the effect of copper, manganese, and zinc deficiencies on parturition in the rat. *Am J Physiol* 215(6) (1968): 1478–1481.

Assaf SY, Chung SH. Release of endogenous Zn^{2+} from brain tissue during activity. *Nature* 308(5961) (1984): 734–736.

Barry-Sterman M, Shouse MN, Fairchild MD, Belsito O. Kindled seizure induction alters and is altered by zinc absorption. *Brain Res* 383(1–2) (1986): 382–386.

Bhatnagar S, Taneja S. Zinc and cognitive development. *Br J Nutr* 85(2) (2001): 139–145.

Bjorklund G. The role of zinc and copper in autism spectrum disorders. *Acta Neurobiol Exp (Wars)* 73(2) (2013): 225–236.

Black MM. Zinc deficiency and child development. *Am J Clin Nutr* 68(2) (1998): 464–469.

Browning JD, O'Dell BL. Low zinc status in guinea pigs impairs calcium uptake by brain synaptosomes. *J Nutr* 124(3) (1994): 436–443.

Caldwell DF, Oberleas D, Clancy JJ, Prasad AS. Behavioral impairment in adult rats following acute zinc deficiency. *Proc Soc Exp Biol Med* 133(4) (1970): 1417–1421.

Chesters JK, Will M. Zinc transport proteins in plasma. *Br J Nutr* 46(1) (1981): 111–118.

Chorin E, Vinograd O, Fleidervish I et al. Upregulation of KCC2 activity by zinc-mediated neurotransmission via the mZnR/GPR39 receptor. *J Neurosci* 31(36) (2011): 12916–12926.

Chowanadisai W, Graham DM, Keen CL, Rucker RB, Messerli MA. A zinc transporter gene required for development of the nervous system. *Commun Integr Biol* 6(6) (2013a): e26207.

Chowanadisai W, Graham DM, Keen CL, Rucker RB, Messerli MA. Neurulation and neurite extension require the zinc transporter ZIP12 (slc39a12). *Proc Natl Acad Sci USA* 110(24) (2013b): 9903–9908.

Cole TB, Robbins CA, Wenzel HJ, Schwartzkroin PA, Palmiter RD. Seizures and neuronal damage in mice lacking vesicular zinc. *Epilepsy Res* 39(2) (2000): 153–169.

Cole TB, Wenzel HJ, Kafer KE, Schwartzkroin PA, Palmiter RD. Elimination of zinc from synaptic vesicles in the intact mouse brain by disruption of the *ZnT3* gene. *Proc Natl Acad Sci USA* 96(4) (1999): 1716–1721.

Connor MA, Chavkin C. Ionic zinc may function as an endogenous ligand for the haloperidol-sensitive sigma 2 receptor in rat brain. *Mol Pharmacol* 42(3) (1992): 471–479.

Cope EC, Levenson CW. Role of zinc in the development and treatment of mood disorders. *Curr Opin Clin Nutr Metab Care* 13(6) (2010): 685–689.

Cousins RJ. Gastrointestinal factors influencing zinc absorption and homeostasis. *Int J Vitam Nutr Res* 80(4–5) (2010): 243–248.

Cousins RJ, McMahon RJ. Integrative aspects of zinc transporters. *J Nutr* 130(5) (2000): 1384–1387.

Crawford IL. Zinc and the hippocampus. In *Neurobiology of the Trace Elements*, Dreosti IE, Smith RM, (eds.), vol. 1. Humana Press, Clifton, NJ (1983), pp. 169–211.

Crawford IL, Connor JD. Zinc in maturing rat brain: Hippocampal concentration and localization. *J Neurochem* 19(6) (1972): 1451–1458.

Davies MF, Maguire PA, Loew GH. Zinc selectively inhibits flux through benzodiazepine-insensitive gamma-aminobutyric acid chloride channels in cortical and cerebellar microsacs. *Mol Pharmacol* 44(4) (1993): 876–881.

Delorme R, Ey E, Toro R, Leboyer M, Gillberg C, Bourgeron T. Progress toward treatments for synaptic defects in autism. *Nat Med* 19(6) (2013): 685–694.

de Moura JE, de Moura EN, Alves CX et al. Oral zinc supplementation may improve cognitive function in schoolchildren. *Biol Trace Elem Res* 155(1) (2013): 23–28.

Dreosti IE, Manuel SJ, Buckley RA, Fraser FJ, Record IR. The effect of late prenatal and/or early postnatal zinc deficiency on the development and some biochemical aspects of the cerebellum and hippocampus in rats. *Life Sci* 28(19) (1981): 2133–2141.

Dreosti IE, Record IR, Manuel SJ. Zinc deficiency and the developing embryo. *Biol Trace Elem Res* 7(2) (1985): 103–122.

Dvergsten CL, Fosmire GJ, Ollerich DA, Sandstead HH. Alterations in the postnatal development of the cerebellar cortex due to zinc deficiency. I. Impaired acquisition of granule cells. *Brain Res* 271 (1983): 217–226.

Dvergsten CL, Fosmire GJ, Ollerich DA, Sandstead HH. Alterations in the postnatal development of the cerebellar cortex due to zinc deficiency. II. Impaired maturation of Purkinje cells. *Brain Res* 318(1) (1984): 11–20.

Elsas SM, Hazany S, Gregory WL, Mody I. Hippocampal zinc infusion delays the development of afterdischarges and seizures in a kindling model of epilepsy. *Epilepsia* 50(4) (2009): 870–879.

Frederickson CJ, Bush AI. Synaptically released zinc: Physiological functions and pathological effects. *Biometals* 14(3–4) (2001): 353–366.

Frederickson CJ, Klitenick MA, Manton WI, Kirkpatrick JB. Cytoarchitectonic distribution of zinc in the hippocampus of man and the rat. *Brain Res* 273(2) (1983): 335–339.

Frederickson CJ, Koh JY, Bush AI. The neurobiology of zinc in health and disease. *Nat Rev Neurosci* 6(6) (2005): 449–462.

Frederickson CJ, Moncrieff DW. Zinc-containing neurons. *Biol Signals* 3(3) (1994): 127–139.

Fukahori M, Itoh M. Effects of dietary zinc status on seizure susceptibility and hippocampal zinc content in the El (epilepsy) mouse. *Brain Res* 529(1–2) (1990): 16–22.

Gao HL, Zheng W, Xin N et al. Zinc deficiency reduces neurogenesis accompanied by neuronal apoptosis through caspase-dependent and -independent signaling pathways. *Neurotox Res* 16(4) (2009): 416–425.

Gewa CA, Weiss RE, Bwibo NO et al. Dietary micronutrients are associated with higher cognitive function gains among primary school children in rural Kenya. *Br J Nutr* 101 (2009): 1378–1387.

Gogia S, Sachdev HS. Zinc supplementation for mental and motor development in children. *Cochrane Database Syst Rev* (12) (2012): CD007991.

Golub MS, Gershwin ME, Vijayan VK. Passive avoidance performance of mice fed marginally or severely zinc deficient diets during post-embryonic brain development. *Physiol Behav* 30(3) (1983): 409–413.

Gower-Winter SD, Corniola RS, Morgan TJ, Levenson CW. Zinc deficiency regulates hippocampal gene expression and impairs neuronal differentiation. *Nutr Neurosci* 16(4) (2013): 174–182.

Gower-Winter SD, Levenson CW. Zinc in the central nervous system: From molecules to behavior. *Biofactors* 38(3) (2012): 186–193.

Grabrucker AM. Environmental factors in autism. *Front Psychiatry* 3 (2012): 118.

Grabrucker AM. A role for synaptic zinc in ProSAP/Shank PSD scaffold malformation in autism spectrum disorders. *Dev Neurobiol* 74(2) (2014): 136–146.

Grabrucker S, Jannetti L, Eckert M et al. Zinc deficiency dysregulates the synaptic ProSAP/Shank scaffold and might contribute to autism spectrum disorders. *Brain* 137(1) (2014): 137–152.

Gropper SS, Smith JL, Groff JL. *Advanced Nutrition and Human Metabolism*, 5th ed. Wadsworth, Bemont, CA (2009), pp. 498–491.

Hagmeyer S, Haderspeck JC, Grabrucker AM. Behavioral impairments in animal models for zinc deficiency. *Front Behav Neurosci* 8 (2014): 443.

Halas ES. Behavioral changes accompanying zinc deficiency in animals. In *Neurobiology of Trace Elements*, Dreosti IE, Smith RM, (eds.), vol. 1. Humana Press, New York (1983), pp. 213–243.

Halas ES, Eberhardt MJ, Diers MA, Sandstead HH. Learning and memory impairment in adult rats due to severe zinc deficiency during lactation. *Physiol Behav* 30(3) (1983): 371–381.

Halas ES, Heinrich MD, Sandstead HH. Long term memory deficits in adult rats due to postnatal malnutrition. *Physiol Behav* 22(5) (1979): 991–997.

Halas ES, Hunt CD, Eberhardt MJ. Learning and memory disabilities in young adult rats from mildly zinc deficient dams. *Physiol Behav* 37(3) (1986): 451–458.

Halas ES, Reynolds GM, Sandstead HH. Intra-uterine nutrition and its effects on aggression. *Physiol Behav* 19(5) (1977): 653–661.

Halas ES, Sandstead HH. Some effects of prenatal zinc deficiency on behavior of the adult rat. *Pediatr Res* 9(2) (1975): 94–97.

Hambidge KM, Neldner KH, Walravens PA. Zinc, acrodermatitis enteropathica and congenital malformations. *Lancet* 305(7906) (1975): 577–578.

Haug FM. Electron microscopical localization of the zinc in hippocampal mossy fibre synapses by a modified sulfide silver procedure. *Histochemie* 8(4) (1967): 355–368.

Hayward LJ, Rodriguez JA, Kim JW et al. Decreased metallation and activity in subsets of mutant superoxide dismutases associated with familial amyotrophic lateral sclerosis. *J Biol Chem* 277(18) (2002): 15923–15931.

Heiliger E, Osmanagic A, Haase H et al. N-Cadherin-mediated cell adhesion is regulated by extracellular Zn(2+). *Metallomics* 7(2) (2015): 355–362.

Henkin RI, Patten BM, Re PK, Bronzert DA. A syndrome of acute zinc loss. Cerebellar dysfunction, mental changes, anorexia, and taste and smell dysfunction. *Arch Neurol* 32(11) (1975): 745–751.

Hidalgo J, Aschner M, Zatta P, Vasák M. Roles of the metallothionein family of proteins in the central nervous system. *Brain Res Bull* 55(2) (2001): 133–145.

Howell GA, Welch MG, Frederickson CJ. Stimulation-induced uptake and release of zinc in hippocampal slices. *Nature* 308(5961) (1984): 736–738.

Huang RC, Peng YW, Yau KW. Zinc modulation of a transient potassium current and histochemical localization of the metal in neurons of the suprachiasmatic nucleus. *Proc Natl Acad Sci USA* 90(24) (1993): 11806–11810.

Huang YZ, Pan E, Xiong ZQ, McNamara JO. Zinc-mediated transactivation of TrkB potentiates the hippocampal mossy fiber-CA3 pyramid synapse. *Neuron* 57(4) (2008): 546–558.

Hübner CA. The KCl-cotransporter KCC2 linked to epilepsy. *EMBO Rep* 15(7) (2014): 732–733.

Hübner CA, Stein V, Hermans-Borgmeyer I, Meyer T, Ballanyi K, Jentsch TJ. Disruption of KCC2 reveals an essential role of K-Cl cotransport already in early synaptic inhibition. *Neuron* 30(2) (2001): 515–524.

Hurley LS. Zinc deficiency and central nervous system malformations in humans. *Am J Clin Nutr* 34(12) (1981): 2864–2865.

Hurley LS, Gowan J, Swenerton H. Teratogenic effects of short-term and transitory zinc deficiency in rats. *Teratology* 4 (1971): 199–204.

Hurley LS, Swenerton H. Congenital malformations resulting from zinc deficiency in rats. *Proc Soc Exp Biol Med* 123(3) (1966): 692–696.

Jan HH, Chen IT, Tsai YY, Chang YC. Structural role of zinc ions bound to postsynaptic densities. *J Neurochem* 83(3) (2002): 525–534.

Jen M, Yan AC. Syndromes associated with nutritional deficiency and excess. *Clin Dermatol* 28(6) (2010): 669–685.

Kasarskis EJ. Zinc metabolism in normal and zinc-deficient rat brain. *Exp Neurol* 85(1) (1984): 114–127.

Kawahara M, Mizuno D, Koyama H, Konoha K, Ohkawara S, Sadakane Y. Disruption of zinc homeostasis and the pathogenesis of senile dementia. *Metallomics* 6(2) (2014): 209–219.

Keen CL, Taubeneck MW, Daston GP, Rogers JM, Gershwin ME. Primary and secondary zinc deficiency as factors underlying abnormal CNS development. *Ann N Y Acad Sci* 678 (1993): 37–47.

Keppen LD, Pysher T, Rennert OM. Zinc deficiency acts as a co-teratogen with alcohol in fetal alcohol syndrome. *Pediatr Res* 19(9) (1985): 944–947.

King JC, Cousins RJ. Zinc. *Modern Nutrition in Health and Disease*, Ross C, Caballero B, Cousins JC, Tucker KL, Ziegler TR, (eds.), 10th ed. Lippincott Williams & Wilkins, Baltimore, MD (2006), pp. 271–285.

Koh JY, Lim J, Byun HR, Yoo MH. Abnormalities in the zinc-metalloprotease-BDNF axis may contribute to megalencephaly and cortical hyperconnectivity in young autism spectrum disorder patients. *Mol Brain* 7(1) (2014): 64.

Kroczka B, Branski P, Palucha A, Pilc A, Nowak G. Antidepressant-like properties of zinc in rodent forced swim test. *Brain Res Bull* 55(2) (2001): 297–300.

Levenson CW. Zinc: The new antidepressant? *Nutr Rev* 64(1) (2006): 39–42.

Levenson CW, Morris D. Zinc and neurogenesis: Making new neurons from development to adulthood. *Adv Nutr* 2(2) (2011): 96–100.

Li Y, Maret W. Human metallothionein metallomics. *J Anal Atom Spectr* 23 (2008): 1055–1062.

Liu H, Oteiza PI, Gershwin ME, Golub MS, Keen CL. Effects of maternal marginal zinc deficiency on myelin protein profiles in the suckling rat and infant rhesus monkey. *Biol Trace Elem Res* 34(1) (1992): 55–66.

Lokken PM, Halas ES, Sandstead HH. Influence of zinc deficiency on behavior. *Proc Soc Exp Biol Med* 144(2) (1973): 680–682.

Maes M, D'Haese PC, Scharpé S, D'Hondt P, Cosyns P, De Broe ME. Hypozincemia in depression. *J Affect Disord* 31(2) (1994): 135–140.

Maret W. The function of zinc metallothionein: A link between cellular zinc and redox state. *J Nutr* 130 (2000): 1455–1458.

Marks PA. Histone deacetylase inhibitors: A chemical genetics approach to understanding cellular functions. *Biochim Biophys Acta* 1799 (2010): 717–725.

Maske H. Über den topochemischen Nachweis von Zink im Ammonshorn verschiedener Säugetiere. *Die Naturwissenschaften* 42 (1955): 424.

Młyniec K, Davies CL, de Agüero Sánchez IG, Pytka K, Budziszewska B, Nowak G. Essential elements in depression and anxiety. Part I. *Pharmacol Rep* 66(4) (2014): 534–544.

Morris DR, Levenson CW. Zinc in traumatic brain injury: From neuroprotection to neurotoxicity. *Curr Opin Clin Nutr Metab Care* 16(6) (2013): 708–711.

Mott DD, Benveniste M, Dingledine RJ. pH-dependent inhibition of kainate receptors by zinc. *J Neurosci* 28(7) (2008): 1659–1671.

Moynahan EJ. Letter: Zinc deficiency and disturbances of mood and visual behaviour. *Lancet* 1(7950) (1976): 91.

Murakami M, Hirano T. Intracellular zinc homeostasis and zinc signaling. *Cancer Sci* 99(8) (2008): 1515–1522.

National Academy of Sciences. Dietary Reference Intakes for vitamin A, vitamin K, arsenic, boron, chromium, copper, iodine, iron, manganese, molybdenum, nickel, silicon, vanadium, and zinc. National Academy Press, Washington, DC (2001).

Nissensohn M, Sánchez-Villegas A, Fuentes Lugo D et al. Effect of zinc intake on mental and motor development in infants: A meta-analysis. *Int J Vitam Nutr Res* 83(4) (2013): 203–215.

Nitzan YB, Sekler I, Hershfinkel M, Moran A, Silverman WF. Postnatal regulation of ZnT-1 expression in the mouse brain. *Brain Res Dev Brain Res* 137(2) (2002): 149–157.

Nuttall JR, Oteiza PI. Zinc and the ERK kinases in the developing brain. *Neurotox Res* 21(1) (2012): 128–141.

O'Dell BL. Roles of zinc and copper in the nervous system. *Prog Clin Biol Res* 380 (1993): 147–162.

O'Dell BL, Browning JD. Impaired calcium entry into cells is associated with pathological signs of zinc deficiency. *Adv Nutr* 4(3) (2013): 287–293.

O'Halloran TV. Transition metals in control of gene expression. *Science* 261 (1993): 715–725.

Oteiza PI, Hurley LS, Lönnerdal B, Keen CL. Marginal zinc deficiency affects maternal brain microtubule assembly in rats. *J Nutr* 118(6) (1988): 735–738.

Oteiza PI, Hurley LS, Lönnerdal B, Keen CL. Effects of marginal zinc deficiency on microtubule polymerization in the developing rat brain. *Biol Trace Elem Res* 24(1) (1990): 13–23.

Palmiter RD, Cole TB, Quaife CJ, Findley SD. ZnT-3, a putative transporter of zinc into synaptic vesicles. *Proc Natl Acad Sci USA* 93(25) (1996): 14934–14939.

Pang W, Leng X, Lu H et al. Depletion of intracellular zinc induces apoptosis of cultured hippocampal neurons through suppression of ERK signaling pathway and activation of caspase-3. *Neurosci Lett* 552 (2013): 140–145.

Pardridge WM. Blood-brain barrier transport of nutrients. *Nutr Rev* 44 (1986): 15–25.

Penland JG, Sandstead HH, Alcock NW et al. A preliminary report: Effects of zinc and micronutrient repletion on growth and neuropsychological function of urban Chinese children. *J Am Coll Nutr* 16 (1997): 268–272.

Peters DP. Effects of prenatal nutritional deficiency on affiliation and aggression in rats. *Physiol Behav* 20(4) (1978): 359–362.

Pfaender S, Grabrucker AM. Characterization of biometal profiles in neurological disorders. *Metallomics* 6(5) (2014): 960–977.

Prasad AS, Bao B, Beck FWJ, Sarkar FH. Zinc-suppressed inflammatory cytokines by induction of A20-medated inhibition of nuclear factor-kB. *Nutrition* 27 (2011): 816–823.

Prasad AS, Halsted JA, Nadimi M. Syndrome of iron deficiency anemia, hepatosplenomegaly, hypogonadism, dwarfism, and geophagia. *Am J Med* 31 (1961): 532–546.

Prasad AS, Miale A, Farid Z, Schulert A, Sandstead HH. Zinc metabolism in patients with the syndrome of iron deficiency anemia, hypogonadism and dwarfism. *J Lab Clin Med* 61 (1963a): 537–549.

Prasad AS, Miale A, Farid Z, Sandstead HH, Schulert AR, Darby WJ. Biochemical studies on dwarfism, hypogonadism, and anemia. *AMA Arch Intern Med* 111 (1963b): 407–428.

Qian J, Xu K, Yoo J, Chen TT, Andrews G, Noebels JL. Knockout of Zn transporters Zip-1 and Zip-3 attenuates seizure-induced CA1 neurodegeneration. *J Neurosci* 31(1) (2011): 97–104.

Richfield EK. Zinc modulation of drug binding, cocaine affinity states, and dopamine uptake on the dopamine uptake complex. *Mol Pharmacol* 43(1) (1993): 100–108.

Roohani N, Hurrell R, Kelishadi R, Schulin R. Zinc and its importance for human health: An integrative review. *J Res Med Sci* 18(2) (2013): 144–157.

Sandstead HH. Subclinical zinc deficiency impairs human brain function. *J Trace Elem Med Biol* 26(2–3) (2012): 70–3.

Sandstead HH, Penland JG, Alcock NW et al. Effects of repletion with zinc and other micronutrients on neuropsychologic performance and growth of Chinese children. *Am J Clin Nutr* 68 (1998): 470–475.

Sandstead HH, Strobel DA, Logan GM, Marks EO, Jacob RA. Zinc deficiency in pregnant rhesus monkeys: Effects on behavior of infants. *Am J Clin Nutr* 31(5) (1978): 844–849.

Selimoglu MA, Ertekin V, Yildirim ZK, Altinkaynak S. Familial hyperzincaemia: A rare entity. *Int J Clin Pract* 60(1) (2006): 108–109.

Shah D, Sachdev HP. Zinc deficiency in pregnancy and fetal outcome. *Nutr Rev* 64(1) (2006): 15–30.

Shuttleworth CW, Weiss JH. Zinc: New clues to diverse roles in brain ischemia. *Trends Pharmacol Sci* 32(8) (2011): 480–486.

Sivasubramanian KN, Henkin RI. Behavioral and dermatologic changes and low serum zinc and copper concentrations in two premature infants after parenteral alimentation. *J Pediatr* 93(5) (1978): 847–851.

Skinner JD, Carruth BR, Houck KS et al. Longitudinal study of nutrient and food intakes of infants aged 2 to 24 months. *J Am Diet Assoc* 97(5) (1997): 496–504.

Smith JC, Zeller JA, Brown ED, Ong SC. Elevated plasma zinc: A heritable anomaly. *Science* 193(4252) (1976): 496–498.

Strobel DA, Sandstead HH. Social and learning changes following prenatal or postnatal zinc deprivation in rhesus monkeys. In *The Neurobiology of Zinc, Part B: Deficiency, Toxicity and Pathology*, Fredericton CJ, Howell GA, Kasarskis EJ, (eds.), Alan R. Liss, New York (1984), pp. 121–138.

Suh SW, Won SJ, Hamby AM et al. Decreased brain zinc availability reduces hippocampal neurogenesis in mice and rats. *J Cereb Blood Flow Metab* 29(9) (2009): 1579–1588.

Swanson CA, King JC. Zinc and pregnancy outcome. *Am J Clin Nutr* 46(5) (1987): 763–771.

Szerdahelyi P, Kása P. Variations in trace metal levels in rat hippocampus during ontogenetic development. *Anat Embryol (Berl)* 167(1) (1983): 141–149.

Szewczyk B, Brański P, Wierońska JM, Pałucha A, Pilc A, Nowak G. Interaction of zinc with antidepressants in the forced swimming test in mice. *Pol J Pharmacol* 54(6) (2002): 681–685.

Tahmasebi Boroujeni S, Naghdi N, Shahbazi M et al. The effect of severe zinc deficiency and zinc supplement on spatial learning and memory. *Biol Trace Elem Res* 130(1) (2009): 48–61.

Takeda A. Movement of zinc and its functional significance in the brain. *Brain Res Brain Res Rev* 34(3) (2000): 137–148.

Takeda A, Hirate M, Tamano H, Nisibaba D, Oku N. Susceptibility to kainate-induced seizures under dietary zinc deficiency. *J Neurochem* 85(6) (2003): 1575–1580.

Takeda A, Takada S, Ando M et al. Impairment of recognition memory and hippocampal long-term potentiation after acute exposure to clioquinol. *Neuroscience* 171(2) (2010): 443–450.

Tapiero H, Tew KD. Trace elements in human physiology and pathology: Zinc and metallothioneins. *Biomed Pharmacother* 57 (2003): 399–411.

Terry CW, Terry BE, Davies J. Transfer of zinc across the placenta and fetal membranes of the rabbit. *Am J Physiol* 198 (1960): 303–308.

Todd WR, Elvehjem CA, Hart EB. Zinc in the nutrition of the rat. *Am J Physiol* 107 (1933): 146–156.

Tupe RP, Chiplonkar SA. Zinc supplementation improved cognitive performance and taste acuity in Indian adolescent girls. *J Am Coll Nutr* 28 (2009): 388–396.

Umamaheswari K, Bhaskaran M, Krishnamurthy G, Hemamalini, Vasudevan K. Effect of iron and zinc deficiency on short-term memory in children. *Indian Pediatr* 48 (2011): 289–293.

Valente T, Auladell C. Developmental expression of ZnT3 in mouse brain: Correlation between the vesicular zinc transporter protein and chelatable vesicular zinc (CVZ) cells. Glial and neuronal CVZ cells interact. *Mol Cell Neurosci* 21(2) (2002): 189–204.

Vela G, Stark P, Socha M, Sauer AK, Hagmeyer S, Grabrucker AM. Zinc in gut-brain interaction in autism and neurological disorders. *Neural Plast* 2015 (2015): Article ID 972791.

Veran J, Kumar J, Pinheiro PS et al. Zinc potentiates GluK3 glutamate receptor function by stabilizing the ligand binding domain dimer interface. *Neuron* 76(3) (2012): 565–578.

Vergnano AM, Rebola N, Savtchenko LP et al. Zinc dynamics and action at excitatory synapses. *Neuron* 82(5) (2014): 1101–1114.

Vincent SR, Semba K. A heavy metal marker of the developing striatal mosaic. *Brain Res Dev Brain Res* 45(1) (1989): 155–159.

Wang FD, Bian W, Kong LW, Zhao FJ, Guo JS, Jing NH. Maternal zinc deficiency impairs brain nestin expression in prenatal and postnatal mice. *Cell Res* 11(2) (2001): 135–141.

Warkany J, Petering HG. Congenital malformations of the central nervous system in rats produced by maternal zinc deficiency. *Teratology* 5(3) (1972): 319–334.

Warthon-Medina M, Moran VH, Stammers AL et al. Zinc intake, status and indices of cognitive function in adults and children: A systematic review and meta-analysis. *Eur J Clin Nutr* 69(6) (2015): 649–661.

Wenk GL, Stemmer KL. Activity of the enzymes dopamine-beta-hydroxylase and phenylethanolamine-N-methyltransferase in discrete brain regions of the copper-zinc deficient rat following aluminum ingestion. *Neurotoxicology* 3(1) (1982): 93–99.

Wessells KR, Brown KH. Estimating the global prevalence of zinc deficiency: Results based on zinc availability in national food supplies and the prevalence of stunting. *PLoS One* 7(11) (2012): e50568.

Willoughby JL, Bowen CN. Zinc deficiency and toxicity in pediatric practice. *Curr Opin Pediatr* 26(5) (2014): 579–584.

Wolf G, Schmidt W. Zinc and glutamate dehydrogenase in putative glutamatergic brain structures. *Acta Histochem* 72(1) (1983): 15–23.

Wolf G, Schütte M, Römhild W. Uptake and subcellular distribution of 65zinc in brain structures during the postnatal development of the rat. *Neurosci Lett* 51(2) (1984): 277–280.

Xie X, Smart TG. Properties of GABA-mediated synaptic potentials induced by zinc in adult rat hippocampal pyramidal neurones. *J Physiol* 460 (1993): 503–523.

Yasuda H, Yoshida K, Yasuda Y, Tsutsui T. Infantile zinc deficiency: Association with autism spectrum disorders. *Sci Rep* 1 (2011): 129.

Yasui M, Ota K, Murphy VA. Role of zinc in the central nervous system. In *Mineral and Metal Neurotoxicology*, Yasui M, Verity A, (eds.), CRC Press, New York (1997), pp. 139–144.

Yu X, Jin L, Zhang X, Yu X. Effects of maternal mild zinc deficiency and zinc supplementation in offspring on spatial memory and hippocampal neuronal ultrastructural changes. *Nutrition* 29(2) (2013): 457–461.

8 Iodine and Brain Development

Sheila A. Skeaff and Shao J. Zhou

CONTENTS

8.1 INTRODUCTION: IODINE METABOLISM AND FUNCTION AS A PART OF THYROID HORMONES

Iodine is an essential micronutrient with a recommended dietary intake in adults of 150 μg/day. To date, the only known function of iodine is in the production of thyroid hormones within the thyroid gland. Iodine in the diet is found in various forms which are reduced to iodide in the gut. Approximately 90% of ingested iodine is absorbed in the stomach and duodenum, the majority of which is excreted in the urine with negligible amounts lost in faeces. The body of a healthy adult contains 15–20 mg of iodine and 70%–80% can be found in the thyroid gland (Zimmermann 2009).

The thyroid gland is made up of two lobes connected by an isthmus. The lobes contain follicles made up of an outer layer of thyroid follicular cells or thyrocytes which surround the follicular lumen or colloid. The transport of iodide from plasma into the thyroid gland occurs via the sodium–iodide symporter (NIS) located at the basolateral membrane of the thyrocyte. The NIS actively transports iodide up its electrochemical gradient while transporting sodium down its electrochemical gradient in the ratio of 1:2. The NIS allows the thyroid gland to concentrate iodide at a level 20–40 times that of the plasma, explaining why the majority of iodide in the body is found in the thyroid gland (Zimmermann 2009). When iodide intake is in excess, the transport of iodide into the thyrocyte is decreased due to reduced expression of the NIS. Conversely, when iodide intake is decreased, such as in iodine deficiency, the expression of the NIS is increased, which leads to an increase in the transport of iodide into the thyrocyte. The expression of NIS is regulated by thyroid-stimulating hormone (TSH). The NIS is found in other tissues such as the mammary gland, which also has the ability to organify iodide.

Within the thyroid gland, iodide is transported across the apical membrane of the thyrocyte into the colloid. In the colloid of the follicle, iodide is stored, attached to thyroglobulin (Tg), a glycoprotein synthesized in the thyrocyte and transported into the follicular lumen where it becomes available for thyroid hormone production. In the follicular lumen, the enzyme thyroid peroxidase (TPO) uses hydrogen peroxide to catalyze the oxidation of iodide to the active form, iodine, and the subsequent binding of iodine to tyrosyl residues of Tg to form mono-iodotyrosine (MIT) or di-iodotyrosine (DIT) (de Vijlder and den Hartog 1998). TPO further catalyzes the coupling of MIT and DIT molecules, still within the Tg molecule, to produce the thyroid hormones 3,5,3′-tri-iodothyronine (T_3) and thyroxine (T_4). T_3 is formed by the coupling of one MIT molecule and one DIT molecule, and T_4 is formed by the coupling of two DIT molecules. Of the tyrosyl residues which form MIT or DIT, only around 30% are used in the thyroid hormone formation. The remaining MIT and DIT are deiodinated in the thyrocyte and the iodide is released transported back to the colloid (Vanderpas 2006).

The release of thyroid hormone from the thyroid gland into the circulation is stimulated via a negative feedback mechanism. When circulating levels of T_4 are low, this causes the hypothalamus to release thyrotropin-releasing hormone (TRH). TRH subsequently stimulates the pituitary gland to secrete TSH, which causes the thyroid to transport Tg into the thyrocyte via pinocytosis of the colloid. Once in the thyrocyte, Tg is proteolyzed by lysosomes to release T_3 and T_4, which are then released into the circulation. An increase in circulating levels of thyroid hormone acts on the hypothalamus and pituitary to inhibit TRH and TSH, respectively, completing the negative feedback loop.

A variety of thyroid diseases can result in abnormal levels of circulating thyroid hormone, but a more common cause is a lack of iodine in the diet. A sustained low intake of iodine will lower thyroid hormone concentrations within 3 months. Low levels of thyroid hormones stimulate the hypothalamus and the pituitary gland to continue to produce TRH and TSH, respectively. TSH stimulates thyroidal uptake of iodide via the NIS and enhances the pinocytosis of Tg from the colloid; however, preferential release of T_3 into the bloodstream and conversion of T_4 to T_3 in peripheral tissues help to conserve the number of iodide atoms used during the period of dietary deficiency (Delange 2000). A small quantity of thyroidal Tg leaks into the circulation, and this is increased when TSH levels are high. TSH also induces hyperplasia and hypertrophy of the thyroid cells, which results in the enlargement of the thyroid gland or goitre. Increased iodide uptake by the thyroid leads to decreased renal clearance, thus a fall in the urinary iodine concentration (UIC). The levels of Tg, T_3, and T_4 in the blood, the amount of iodine in the urine, and thyroid volume can all be used to assess iodine status in humans and to ascertain the severity of iodine deficiency in a population (WHO et al. 2007). However, the mechanisms described earlier that enable the body to more efficiently use dietary iodine and to maintain, as long as possible, normal circulating concentrations of T_4 and T_3 means that only in severe iodine deficiency do the concentrations of T_4 and T_3 fall outside the normal reference range.

Thyroid hormone is transported within the circulation primarily bound to transport hormones with the majority bound to thyroxine-binding globulin and the remainder bound to transthyretin, albumin, and lipoproteins (Zimmermann 2009). The fraction of total T_4 and T_3 that can be found free in the circulation is approximately 0.03% and 0.3%, respectively (Bianco & Larsen 2005). Once in the circulation, degradation of thyroid hormones eventually occurs with T_3 having a half-life of approximately 1 day and T_4 a half-life of approximately 7 days. The majority of thyroid hormone released from the thyroid gland is in the form of T_4, a prohormone for the more active form of thyroid hormone, T_3. Approximately 80% of T_3 produced each day is done so extrathyroidally. Nearly all of T_4 in the circulation is converted into T_3 by Type I iodothyronine 5′-deiodinase (D1) in the liver and kidney. Type II iodothyronine 5′-deiodinase (D2) found in the brain and the pituitary also converts T_4 into T_3, primarily for intracellular use (Richardson et al. 2015). Iodine released into plasma during deiodination of T_4 or due to thyroid hormone degradation may be reabsorbed by the thyroid gland or be excreted in the urine.

T_3 exerts its effect on a number of target tissues where it acts at a genomic level by binding to thyroid hormone receptors (TRs) within the nucleus. There are two isotypes of TR: TRα and TRβ (Preau et al. 2015). TRs are found throughout the body, but particularly in the liver, kidney, heart, skeletal muscle, pituitary, and brain. In the liver, thyroid hormone causes changes in gene transcription, affecting carbohydrate metabolism and lipogenesis. Cardiac and skeletal muscles are affected by thyroid hormone through changes in muscle tissue production. Thyroid hormone affects muscle contraction due to genetic alteration of calcium uptake by muscle cells. Thyroid hormone exerts its function in the pituitary gland through regulation of the synthesis and secretion of growth hormone via gene transcription. Indeed, thyroid hormones are involved in many aspects of carbohydrate and protein metabolism (Delange 1993). The most well-known function of thyroid hormone, however, is in the development of the central nervous system, more specifically in the developing brain. For many decades, a lack of iodine in the diet was the single most preventable cause of mental retardation in the world.

8.2 ROLE OF IODINE IN THE DEVELOPING BRAIN

There is good evidence that the timing of iodine deficiency during human development has different effects on the brain; this is logical when one considers how the brain grows and develops through the lifespan. The embryonic period of brain development begins at conception until gestation week 8. During this period, the basic structures of the brain and central nervous system, such as the neural tube and ventricles, are formed. The next phase is fetal development, which takes place from gestation week 9 until the end of gestation. This phase is characterized by neuronal production (i.e. neurogenesis), migration, and differentiation. Later in gestation and into the postnatal period, other developments occur including myelination. Myelination begins about 16 weeks gestation with different parts of the central nervous undergoing myelination at different time points in gestation. The frontal cortex is the area of the brain that is the slowest to fully myelinate, with spurts of increased development between birth and 2 years, 7–9 years, and again in the mid-teens (Hughes & Bryan 2003; Stiles & Jernigan 2010).

The first parts of the brain to mature are those involved in visual control, balance, and motor function (Hughes & Bryan 2003). The next parts of the brain to mature include the hippocampus, left temporal lobes, and the right hemisphere: areas of the brain needed for learning, memory, language, and spatial ability. The last parts of the brain to mature are the frontal lobes, which are required for higher-order cognitive abilities such as executive functioning (Hughes & Bryan 2003). Thus, although the most significant and rapid development of the brain occurs in the first half of gestation and any insults to this process are likely to have irreversible and lasting effects, the brain continues to grow and develop, albeit more slowly, throughout childhood and adulthood. Thus, nutrition can affect the brain's macrostructure (e.g. the gross nuclei constituting the hippocampus and frontal lobes), microstructure (i.e. cellular architecture and subcellular structures such as myelin), and affect neurotransmitters. Evidence suggests that iodine, in the form of thyroid hormone, is needed at all stages of brain development (Bernal et al. 2003).

Much of the evidence for the role of iodine and thyroid hormones in brain development comes from three different sources: first, studies of animal models including sheep, marmosets, chickens, rodents, and non-mammalian creatures such as fish, amphibians, and birds (Hetzel & Dunn 1989); second, observational studies and randomized controlled trials of populations living in areas of iodine deficiency; and third, studies of women and children with thyroid disease. The use of animal models is important, because it is ethically not possible to induce iodine deficiency in pregnant women, or to study the brains of their children. Of course, brain development in animal models does not directly mimic human brain development; in sheep, more brain development occurs in utero compared to humans, while the brains of newborn rats are not as developed as human brains at birth. However, thyroid hormones and their synthesis are exactly the same in mammalian and non-mammalian models and all aspects of thyroid hormone signalling, receptors, transporters, and deiodinases are present in early embryogenesis in these models (Preau et al. 2015). A combination of models, human studies, and the use of new tools to study the human brain, for example, functional magnetic resonance imaging, is helping to elucidate the role of iodine and thyroid hormone in brain development. The next section provides some specific examples using both animal and human research illustrating the involvement of the thyroid hormone in the developing brain.

8.2.1 Thyroid Hormones and Brain Development during the Prenatal and Perinatal Period

The effect of thyroid hormones on fetal brain development is influenced by an interplay between maternal and fetal thyroid hormones, the concentrations of which should be neither too high or too low, and deiodinase enzymes (Zoeller & Rovet 2004). Maternal T_4 is found in the embryonic cavities soon after conception and maternal thyroid hormones cross the placenta (Morreale de Escobar et al. 2007). Before mid-gestation, the mother is the only source of cerebral T_3, which is generated locally by the conversion of maternal free T_4 by type II 5′ iodothyronine deiodinase (D2). D2 has been shown to occur in the cerebral cortex of the human brain in the first trimester and the concentration of D2 is the highest in the cerebral cortex of the fetus before mid-gestation. Between 13 and 20 weeks' gestation, the levels of T_3 in the fetal cortex are higher than in the mother (Morreale de Escobar et al. 2004). The surge of maternal free T_4 in the first trimester is thought to ensure an adequate supply of T_3 for the developing cortex. Type 3 deiodinase (D3) is another enzyme and the major physiological deactivator of thyroid hormones (i.e. converts T_4 to T_2 and T_3 to reverse T_3). D3 is thought to be important to prevent a surge in maternal free T_4 that might hinder fetal brain development. D3 is found in high concentrations in the mid-brain, basal ganglia, brain stem, spinal cord, and hippocampus until mid-gestation, from which time it declines. Morreale de Escobar et al. (2007) suggest that D3 protects brain regions from excessive T_3 until differentiation is required. The differences in the concentration and activity of the deiodinase enzymes in the various parts of the developing brain indicate they play an essential role in normal brain development. The secretion of thyroid hormones by the fetal thyroid takes place around 18–20 weeks gestation, although the fetus does synthesize thyroid hormones, albeit at low levels, prior to this time (Williams 2008). However, even after the onset of fetal thyroid function, the fetus continues to rely on maternal thyroid hormones. Fetal levels of T_4 and free T_4 concentrations steadily increase with gestational age, reaching maternal and adult concentrations by the beginning of the third trimester.

Throughout pregnancy, the fetus is reliant on an adequate supply of maternal T_4 (not T_3) for normal brain development. As discussed in more detail later, low maternal T_4 can be caused by thyroid dysfunction or iodine deficiency (Williams 2008). After birth, the child can no longer rely on their mother for a source of thyroid hormone. In children born prematurely, alterations in the normal supply of thyroid hormone to the developing brain are believed to contribute to the developmental delays often observed in premature children (Zoeller & Rovet 2004). The earlier the preterm birth, the more severe the consequences, because the child's thyroid is not mature enough to produce adequate amounts of T_4 needed for normal neurodevelopment. Because the brain continues to develop after birth, children born at term but with congenital hypothyroidism will also display neurological damage and mental impairment. An elevated TSH concentration in blood spots collected as part of routine neonatal screening programmes is used for the early diagnosis of congenital hypothyroidism so that early treatment (i.e. with thyroxine) of affected children enables normal growth and development (Horn & Heuer 2010).

In order to influence the brain, thyroid hormones must be transported through the blood. They can then enter the brain either through the blood–brain barrier (80%) or the blood–cerebrospinal fluid barrier (20%); both T_3 and T_4 can cross these barriers (Horn & Heuer 2010; Richardson et al. 2015). Thyroid hormones enter the cells using a number of different membrane transporters. The monocarboxylate anion transporters (MCT) MCT8 and MCT10 have specificity for the thyroid hormones and have slightly higher affinity for T_3 than T_4 (Bernal 2012; Horn & Heuer 2010). Other transporters include the organic anion transporters 2 and 3 that also actively transport thyroid hormones across the cell membrane. Once in the cell, after deiodination, T_3 binds to a nuclear receptor, which subsequently affects gene expression. Bernal (2012) states that the primary role of thyroid hormone is to accelerate the rate of gene expression. Increasing numbers of genes have been identified, which have been shown to have a role in neuron development and migration (Bernal et al. 2003). What is also becoming clear is that the impact of thyroid hormone–regulated gene expression is influenced by many factors including dose of thyroid hormones, timing, and brain region. Of course, the findings of new research in this area, using increasingly sophisticated models and techniques, reinforce observational studies in humans that the consequences of a lack of iodine in the diet, and hence thyroid hormones, vary considerably with the degree of iodine deficiency and the timing of the deficiency in the life cycle.

Rat and human studies have shown that nuclear TRs are present in the cerebral cortex of the fetal brain from around 8 to 9 weeks gestation and reach adult levels by 18 weeks gestation. The early presence of TR in the brain supports the view that thyroid hormones are needed for early brain development (de Escobar et al. 2008; Williams 2008). T_3 binds to nuclear thyroid receptors affecting neurogenesis, cell migration, synaptogenesis, and differentiation of glial and neuronal cells. In rats and chickens, TRα are expressed early in development and seen in the neural tube, hippocampus, cerebellum, and midbrain (Preau et al. 2015). Compared to matched controls, fetuses of iodine-deficient sheep were found to have a morphologically altered cerebellum and cerebral hemispheres, indicating poor maturation; brain weights were also lower (Hetzel et al. 1990; Morreale de Escobar et al. 2007). Similar findings were found in marmosets. In the chicken, TRβ is expressed in more specific areas during embryogenesis, for example, developing sensory organs such as the eye. Most of the neurons in the human brain are produced mid-gestation, a time when the levels of T_4 are the highest in the fetal brain. During brain development, neurons are produced in the walls of the ventricles (i.e. ventricular zone) and subsequently migrate radially from the centre of the brain out to the developing cortex, to form six discrete layers. Simultaneously, the neurons differentiate and the various layers of the cortex contain different types of neurons. Thyroid hormones appear to play a role in most of these processes (Henrichs et al. 2013). Experimentally induced thyroid hormone deficiency in animal models interferes with neural proliferation and alters cell migration into the neocortex and hippocampus (Bernal 2012). Thyroid hormones have also been shown to regulate the differentiation of neurons as well as other cells such as oligodendrytes, astrocytes, and microglia. Myelination is another aspect of brain development affected by iodine. Thyroid hormones are essential for myelin development and maintenance, including control of myelin composition and metabolism. In hypothyroid rats, there is a reduction in myelin, whereas in hyperthyroid rats, there is an increase in myelin. Thyroid hormone also influences both oligodendrocyte maturation (the cells that wrap myelin around axons of neurons) and the level of myelin production from the oligodendrocyte (Stenzel & Huttner 2013). In rats, neural maturation and myelination, axon and dendrite formation, as well as synaptogenesis reach its peak in the first few weeks after birth, which corresponds to the third trimester in humans and exposure by the fetus to maternal thyroid hormone (Stenzel & Huttner 2013). Stenzel & Huttner (2013) suggest that the relatively longer exposure of the human brain to maternal thyroid hormones may explain, in part, the 'evolutionary expansion of the human brain and (its) increased cognitive abilities'.

It is clear that thyroid hormones are required for normal brain development; however, both the extent and exact mechanisms involved require further investigation. There is little doubt that iodine deficiency results in a range of impairments in human cognitive function (Table 8.1). Iodine in its role in the thyroid hormones has been associated with the following cognitive abilities: attention, information processing, hearing, learning and memory, executive functioning (i.e. a cluster of abilities that are needed for higher-level thinking particularly in response to novel situations and stimuli), and intelligence.

TABLE 8.1
Categorization of Iodine Deficiency during the Life Cycle and Effects on Brain Development

	Index to Assess Iodine Deficiency		Evidence of Effect on Brain	
Categorization of Iodine Deficiency	**Median Urinary Iodine Concentration of Group**	**Thyroid Indices in Blood**	**Adverse Effect on Brain and Cognition**	**Evidence[a]**
Pregnant women				
Mild	<150 μg/L	±TSH	✓ in child	+
Moderate		↑ TSH & ±T_4	✓ in child	++
Severe		↑ TSH & ↓ T_4	✓ in child	+++
Children				
Mild	50–99 μg/L	↑ Tg	✓	+
Moderate	20–49 μg/L	↑ Tg, TSH & ↓ T_4	✓	+
Severe	<20 μg/L	↑ Tg, TSH & ↓ T_4	✓	+++
Adolescents	<100 μg/L	?	?	Little
Adults	<100 μg/L	Varies with severity	✓	+

TSH, thyroid-stimulating hormone; T_4, thyroxine; Tg, thyroglobulin.

[a] Increasing + indicates increasing quality and quantity of evidence.

8.3 EFFECT OF IODINE DEFICIENCY AND THYROID DYSFUNCTION ON BRAIN DEVELOPMENT AT DIFFERENT STAGES OF THE LIFE CYCLE

During the life cycle, two factors determine the impact of iodine deficiency in brain development: the severity of the iodine deficiency and the timing of the iodine deficiency. The importance of these factors on cognition is well illustrated by reviewing studies conducted in human populations.

8.3.1 Pregnancy

8.3.1.1 Abnormal Thyroid Hormones in Pregnancy without Iodine Deficiency and the Effect on the Brains of Offspring

For many decades, endocrinologists have expressed concern that hypothyroidism in pregnancy and other milder forms of maternal thyroid dysfunction including hypothyroxinaemia can affect cognitive development in the offspring of these women (Kilby 2003). Dutch women with free T_4 levels (fT_4) less than the 10th percentile at 12 weeks gestation had infants with Bayley scores of infant development 7–8 points lower at 10 months of age than children whose mothers had free T_4 levels above the 10th percentile (Pop et al. 1999); similar differences were noted at 1 and 2 years of age (Pop et al. 2003) and in another more recent study, in 5 to 6-year-old children (Finken et al. 2013). Low fT_4 concentrations (<10th percentile) at 12 weeks gestation have also been linked with neurodevelopmental difficulties in early infancy (Kooistra et al. 2006). American women with serum thyroid-stimulating hormone (TSH) concentrations higher than the 98th percentile in pregnancy had children with IQ scores 4 points lower at age 7–9 years than similarly aged children of matched women with normal TSH values (Haddow et al. 1999). If maternal hypothyroidism remained untreated in pregnancy, the IQ scores of their 7 to 9-year-old children were 7 points lower than those of matched control children. Including these studies, of the almost dozen similar observational studies, most with relatively small sample sizes, around half have reported an association between maternal hypothyroxinaemia in the first half of pregnancy and impaired cognitive development. However, the Generation R study included a cohort of 3659 children and their mothers and found no association between maternal TSH at 13 weeks gestation and any cognitive outcomes in offspring at 18 and 30 months. Low maternal free T_4 concentration (<10th percentile) at 13 weeks was associated with language delay at both ages (Henrichs et al. 2013). Confirmation of the importance of adequate thyroid hormones in pregnancy was expected with the results of a large randomized controlled trial known as the CATS (Controlled Antenatal Thyroid Screening) study; however, no difference was found between the IQ of children at 3 years born to women with reduced thyroid function in early pregnancy (i.e. elevated TSH and low free T_4) who were treated with levothyroxine before 20 weeks gestation compared to the children of women who were untreated (Lazarus et al. 2012). The authors suggest that treatment with thyroid hormone may have been started too late in gestation; however, it is also possible that subtle reductions in thyroid function seen in these women do not have an adverse effect on neurodevelopment in the child. Other clinical trials are currently underway, but the results are not yet available.

It is important to note that many of these studies were conducted in the areas of adequate iodine status (i.e. in women who were not iodine deficient) or, in the case of the CATS study, iodine status was not measured in the women taking part in the studies. These studies are often included in chapters such as this because of the assumption that the effects of altered thyroid hormones on the developing fetal brain are similar regardless of whether the cause of the lowered thyroid hormones is a result of thyroid disease or iodine deficiency. Retrospective measurement of the thyroid hormone status and iodine status in stored samples of blood and urine samples collected from pregnant women participating in either observational or randomized trials, many of which already have measures of cognitive development in the child, are likely to be forthcoming in the literature over the next 5–10 years as a result of the increased focus on the role of thyroid hormones and/or iodine status on child development (Trumpff et al. 2013).

8.3.1.2 Pregnancy with Iodine Deficiency and the Effect on the Brains of Offspring

Approximately 5%–10% of pregnant women who are severely iodine deficient give birth to a child with cretinism. Cretinism is always associated with a significant impairment in mental function and/or defects in hearing, speech, stance, gait, hypothyroidism, and growth. There are two types of cretinism: myxoedematous cretinism and neurological cretinism (Halpern et al. 1991). Myxoedematous cretinism results from thyroid gland dysfunction of the fetus in the last trimester of pregnancy, whereas neurological cretinism results from low maternal thyroid hormone concentration early in pregnancy. Given the widespread prevalence of iodine deficiency worldwide, it is not surprising that neurological cretinism is the more common form. Neurological cretinism is characterized by mental retardation, deaf mutism, squint, spastic displegia, and disorders of the stance and gait. Myxoedematous or hypothyroid cretinism is characterized by less severe mental retardation, dwarfism, hypothyroidism, and a variety of other physical symptoms such as coarse and dry skin, a husky voice, and delayed sexual maturation. The IQ of cretins living in Thailand was reported to be 30, well below the 100-point IQ of a normal population (Rajatanavin et al. 1997). In areas with endemic cretinism, around 5%–15% of children who are not overt cretins will also have impaired mental function with an IQ of 50–69; these children are sometimes referred to as 'sub-cretins' (Chen & Hetzel 2010).

8.3.1.3 Observational Studies of the Effects of Iodine Deficiency in Pregnancy on Brain Development

There are a number of observational studies investigating the association between iodine status in pregnancy and aspects of brain development in the offspring with mixed results. In a small study of Spanish pregnant women, there was no association between urinary iodine concentration of women in pregnancy and Bayley's scores in their children (Costeira et al. 2011). Similar results were observed in a larger study, also conducted in Spain, finding no association between urinary iodine concentration in samples obtained in the first trimester of pregnancy and neurological development in their 1-year-old infants (Rebagliato et al. 2013). The iodine status of a subsample of women from the Generation R study was measured in early pregnancy and executive functioning was assessed in their children at 4 years of age finding that a low urinary iodine concentration in pregnancy was associated with impaired executive functioning in children (van Mil et al. 2012). The authors of this study note that impairment in executive functioning is associated with attention-deficit hyperactivity disorder (ADHD), supporting another study, often cited, by Vermiglio et al. (2004) who reported a higher prevalence of children with ADHD born to mothers living in a mild to moderate area of iodine deficiency in Italy compared to children born to mothers living in an area with adequate iodine status. Pregnant women participating in the Avon Longitudinal Study of Parents and Children had their iodine status retrospectively assessed by measuring the iodine concentration of urine samples collected in the first trimester of pregnancy (Bath et al. 2013). Their children were assessed using the Wechsler Intelligence Scale for Children at 8 years, and reading ability of the children were also assessed at 9 years of age. After adjusting for 21 factors, there was a significant association between maternal iodine status and cognitive performance in the child. Children born to the group of mothers categorized as mildly iodine deficient in early pregnancy had poorer verbal IQ, reading comprehension, and reading accuracy than the group of children born to mothers with better iodine status in pregnancy; the results of the study were further strengthened by the finding that the association was dose dependent. Similar results were found in a smaller Australian study (Hynes et al. 2013). Maternal iodine status was also assessed via a first trimester urine sample and children tested at 9 years via Australia's standardized National Assessment Programme. Children born to mothers with mild iodine deficiency had poorer spelling and grammar, compared to the children of mothers who were iodine sufficient during pregnancy with the authors suggesting that processing speed and working memory may be affected by the maternal iodine status. A major limitation of observational studies of this nature is the use of urinary iodine concentration as an index of iodine status in pregnancy, particularly when measured in single spot (i.e. one-off) urine sample; the large inter- and intra-individual variation associated with both spot and 24-hour urine samples means such studies should be interpreted with caution.

8.3.1.4 Randomized Controlled Trials of the Effects of Iodine Deficiency in Pregnancy on Brain Development

The importance of adequate dietary iodine in preventing cretinism was highlighted in the 1960s in a large trial of 165,000 people living in a part of Papua New Guinea with severe iodine deficiency and endemic cretinism (Pharoah et al. 2012). This study is considered the first randomized controlled trial of iodine supplementation in pregnant women. The authors found that an injection of iodized oil before conception or in early pregnancy reduced the number of cretins and improve motor function of their children compared with those women who received the placebo. This study is one of two (the other from Peru; Kevany et al. 1969) well-conducted randomized controlled trials of iodine supplementation of pregnant women living in areas of severe iodine deficiency. Both studies found that iodine supplementation reduced cretinism, but there were no other improvements in cognition. These studies were conducted more than 50 years ago, a time when research in this area focused on the overt and most serious consequence of severe iodine deficiency, that is, the elimination of cretinism.

Two systematic reviews have been recently published trying to assess the effect of iodine deficiency in pregnancy on development in the child. Bougma et al. (2013) included a variety of study designs in their review (e.g. randomized controlled trial, quasi-randomized and prospective cohort studies), estimating that iodine deficiency lowers IQ in children under the age of 5 years by 7.4 IQ points. In contrast, a recent review was only able to identify six well-conducted randomized controlled trials conducted in pregnant women living in regions of moderate to mild iodine deficiency of which none measured childhood development (Zhou et al. 2013). It is clear that randomized controlled trials are urgently required in areas of moderate to mild iodine deficiency to determine the effect of iodine supplementation in pregnancy on child development.

8.3.2 Childhood

The development of the brain is associated with the development of cognitive abilities or functions (Schmitt et al. 2005). At a general level, overall intellectual ability is often measured by 'intelligence quotient' or IQ; however, specific cognitive abilities can also be assessed, such as memory, hearing, visual, language, and executive functions (Isaacs & Oates 2008). The following texts review studies using a range of cognitive tests designed to assess the impact of iodine on the brain in children.

8.3.2.1 Meta-Analyses of Observational Studies of the Effects of Iodine Deficiency on Brain Development in Children

Two meta-analyses have examined the effect of severe to moderate iodine deficiency on IQ in children. The first was published in 1994 and included both observational and intervention studies of children aged 2 months to 15 years; 18 of 21 studies met the inclusion criteria (Bleichrodt & Born 1994). The authors estimated that children who lived in moderately to severely iodine deficient areas had IQ scores 13.5 IQ points lower than children who lived in the areas of iodine sufficiency. The studies included in this meta-analysis used a wide range of cognitive tests; thus, the results should be interpreted with caution (Bleichrodt & Born 1994). The second meta-analysis included 37 observational studies, published in Chinese journals, of children aged 4.5–15 years using two intelligence scales modified for use in China (Qian et al. 2005). Children living in iodine-deficient areas were compared with children living in iodine-sufficient areas, and children living in iodine-deficient areas were compared before and after iodine prophylaxis had been implemented; for both comparisons, a 12–13 point lower IQ score was estimated in the children with poorer iodine status.

8.3.2.2 Observational Studies of the Effects of Iodine Deficiency on Brain Development in Children

A number of additional observational studies have compared the cognitive abilities of children from iodine-sufficient areas to children from the areas of iodine deficiency. Four studies have reported differences in IQ between groups of children with varying degrees of iodine deficiency. Boyages et al. (1989) found that rural children from an iodine-deficient area had a significantly lower IQ when compared with controls from one rural and two urban iodine-sufficient areas in central China; 15% of iodine-deficient children had IQ scores between 90 and 109 compared with 33% of rural iodine-sufficient children; and 44% of iodine-deficient children had IQ scores less than 70 compared with 18% of rural iodine-sufficient children. Azizi et al. (1995) and Tang et al. (2007) compared children from mild, moderate, and severely iodine-deficient areas of Iran and China, respectively. Both studies found IQ to be significantly higher in children living in areas with mild iodine deficiency compared with children who lived in moderately or severely iodine-deficient areas. The fourth study was a large cross-sectional Spanish study reporting that children with a urinary iodine concentration <100 μg/L (i.e. categorized as mildly iodine deficient) had a lower IQ than those classed as iodine sufficient (i.e. >100 μg/L) (Santiago-Fernandez et al. 2004). Rather than using urinary iodine concentration as a measure of iodine status, a study conducted in Ethiopia used the presence of goitre as a proxy for iodine status; Wolka et al. (2014) reported that children with goitre had a 1.8 times greater odds of having a below average academic achievement than children who did not have goitre (Figure 8.1).

Another group of studies have compared children from areas with varying degrees of iodine deficiency and assessed specific aspects of cognition. Tiwari et al. (1996) administered learning tasks to boys from mild or severely iodine-deficient areas in India. Children from the mildly iodine-deficient area performed better on two of three cognitive tests compared with children from the severely iodine-deficient area.

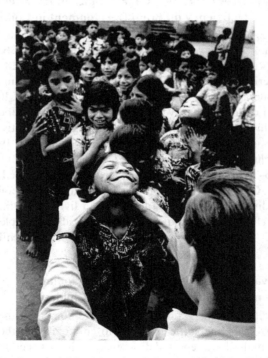

FIGURE 8.1 School-aged child with goitre being examined by Dr. Nevin Scrimshaw. (Photo courtesy of Getty Images.)

Vermiglio et al. (1990) compared iodine-deficient children from areas with and without endemic cretinism with iodine-sufficient controls in Sicily using the Bender Gestalt test, which measures visual perception and assesses memory, spatial abilities, and aspects of executive functioning. A greater proportion of iodine-deficient children had poor performance on the Bender Gestalt test compared with iodine-sufficient children. The study of Azizi et al. (1995) mentioned earlier, in addition to assessing IQ, found similar results to Vermiglio et al. (1990); mildly iodine-deficient children performed better on the Bender Gestalt test than moderately and severely iodine-deficient children.

There are a handful of observational studies which have assessed the effect of iodine deficiency on auditory function in children. Valeix et al. (1994) found that hearing loss and hearing impairment were more severe in a group of French preschool children categorized as iodine deficient compared to a group of children who were iodine sufficient. In a study of Spanish children aged 6–14 years, a significant association between poorer iodine status characterized by urinary iodine concentration, goitre, and thyroglobulin concentration and higher auditory thresholds was observed (Soriguer et al. 2000). There is evidence in animal models that thyroid hormones are needed during pregnancy for auditory function, and indeed, deaf mutism is a symptom of cretinism, so findings of such a relationship are plausible. Despite this, there are little recent data further examining the relationship between iodine status and hearing.

In summary, over two dozen observational studies from a large number of countries in the last 50 years have reported that children living in areas of moderate to severe iodine deficiency have poorer cognition than children with better iodine status. One difficulty in evaluating this research is the inability of such studies to separate the impact of iodine deficiency on the child's brain before birth and after birth, as well as other sociodemographic and environmental factors which may be associated with living in regions with severe to moderate iodine deficiency. To further evaluate the effect of iodine deficiency on brain development in children, evidence from intervention studies must be needed.

8.3.2.3 Intervention Studies of the Effects of Iodine Deficiency on Brain Development in Children

Most intervention trials looking at the effect of iodine supplementation on cognition have been carried out in moderately to severely iodine-deficient children. Typically in such studies, children are treated with a bolus (i.e. one-off) dose of iodized oil containing 400,000–540,000 µg of iodine although in some studies iodized salt has been used. Results from many of these studies have been inconsistent due to a number of methodological problems, including contamination of the control group with iodine resulting in improved iodine status in both the treated and untreated children (Bautista et al. 1982; Isa et al. 2000; van den Briel et al. 2000), or failure of the treatment to improve iodine status in the children (Huda et al. 2001; Shrestha 1994).

A Cochrane review by Angermayr and Clar published in 2004 examined the effect on iodine supplementation in children under the age of 18 years in reducing a range of iodine deficiency disorders such as goitre, physical development, and mental development; only four studies assessing the aspects of cognition met the strict inclusion criteria required by the Cochrane process (Angermayr & Clar 2004). In a study by Bautista et al. (1982), Bolivian children aged 5–12 years were given a dose of iodized oil or non-iodized mineral oil (i.e. control), with IQ, school grades, and psychomotor development measured 22 months later. Both the treated children and the control children had improvements in all measurements; however, the differences between the two groups were not statistically significant. Shrestha (1994) utilized a range of mental tests including those for verbal fluency and memory in 6 to 8-year-old children from Malawi. Ten months after a dose of iodized oil, treated children had significant improvements in motor skills as well as in six out of seven cognitive tests compared to control children who received non-iodized oil; however, baseline values for each group of children were not reported. A trial in Indonesian children aged 8–10 years (Untoro et al. 2007) also reported improvements in cognitive performance using the Cattell's Culture-Fair Intelligence Test in the treated children 22 months after their bolus dose; however, the improvements were not significantly different from the untreated children. A study of 8 to 10-year-old children living in a severely iodine-deficient area of Bangladesh given a bolus dose of iodized oil found that there were no differences in any of 12 different cognitive or motor tests 4 months after the children had been treated compared with the controls (Huda et al. 2001); the short duration of this study may, in part, explain the findings.

In contrast to the variable results of the studies described earlier, two more recent well-conducted, double-blind, randomized, placebo-controlled trials have shown that iodine supplementation significantly improves cognition in schoolchildren. Zimmermann et al. (2006) randomized moderately iodine-deficient 10 to 12-year-old schoolchildren in Albania to receive a bolus dose of iodized oil or sunflower oil and administered seven cognitive tests at baseline and 24 weeks. After 24 weeks, the iodine status of the treatment group had improved such that they were classified as having adequate iodine status, while the control group was still moderately iodine deficient. Treated children had significantly improved performance in four of the seven cognitive tests compared with controls. One of these tests was a measure of reasoning and problem-solving, while the remaining three tests measured processing speed. Gordon et al. (2009) conducted the first randomized controlled trial to investigate the effect of iodine supplementation on cognition in mildly iodine-deficient children using a daily iodine supplement. The intervention was carried out in New Zealand, and participating 10 to 13-year-old children were randomized to receive either a supplement of 150 μg/day iodine or placebo for 28 weeks. Children were administered four cognitive tests at baseline and 28 weeks. Like the study of Zimmermann et al. (2006), these tests were specifically chosen based on the likelihood (from previous research and the parts of the brain experiencing a surge in development at this age) that they would respond to iodine supplementation. After 28 weeks, children taking the iodine supplement were categorized as iodine sufficient, while children taking the placebo remained mildly iodine deficient. Iodine supplementation significantly improved scores on two of the four cognitive tests, both of which measured perceptual reasoning; however, in contrast to Zimmermann et al., there was no effect on processing speed.

A recent pooled analysis conducted by Taylor et al. (2014) was only able to use the studies of Zimmerman and Gordon finding 'modest' benefits of iodine supplementation with respect to perceptual reasoning and a global cognitive index.

More high-quality trials are needed to confirm these results, particularly in children from a wider range of countries. Such trials, however, are becoming increasingly difficult to conduct as many countries, including New Zealand, have implemented strategies to improve iodine status. In 1990, the elimination of iodine deficiency by the year 2000 was adopted as a goal by the World Summit for Children and the World Health Assembly. Although progress has been slower than planned, there has been a remarkable improvement in the iodine status of the world's population through the promotion of iodized salt; cretinism is non-existent and the number of countries with iodine deficiency has fallen from 110 in 1993 to 25 in 2015. Thus, finding populations of iodine-deficient children for intervention trials to assess the effect of iodine deficiency on brain function is now difficult. At the same time, iodine research has become less focused on schoolchildren and more concerned with investigating the effect of iodine deficiency in pregnancy on neurodevelopment in the child.

8.3.3 Adulthood

Not much is known about the effect of iodine deficiency on adolescents or adults. Indeed, for many decades, it was believed that alterations in thyroid hormones in adults had little effect on the brain, and if such effects were observed, they were likely to be reversible. It is now accepted that adult neurogenesis is sensitive to changes in hormones, including thyroid hormones (Kapoor et al. 2015). The impact of thyroid hormone on the brains of adults has been well studied in rodent models, but there is parallel research in humans. Hypothyroidism in adults is associated with an increased susceptibility for depression, and thyroid hormone is used as adjunct to antidepressant therapy (Constant et al. 2001). Prinz et al. (1999) have reported a positive association between thyroid hormone levels and cognitive scores in older adults.

In contrast to studies focusing on thyroid hormones, there are few studies which directly report the effect of iodine deficiency in adults. Chen & Hetzel (2010) stated that Indonesian villages with severe iodine deficiency were quiet, with adults appearing lethargic and apathetic. When all villagers received an injection of iodized oil, within a year, adults were more animated and the level of activity in the community, as evidenced by outdoor games, had increased. Furthermore, economic productivity also improved in these villages. In 2013, the National Bureau of Economic Research published a report which examined the effect of iodized salt on cognitive outcomes measured using military data (Feyrer et al. 2013). Iodized salt was first used in the United States in 1924, after studies found a high prevalence of goitre in many parts of the United States. Iodized salt was introduced in the United States over a short time frame, allowing the authors to compare IQ in the cohorts of men serving in WW I (before salt iodization) and WW II (after salt iodization); they estimate that additional iodine in the diet through iodized salt was responsible for a 3.5 increase in IQ score. To our knowledge, there is only one randomized, placebo-controlled, double-blind study investigating the impact of mild iodine deficiency on adults. Daily iodine supplementation for 28 weeks significantly improved iodine status in the treated group compared to those receiving a placebo but did not improve scores for any of the seven cognitive tests used, which suggests that mild iodine deficiency has no observable adverse consequences on cognition in young adults (Fitzgerald 2011) (Figure 8.2).

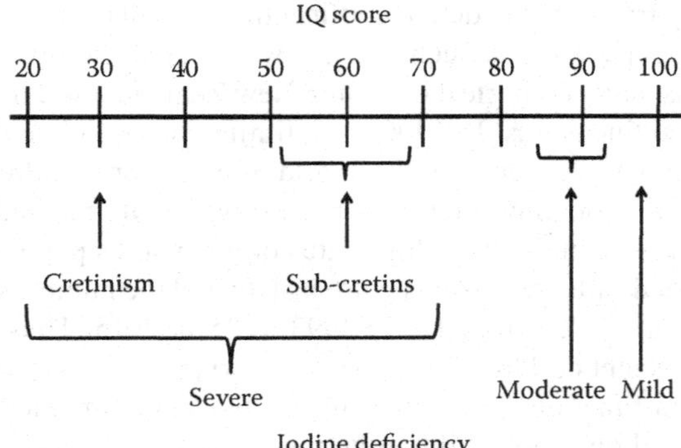

FIGURE 8.2 The effect of varying degrees of iodine deficiency on IQ.

8.4 CONCLUSION

Iodine is an essential micronutrient needed for the synthesis of thyroid hormones. Thyroid hormones are involved in almost all aspects of brain development. Maternal thyroid hormones, and thus an adequate iodine status, are both important and necessary for normal brain development. Severe iodine deficiency during pregnancy is a known cause of cretinism, which is characterized by profound mental retardation. There is growing evidence that less severe iodine deficiency in pregnancy can also have subtle but detrimental effects on the growing brain, but more evidence, particularly randomized clinical trials are needed to confirm observational studies. There is also a dearth of good-quality research examining the role of iodine in brain function and cognitive abilities in children and adults. The increasing acceptance by scientists that varying degrees of iodine deficiency causes a spectrum of disorders across the life cycle is a step forward. A lack of iodine in the diet reduces cognitive abilities in all age groups; in children, a lowered cognitive capacity limits a child's future, and eventually the capacity of the country. In 2008, the Copenhagen Consensus Center invited a panel of eight economic experts, including five Nobel Prize winners, to prioritize the most cost-effective solutions for the great global challenges. The elimination of iodine deficiency was ranked as the world's third best economic investment, highlighting the importance of nutritional strategies to strengthen human capital.

REFERENCES

Angermayr, L. and C. Clar. Iodine supplementation for preventing iodine deficiency disorders in children. *Cochrane Database Syst Rev* 2004; (2):CD003819.

Azizi, F., H. Kalani, M. Kimiagar, A. Ghazi, A. Sarshar, M. Nafarabadi, N. Rahbar, S. Noohi, M. Mohajer, and M. Yassai. Physical, neuromotor and intellectual impairment in non-cretinous schoolchildren with iodine deficiency. *Int J Vitam Nutr Res* 1995; 65:199–205.

Bath, S.C., C.D. Steer, J. Golding, P. Emmet, and M.P. Rayman. Effect of inadequate iodine status in UK pregnant women on cognitive outcomes in their children: Results from the Avon Longitudinal Study of Parents and Children (ALSPAC). *Lancet* 2013; 382:331–337.

Bautista, A., P.A. Barker, J.T. Dunn, M. Sanchez, and D.L. Kaiser. The effects of oral iodised oil on intelligence, thyroid status, and somatic growth in school-age children from an area of endemic goiter. *Am J Clin Nutr* 1982; 35:127–134.

Bernal, J. 2012. Thyroid hormones in brain development and function. South Darmouth, MA: Endocrine Education. http://www.thyroidmanager.org. Accessed on April 5, 2016.

Bernal, J., A. Guadano-Ferraz, and B. Morte. Perspectives in the study of thyroid hormone action on brain development and function. *Thyroid* 2003; 13:1005–1012.

Bianco, A.C. and P.R. Larsen. 2005. Intracellular pathways of iodothyronine metabolism. In *Werner and Ingbar's—The Thyroid: A Fundamental and Clinical Text*, L.E. Braverman and R.D. Utiger (eds.). Philadelphia, PA: Lippincott Williams & Wilkins.

Bleichrodt, N. and M.P. Born. 1994. A meta-analysis on iodine and its relationship to cognitive development. In *The Damaged Brain of Iodine Deficiency*, J.B. Stanbury (ed.), pp. 195–200. New York: Cognizant Communications.

Bougma, K., F.E. Aboud, K.B. Harding, and G.S. Marquis. Iodine and mental development of children 5 years old and under: A systematic review and meta-analysis. *Nutrients* 2013; 5:1384–1416.

Boyages, S., J.K. Collins, G.F. Maberly, J.J. Jupp, J. Morris, and C.J. Eastman. Iodine deficiency impairs intellectual and neuromotor development in apparently-normal persons. *Med J Aust* 1989; 150:676–682.

Chen, Z.-P. and B.S. Hetzel. Cretinism revisited. *Best Pract Res Clin Endocrin Metabol* 2010; 24:39–50.

Constant, E.L., A.G. de Volder, A. Ivanoiu, A. Bol, D. Labar, A. Seghers, G. Cosnard, J. Melin, and C. Daumerie. Cerebral blood flow and glucose metabolism in hypothyroidism: A positron emission tomography study. *J Clin Endocrinol Metab* 2001; 86:3864–3870.

Costeira, M.J., P. Oliveira, N.C. Santos, S. Ares, B. Saenz-Rico, G. Morreale de Escobar, and J.A. Palha. Psychomotor development of children from an iodine-deficient region. *J Pediatr* 2011; 159:447–453.

de Escobar, G.M., S. Ares, P. Berbel, M.J. Obregon, and F.E. del Rey. The changing role of maternal thyroid hormone in fetal brain development. *Semin Perinatol* 2008; 32:380–386.

Delange, F. 1993. Requirements of iodine in humans. In *Iodine Deficiency in Europe: A Continuing Concern*, F. Delange, J.T. Dunn, and D. Glinoer (eds.), pp. 5–16. New York: Plenum Press.

Delange, F. 2000. Iodine deficiency. In *Werner and Ingbar's—The Thyroid: A Fundamental and Clinical Text*, L. Braverman and R.D. Utiger (eds.), pp. 295–316. Philadelphia, PA: Lippincott Williams and Wilkins.

de Vijlder, J.J. and M.T. den Hartog. Anionic iodotyrosine residues are required for iodothyronine synthesis. *Eur J Endocrinol* 1998; 138:227–231.

Feyrer, F., D. Politi, and D.N. Weil. 2013. The cognitive effects of micronutrient deficiency: Evidence from salt iodization in the United States. NBER Working Paper No. 19233. Cambridge, MA: National Bureau of Economic Research.

Finken, M.J., M. van Eijsden, E.M. Loomans, T.G. Vrijkotte, and J. Rotteveel. Maternal hypothyroxinemia in early pregnancy predicts reduced performance in reaction time tests in 5- to 6-year-old offspring. *J Clin Endocrinol Metab* 2013; 98:1417–1426.

Fitzgerald, P. 2011. The effect of iodine supplementation on cognition in mildly deficiency young New Zealand adults. MSc, Human Nutrition, University of Otago, Dunedin, New Zealand.

Gordon, R.C., M.C. Rose, S. Skeaff, A. Gray, K. Morgan, and T. Ruffman. Iodine supplementation improves cognition in mildly iodine deficient children *Am J Clin Nutr* 2009; 90:1264–1271.

Haddow, J.E., G.E. Palomaki, W.C. Allan et al. Maternal thyroid deficiency during pregnancy and subsequent neuropsychological development of the child. *N Eng J Med* 1999; 341:549–555.

Halpern, J.P., S.C. Boyages, G.F. Maberly, J.K. Collins, C.J. Eastman, and J.G. Morris. The neurology of endemic cretinism. A study of two endemias. *Brain* 1991; 114(Pt 2):825–841.

Henrichs, J., A. Ghassabian, R.P. Peeters, and H. Tiemeier. Maternal hypothyroxinemia and effects on cognitive functioning in childhood: How and why? *Clin Endocrinol (Oxf)* 2013; 79:152–162.

Hetzel, B.S. and J.T. Dunn. The iodine deficiency disorders: Their nature and prevention. *Ann Rev Nutr* 1989; 9:21–38.

Hetzel, B.S., J.D. Potter, and E.M. Dulberg. The iodine deficiency disorders: Nature, pathogenesis and epidemiology. *World Rev Nutr Diet* 1990; 62:59–119.

Horn, S. and H. Heuer. Thyroid hormone action during brain development: More questions than answers. *Mol Cell Endocrinol* 2010; 315:19–26.

Huda, S.N., S.M. Grantham-McGregor, and A. Tomkins. Cognitive and motor functions of iodine-deficient but euthyroid children in Bangladesh do not benefit from iodized poppy seed oil (Lipiodol). *J Nutr* 2001; 131:72–77.

Hughes, D. and J. Bryan. The assessment of cognitive performance in children: Considerations for detecting nutritional influences. *Nutr Rev* 2003; 61:413–422.

Hynes, K.L., P. Otahal, I. Hay, and J.R. Burgess. Mild iodine deficiency during pregnancy is associated with reduced educational outcomes in the offspring: 9-year follow-up of the gestational iodine cohort. *J Clin Endocrinol Metab* 2013; 98:1954–1962.

Isa, Z.M., I.Z. Alias, K.A. Kadir, and O. Ali. Effect of iodized oil supplementation on thyroid hormone levels and mental performance among Orang Asli schoolchildren and pregnant mothers in an endemic goitre area of Peninsular Malaysia. *Asia Pac J Clin Nutr* 2000; 9:274–281.

Isaacs, E. and J. Oates. Nutrition and cognition: Assessing cognitive abilities in children and young people. *Eur J Nutr* 2008; 47:4–24.

Kapoor, R., S.E. Fanibunda, L.A. Desouza, S.K. Guha, and V.A. Vaidya. Perspectives on thyroid hormone action in adult neurogenesis. *J Neurochem* 2015; 133:599–616.

Kevany, J., R. Fierro-Benitez, E.A. Pretell, and J.B. Stanbury. Prophylaxis and treatment of endemic goiter with iodized oil in rural Ecuador and Peru. *Am J Clin Nutr* 1969; 22:1597–1607.

Kilby, M.D. Thyroid hormones and fetal brain development. *Clin Endocrinol* 2003; 59:280–281.

Kooistra, L., S. Crawford, A.L. van Baar, E.P. Brouwers, and V.J. Pop. Neonatal effects of maternal hypothyroxinemia during early pregnancy. *Pediatrics* 2006; 117:161–167.

Lazarus, J.H., J.P. Bestwick, S. Channon et al. Antenatal thyroid screening and childhood cognitive function. *N Engl J Med* 2012; 366:493–501.

Morreale de Escobar, G., M. Jesus Obregon, and F. Escobar del Rey. Role of thyroid hormone during early brain development. *Eur J Endocrinol* 2004; 151:U25–U37.

Morreale de Escobar, G., M. Jesus Obregon, and F. Escobar del Rey. Iodine deficiency and brain development in the first half of pregnancy. *Public Health Nutr* 2007; 10:1554–1570.

Pharoah, P., I.H. Buttfield, and B.S. Hetzel. Neurological damage to the fetus resulting from severe iodine deficiency during pregnancy. *Int J Epidemiol* 2012; 41:589–592.

Pop, V.J., E.P. Brouwers, H.L. Vader, T. Vulsma, A.L. van Baar, and J.J. Vijlder. Maternal hypothyroxinaemia during early pregnancy and subsequent child development: A 3 year follow-up study. *Clin Endocrinol* 2003; 59:282–288.

Pop, V.J., J.L. Kuijpens, A.L. van Baar, G. Verkerk, M.M. van Son, J.J. Vijlder, T. Vulsma, W.M. Wiersinga, H.A. Drexhage, and H.L. Vader. Low maternal free thyroxine concentrations during early pregnancy are associated with impaired psychomotor development in infancy. *Clin Endocrinol* 1999; 50:149–155.

Preau, L., J.B. Fini, G. Morvan-Dubois, and B. Demeneix. Thyroid hormone signaling during early neurogenesis and its significance as a vulnerable window for endocrine disruption. *Biochim Biophys Acta* 2015; 1849:112–121.

Prinz, P.N., J.M. Scanlan, P.P. Vitaliano, K.E. Moe, S. Borson, B. Toivola, G.R. Merriam, L.H. Larsen, and H.L. Reed. Thyroid hormones: Positive relationships with cognition in healthy, euthyroid older men. *J Gerontol Biol Sci Med Sci* 1999; 54:111–116.

Qian, M., D. Wang, W.E. Watkins, V. Gebski, Y.Q. Yan, M. Li, and Z.P. Chen. The effects of iodine on intelligence in children: A meta-analysis of studies conducted in China. *Asia Pac J Clin Nutr* 2005; 14:32–42.

Rajatanavin, R., L. Chailurkit, P. Winichakoon, P. Mahachoklertwattana, S. Soranasataporn, R. Wacharasin, V. Chaisongkram, P. Amatyakul, and L. Wanarata. Endemic cretinism in Thailand: A multidisciplinary study. *Eur J Endocrinol* 1997; 137:349–355.

Rebagliato, M., J. Vioque, and J.J. Arrizabalaga. Iodine supplements during and after pregnancy. *JAMA* 2013; 309:1345–1346.

Richardson, S.J., R.C. Wijayagunaratne, D.G. D'Souza, V.M. Darras, and S.L. Van Herck. Transport of thyroid hormones via the choroid plexus into the brain: the roles of transthyretin and thyroid hormone transmembrane transporters. *Front Neurosci* 2015; 9:66.

Santiago-Fernandez, P., R. Torres-Barahona, J.A. Muela-Martinez, G. Rojo-Martinez, E. Garcia-Fuentes, M.J. Garriga, A. Garcia Leon, and F. Soriguer. Intelligence quotient and iodine intake: A cross-sectional study in children. *J Clin Endocrinol Metabol* 2004; 89:3851–3857.

Schmitt, J.A.J., D. Benton, and K.W. Kallus. General methodological considerations for the assessment of nutritional influences on human cognitive functions. *Eur J Nutr* 2005; 44:459–464.

Shrestha, R.M. 1994. Effect of iodine and iron supplementation on physical, psychomotor and mental development in primary school children in Malawi. PhD, University of Wageningen, Wageningen, the Netherlands.

Soriguer, F., M.C. Millon, R. Munoz et al. The auditory threshold in a school-age population is related to iodine intake and thyroid function. *Thyroid* 2000; 10:991–999.

Stenzel, D. and W.B. Huttner. Role of maternal thyroid hormones in the developing neocortex and during human evolution. *Front Neuroanat* 2013; 7:19.

Stiles, J. and T.L. Jernigan. The basics of brain development. *Neuropsychol Rev* 2010; 20:327–348.

Tang, Z., W. Lui, H. Yin, P. Wang, J. Dong, Y. Wang, and J. Chen. Investigation of intelligence quotient and psychomotor development in schoolchildren in areas with different degrees of iodine deficiency. *Asia Pac J Clin Nutr* 2007; 16:731–737.

Taylor, P.N., O.E. Okosieme, C.M. Dayan, and J.H. Lazarus. Therapy of endocrine disease: Impact of iodine supplementation in mild-to-moderate iodine deficiency: Systematic review and meta-analysis. *Eur J Endocrinol* 2014; 170:R1–R15.

Tiwari, B.D., M.M. Godbole, N. Chattopadhyay, A. Mandal, and A. Mithal. Learning disabilities and poor motivation to achieve due to prolonged iodine deficiency. *Am J Clin Nutr* 1996; 63:782–786.

Trumpff, C., J. De Schepper, J. Tafforeau, H. Van Oyen, J. Vanderfaeillie, and S. Vandevijvere. Mild iodine deficiency in pregnancy in Europe and its consequences for cognitive and psychomotor development of children: A review. *J Trace Elem Med Biol* 2013; 27:174–183.

Untoro, J., N. Mangasaryan, B. de Benoist, and I. Darnton-Hill. Reaching optimal iodine nutrition in pregnant and lactating women and young children: Programmatic recommendations. *Public Health Nutr* 2007; 10:1527–1529.

Valeix, P., P. Preziosi, C. Rossignol, M.A. Farnier, and S. Hercberg. Relationship between urinary iodine concentration and hearing capacity in children. *Eur J Clin Nutr* 1994; 48:54–59.

van den Briel, T., C.E. West, N. Bleichrodt, F.J.R. van de Vijver, E.A. Ategbo, and J.G.A.J. Hautvast. Improved iodine status is associated with improved mental performance of schoolchildren in Benin. *Am J Clin Nutr* 2000; 72:1179–1185.

van Mil, N.H., H. Tiemeier, J.J. Bongers-Schokking et al. Low urinary iodine excretion during early pregnancy is associated with alterations in executive functioning in children. *J Nutr* 2012; 142:2167–2174.

Vanderpas, J. Nutritional epidemiology and thyroid hormone metabolism. *Annu Rev Nutr* 2006; 26:293–322.

Vermiglio, F., V.P. Lo Presti, M. Moleti et al. Attention deficit and hyperactivity disorders in the offspring of mothers exposed to mild-moderate iodine deficiency: A possible novel iodine deficiency disorder in developed countries. *J Clin Endocrinol Metab* 2004; 89:6054–6060.

Vermiglio, F., M. Sidoti, M.D. Finocchiaro, S. Battiato, V.P.L. Presti, S. Benvenga, and F. Trimarchi. Defective neuromotor and cognitive ability in iodine-deficiency schoolchildren of an endemic goiter region of Sicily. *J Clin Endocrinol Metabol* 1990; 70:379–384.

WHO, UNICEF, and ICCIDD. 2007. *Assessment of Iodine Deficiency Disorders and Monitoring Their Elimination: A Guide for Programme Managers*, 3rd edn. Geneva, Switzerland: World Health Organization.

Williams, G.R. Neurodevelopmental and neurophysiological actions of thyroid hormones. *J Neuroendocrinol* 2008; 20:784–794.

Wolka, E., S. Shiferaw, and S. Biadgilign. Epidemiological study of risk factors for goiter among primary schoolchildren in southern Ethiopia. *Food Nutr Bull* 2014; 35:20–27.

Zhou, S.J., A.J. Anderson, R.A. Gibson, and M. Makrides. Effect of iodine supplementation in pregnancy on children development and other clinical outcomes: A systematic review of randomized controlled trials. *Am J Clin Nutr* 2013; 98:1241–1254.

Zimmermann, M.B. Iodine deficiency. *Endocr Rev* 2009; 30:376–408.

Zimmermann, M.B., K.J. Connolly, M. Bozo, J. Bridson, F. Rohner, and L. Grimci. Iodine supplementation improves cognition in iodine-deficient schoolchildren in Albania: A randomized, controlled, double-blind study. *Am J Clin Nutr* 2006; 83:108–114.

Zoeller, R.T. and J. Rovet. Timing of thyroid hormone action in the developing brain: Clinical observations and experimental findings. *J Neuroendocrinol* 2004; 16:809–818.

9 Copper and Selenium and the Developing Brain

Nicola M. Lowe

CONTENTS

9.1 INTRODUCTION

Trace elements, including iron, zinc, copper, and selenium, are all found in the central nervous system (CNS), particularly within the limbic system, an interconnected series of structures which form the inner border of the cortex (Figure 9.1). The limbic system supports a range of functions related to motor coordination, emotions, behaviour, memory, and olfaction and is particularly vulnerable to nutritional and other disruptions during the gestational period and the first year of life (Rice & Barone 2000; Torres-Vega et al. 2012). This chapter will describe the role of copper and selenium in brain development and function, drawing on knowledge gained from animal studies, and those of humans with defects of copper and selenium metabolism. Iron and zinc are discussed separately in Chapters 6 and 7, respectively.

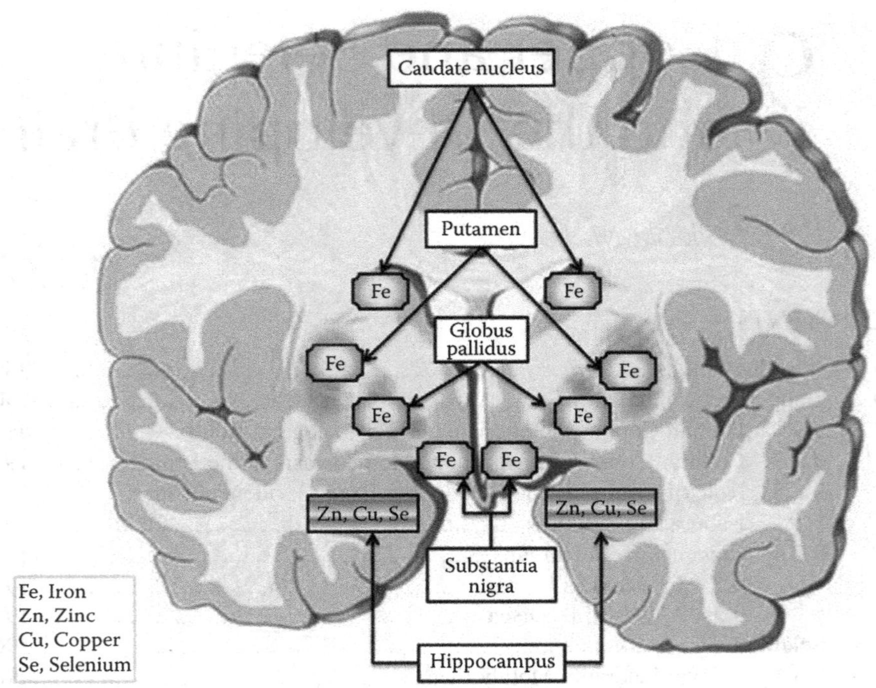

FIGURE 9.1 Distribution of trace elements in the limbic system. The hippocampus shows the highest concentrations of zinc (Zn) (Walsh et al. 1994); copper (Cu) (White et al. 2008, Bekris et al. 2010); and selenium (Se) (Zhang et al. 2008). (Reproduced from Torres-Vega, A. et al., *Nutr. Rev.*, 70, 679, 2012. With permission.)

9.2 COPPER

Copper is the third most abundant trace element in the body, after iron and zinc. It plays a number of essential biochemical roles, most notably as a cofactor for copper-dependent enzymes. Copper is essential for normal brain development and function and was first recognized as essential in the mammalian brain in 1937 in sheep grazing in pastures with a low soil copper content. Lambs born to these ewes often died before birth, or had enzootic ataxia (swayback), manifested as reduced nerve myelination in the spinal cord, affecting motor coordination such that the lambs had difficulty walking or were unable to stand. Lambs with this condition ultimately die of starvation, unless treated with copper supplements. Since the 1930s, numerous studies in laboratory animals and observations in humans with genetic abnormalities of copper metabolism have confirmed the essential role of copper in brain development and function. The pathology of the metabolic changes associated with copper deficiency can be influenced by the timing and duration of the deficiency, and the degree of response can be different depending on the species (Uriu-Adams et al. 2010).

9.2.1 Human Copper Metabolism and Physiological Roles

The adult body contains around 100 mg copper (Turnlund 1998). The highest copper concentrations are in the liver (containing around 10 mg), followed by the brain (containing around 8.8 mg), kidney, and heart (Linder et al. 1998). In the brain, the highest copper concentrations are found in substantia nigra, rich in dopamine-producing neurones and responsible for motor coordination (59.9 μg/g), cerebellar cortex (33.1 μg/g), and putamen (32.9 μg/g). Numerous neurological disorders have been linked to the abnormalities of copper metabolism, and have been reviewed by Desai & Kaler (2008). These include aceruloplasminemia, Alzheimer's disease, amyotrophic, lateral sclerosis, Huntington's disease, Menkes disease, occipital horn syndrome, Parkinson's disease, prion disease, and Wilson's disease. Much of our understanding of the role of copper in neurological function comes from the study of these disorders.

The UK Dietary Reference Value for copper is 1.2 mg/day for adult males and females, with an increase of 0.3 mg/day during lactation. Rich sources of copper include organ meats, seafood and whole grain and cocoa products, nuts, and seeds. The percentage of dietary copper absorbed can range from 15% to 55% (over an intake range of 1–8 mg) and is inversely related to the amount of copper consumed (Turnlund 1998). Excretion of endogenous copper is primarily via the bile, with small amounts lost via sweat and skin. Most cases of copper deficiency are reported in malnourished children (Olivares & Uauy 1996), but whether or not copper deficiency is a significant public health concern more generally is difficult to discern due to the lack of a specific biomarker for copper status (Arredondo & Nunez 2005). There is evidence from the United States and the United Kingdom that dietary intake in women aged 19–24 years is frequently below recommended levels (Board 2001; Henderson et al. 2004), and there are data suggesting that this is more of a problem during pregnancy, when requirements increase. Secondary copper deficiency may be a result of malabsorption (e.g. bariatric surgery, diarrhoea) or drug interactions (e.g. use of copper chelators such as D-penicillamine), genetic mutations or polymorphisms in copper transporters (e.g. Menkes syndrome), diseases (e.g. celiac), and prematurity and low birthweight (Uriu-Adams et al. 2010), particularly in those receiving copper-free total parenteral nutrition (Uauy et al. 1998). A crucial period in human fetal development appears to be towards the end of gestation when accumulation of copper (as well as zinc and iron) in the fetal liver occurs, to provide copper for the early months when the copper content of the breast milk is low. Therefore, infants born prematurely are born with low copper stores and are at increased risk of deficiency (Uriu-Adams et al. 2010).

Copper is absorbed via the small intestine and transported via the portal vein to the liver, where most of it is bound to not only ceruloplasmin but also albumin and histidine. The bound copper is then released into the circulation and delivered to the tissues where it acts as a cofactor for enzymes involved in oxidation/reduction reactions, for example, cytochrome-c oxidase (the terminal enzyme of electron transport and oxidative phosphorylation) and superoxide dismutase. Another well-documented role is as a cofactor for lysyl oxidase which is responsible for the maturation of collagen cross-links during collagen synthesis in bone and connective tissue. Copper plays additional roles which are less well understood and may be in part non-enzymatic, such as in angiogenesis, nerve myelination, and endorphin action (Linder et al. 1998). In the brain, Cu is linked to enzymes related to CNS transmission, for example dopamine beta-hydroxylase, a catecholamine-synthesizing enzyme which requires two units of copper per unit of enzyme for optimal activity. Copper also plays a role in iron accretion in the fetal and neonatal brain as described in Chapter 6.

9.2.2 Cellular Copper Transport and Homeostasis in the Brain

Copper is transported across the plasma membrane by a high-affinity carrier, CTR1. Within the cytoplasm, copper is bound to metal-binding proteins metallothionein and glutathione and to chaperone proteins (cytochrome-c oxidase [COX17], anti-oxidant 1 [ATOX-1], and copper chaperone for superoxide dismutase CCS), which ensure the safe delivery of the copper ion, either out of the cell via the membrane-bound Cu-ATPase ATP7A or to the trans-Golgi network (TGN) for incorporation into copper-dependent enzymes. ATP7A is expressed in most tissues, except the liver where a homologous protein, ATP7B, undertakes the same role (Gybina et al. 2009). Similarly, during pregnancy, copper is transported across the placenta to the fetal circulation via the same system of transporter proteins and copper-specific chaperones (McArdle et al. 2008). The rate of transfer of copper to the fetus increases with gestational age.

Brain copper homeostasis is thought to be achieved through the control of the movement of copper across the blood–brain barrier (BBB) at the cerebral endothelium and the blood–cerebrospinal fluid barrier (BCB) at the choroid plexus; however, the precise mechanisms involved are not fully elucidated (Fu et al. 2014). As described earlier for placental transfer, copper transport into the cells of the BBB or BCB is mediated by CPR1 and divalent metal transporterl (DMT1). CPR1 is expressed throughout CNS and its lack of expression is fatal, leading to embryonic death (Gupta & Lutsenko 2009; Prohaska 2008). Studies in mice have shown that when the dietary availability of copper is low, the brain responds with compensatory mechanisms to increase the expression of Crt1 receptors in the choroid plexus, which increases copper uptake into the brain (Kuo et al. 2006).

Both Cu-ATPases, ATP7A and ATP7B, have been shown to be expressed in the brain capillary endothelia (Qian et al. 1998) and choroidal epithelia (Choi & Zheng 2009; Iwase et al. 1996). These transport proteins are located both within the endoplasmic reticulum (ER) and the cell membrane and responsible for moving excess copper ions into vesicles for the exocytosis and also transporting copper into the ER for incorporation into newly synthesized proteins (Arredondo et al. 2003; Petris et al. 1996).

Copper moves from interstitial space between neurons and glial cells into the CSF, by diffusion. Copper is found in all regions of the brain. Enzymes in the central nervous system, which depend on copper for their function, include tyrosinase, peptidylglycine α-amidating monooxygenase, copper/zinc superoxide dismutase, ceruloplasmin, hephaestin, dopamine-β-hydroxylase, and cytochrome-c oxidase (Desai & Kaler 2008; Zucconi et al. 2007).

9.2.3 Role of Copper in the Developing Brain: Evidence from Laboratory Animals

Much of what we know about the role of copper in the brain comes from the study of copper deficiency in laboratory animals. Copper-deficient rats experience blunted brain development, particularly of cerebellum, marked by reduced myelination and synaptogenesis, as well as motor function disturbances. Delayed development of the hippocampus has also been reported in copper-deficient rat pups. The mechanism is not fully understood; however, it is hypothesized that copper deficiency impairs brain development by disturbing brain energy metabolism via mitochondrial dysfunction where the cytochrome oxidase component of the electron transport chain requires copper as a cofactor. Thus, the activity of the mitochondria in brain tissue is impaired by copper deficiency (Gybina et al. 2009). Studies in laboratory animals reveal that copper deficiency of the dam results in low copper concentration of the neonatal brain which has long-term effects on motor function, balance, and coordination that cannot be reversed by feeding a high-copper diet post-partum.

9.2.4 Evidence from Humans

There are two well-documented genetic conditions of altered copper metabolism that provide an insight into the role of copper in cognitive development and function: Menkes disease in which copper accumulates in some organs (intestine and kidney) and is low in others (liver and brain) and Wilson's disease, where copper distribution fails and copper accumulates (Prohaska 1986). Both diseases are caused by mutations of the genes encoding copper-dependent ATPase transporters which are responsible for the movement of copper out of cells and into the cellular compartments for incorporation into copper-dependent proteins.

9.2.4.1 Menkes Disease

Menkes disease is an X-linked chromosomal mutation of gene ATP7A. The mutation means that the transport of copper out of cells and the movement of copper into intracellular compartments for incorporation into copper-dependent proteins are disrupted (Tumer & Moller 2010). If the mutation results in little to no residual ATP7A activity, the infant will not survive beyond 3 years of age (Tumer & Moller 2010; Uriu-Adams et al. 2010). Menkes disease is not often diagnosed until the infant is least 5 months old. The pregnancy is usually uncomplicated, and infants are born at term (Tumer & Moller 2010). Early in the neonatal period, the physical symptoms are not immediately obvious; however, the appearance of wirey, depigmented, brittle hair at the age of 1–2 months is a characteristic symptom of the condition, along with pale skin, feeding difficulties, and sometimes bone abnormalities including sunken chest and susceptibility to fracture. Neurological motor development appears normal until 2–4 months, after which signs of developmental regression become apparent, with previously learned skills, such as smiling, being lost. Due to the lack of functionality of the ATP7A protein, it is thought that copper is trapped in both the BBB and the BCB, depriving the neurones and glial cells of copper (Tumer & Moller 2010). The lack of the catalytic activity of copper-dependent enzymes leads to neuronal degeneration and altered neurotransmitter metabolism, which is manifested as motor dysfunction and loss of muscular tone, with the limbs eventually becoming spastic. The copper-dependent enzymes and their roles that contribute to the symptoms observed in Menkes patients are shown in Table 9.1. In addition, there is an evidence of abnormalities of mitochondrial function in Menkes patients, manifested as elevated levels of brain lactate, and low levels of NAA (*N*-acetylaspartate), a neurone-specific metabolite synthesized in the brain mitochondria, which are reversed by copper supplementation (Gybina et al. 2009).

TABLE 9.1
Mammalian Copper Enzymes and Their Suggestive Relationship with Menkes Disease Symptoms

Enzyme	Biological Activity	Symptom
Cytochrome-c oxidase	Cellular respiration	CNS degeneration Ataxia Muscle weakness Respiratory failure
Superoxide dismutase	Free radical scavenging	CNS degeneration
Ceruloplasmin	Iron and copper transport	Anaemia
Hephaestin	Iron transport	Anaemia
Tyrosinase	Pigment formation	Hypopigmentation
Dopamine beta-hydroxylase	Catecholamine production	Ataxia
Peptidyl alpha-amidating enzyme	Activation of peptide hormones	Widespread effects
Lysyl oxidase	Collagen and elastin cross-linking	Premature rupture of fetal membranes Cephalohematoma Abnormal facies High-arched palate Emphysema Hernias Bladder diverticula Arterial aneurysms Loose skin and joints Osteoporosis Petechial haemorrhage Poor wound healing CNS degeneration
Sulfhydryl oxidase	Cross-linking of keratin	Abnormal hair Dry skin

Source: Reproduced from Tumer, Z. & Moller, L.B., *Eur. J. Hum. Genet.*, 18, 511, 2010. (With permission.)

9.2.4.2 Wilson's Disease

Wilson's disease was first described by Kinnier Wilson in 1912 (Wilson 1912). It is a rare autosomal recessive genetic disorder and is caused by a mutation of the ATP7B gene which resides on chromosome 13. The condition is characterized by hepatic and neuronal dysfunctions, and the symptoms usually appear in young people aged in their teens and early twenties, although any time between 5 and 45 years old is possible. This gene codes for a copper-dependent ATPase, which is expressed predominantly not only in the liver but also in the kidney, brain, cornea, and placenta. This transporter is responsible for both movement of copper out of the cell and also intracellular transport into the trans-Golgi compartment for incorporation into the plasma protein ceruloplasmin and into the bile for the excretion of excess stores (Ala et al. 2007). Thus, mutations of this gene result in the accumulation of copper in the kidney, eye, liver, and brain tissues (Ala et al. 2007; Dziezyc et al. 2014) and a reduced copper excretion in the bile.

Copper deposits in the eye that result in coppery brown colouration visible around the outer margins of the cornea, known as Kayser–Fleischer rings, are diagnostic for Wilson's disease, along with decreased ceruloplasmin concentrations. In terms of the neurological and psychiatric symptoms, these include motor dysfunction and depression and are summarized in Table 9.2. Between 40% and 50% of patients present with these symptoms (Walshe 1962).

TABLE 9.2
Neurological and Psychiatric Symptoms of Wilson's Disease

Neurological Symptoms	Psychiatric Symptoms
Movement disorders	Depression
Tremors	Neurotic behaviours
Poor coordination	Psychosis
Loss of fine-motor control	Personality changes
Cramped hand writing	Aggressive/antisocial behaviour
Choreic/choreoathetoid movements with dystonia	Emotional lability/impulsive behaviour
Rigid dystonia	Poor memory and/or difficulty in abstract thinking
Mask-like facies	
Rigidity	
Gait disturbance	
Pseudobulbar symptoms, e.g. dysarthria, drooling, difficulty swallowing.	
Migraine headaches	
Insomnia	
Seizures	

Sources: Adapted from Roberts, E.A., *Medicine*, 39, 602, 2011; Ala, A. et al., *Lancet*, 369, 397, 2007.

In terms of the developing brain, both Wilson's disease and Menkes disease provide an insight into the consequences of copper deprivation (deficiency) or copper accumulation (toxicity) at the cellular level. Both have neurological implications that impact on cognitive and motor function; however, further research is needed to elucidate the mechanisms through which copper exerts its effects.

9.3 SELENIUM

Selenium was first recognized as an essential trace element in 1957 (Schwarz & Foltz 1999). Selenium plays a vital role within mammalian enzymes, perhaps one of the most well-documented enzymes is the glutathione peroxidase family (GPxs) which plays a crucial antioxidant role in human tissues, including the brain. The highest concentration of selenium in the brain is found in regions rich in grey matter, particularly the putamen. Selenium deficiency during pregnancy may lead to damage of the nervous system of the fetus. Studies in rats revealed that the selenium concentration in the brain is highly conserved, even in conditions of selenium deficiency when other tissue selenium concentrations decline, and is the first tissue to be re-supplied when selenium is introduced back into the diet after a period of deficiency (Burk et al. 1972). The theory is that during selenium shortage, it is relocated from less critical tissues to meet the requirements of the critical organs, with the implication that the role of selenium in the brain is of primary importance. A link has been suggested between selenium deficiency and several neuronal and neuromuscular disorders, including epileptic seizures, Parkinson's disease, Duchenne muscular dystrophy, and Alzheimer's disease. Oxidative stress and the generation of reactive oxygen species are strongly implicated in the aetiology of these conditions; therefore, a possible link to selenium may be via its antioxidant role within the GPxs and selenoprotein P (Chen & Berry 2003; Schweizer et al. 2004). In addition to its role as an antioxidant, selenium also plays a central role along with iodine in the metabolism of thyroid hormones. As described in Chapter 8, iodine deficiency combined with selenium deficiency results in neurodevelopmental defects that characterize both neurological and myxoedematous cretinism due to impaired thyroid hormone synthesis during fetal development and early infancy (Aghini Lombardi et al. 1995; Mitchell et al. 1998).

9.3.1 Human Selenium Metabolism

Rich sources of dietary selenium include cereals, seafood, and meat, where it is present in the organic selenomethionine form which is more bioavailable than the inorganic form. The entry of selenium into the human food chain is highly dependent upon soil selenium levels, such that there are regions in the world (e.g. in China) where endemic selenium deficiency occurs due to extremely low soil selenium content and reliance on locally produced foods (Fairweather-Tait et al. 2011). The most well-documented example of this was in Keshan county of Heilongjiang Province in China in 1935. The selenium deficiency came to be known as 'Keshan disease' and was characterized by acute chronic heart disease, with symptoms including an enlarged heart, congestive heart failure, cardiac arrhythmias, and ECG changes.

It was often fatal, and primarily affected children aged 2–7 years old and women of childbearing age. Initially, it was thought that the disease was caused by an infectious agent; however, extensive epidemiological studies conducted in the 1960s and 1970s provided the evidence that established the causal relationship between selenium deficiency and Keshan disease (Chen 2012).

Recommendations for selenium intake average 60 μg/day for men and 53 μg/day for women; however, intakes required to maximize plasma GPX activity may be higher at 80–100 μg/day, with upper limits in the region of 400 μg/day (Rayman 2004). The European Food Safety Authority published revised intake guidelines recommending intakes of 70 μg/day (EFSA Panel on Dietetic Products 2014). Additional intakes during pregnancy and lactation of 15 μg/day in the United Kingdom and Europe are indicated or up to an additional 60 or 70 μg/day during pregnancy and lactation, respectively, according to the U.S. RDA (Institute of Medicine 2000). Most Europeans have a mean intake of only 40 μg/day (Rayman 2012), whereas in the United States, mean intakes are 106 μg/day (Rayman 2008), the difference due primarily to the variation in the selenium content of the soil in which the dietary staples are grown. For example, the selenium contents of breakfast cereal cornflakes in Denmark, Finland, and Canada are 5, 2.9, and 15 μgSe/100 g, respectively (Pieczynska & Grajeta 2015). It is estimated that approximately one billion people worldwide are selenium deficient (Haug et al. 2007), and this will clearly have an impact on fetal and infant development.

Breast milk selenium concentration varies with time post-partum, with colostrum containing high levels of selenium (26 μg/L) that decreases as lactation progresses to mature milk (15 μg/L) (Dorea 2002). Despite the regulation of selenium incorporation into milk proteins by the mammary gland, the concentration of selenium in breast milk is highly influenced by maternal dietary intake and has been shown to increase following a national soil selenium fertilization program in Finland (Kantola & Vartiainen 1991). The relationship between maternal selenium intake and breast milk concentration globally has been extensively reviewed (Dorea 2002).

More than half (50%–70%) of the selenium entering the blood from the gastrointestinal tract is taken up by erythrocytes within 1 minute and distributed by binding proteins throughout the body (Brtkova & Brtko 1996). Selenoprotein P, a glycoprotein synthesized in the liver, is the primary selenium transport protein, accounting for up to 60% of the selenium circulating in the plasma (Torres-Vega et al. 2012). It binds 10–12 atoms of selenium per molecule, with the selenium bound to cysteine within the protein. There are 25 selenoproteins which have selenocysteine at their active site, many of which can be grouped into families including the glutathione peroxidases (GPxs), iodothyronine deiodinases, and thioredoxin reductases (TrxR). The roles of some of these selenoproteins which are relevant to human health are summarized in a recent review (Rayman 2012). The total amount of selenium in the adult body varies greatly depending upon dietary intake, but has been reported to be between 2 and 20.3 mg, with the highest concentrations in the kidney, followed by the liver, spleen, pancreas, heart, brain, lung, bone, and skeletal muscle (Oster et al. 1988; Zachara et al. 2001). Selenium transport across the human placenta is not well understood; however, *in vitro* studies suggest that it is transported by passive diffusion down a concentration gradient (Nandakumaran et al. 2002), which is highly likely to be influenced by maternal selenium intake. Maternal deficiency of selenium during pregnancy has been postulated to lead to dysfunctions in the nervous system of the developing fetus (Cengiz et al. 2004). Examination of the brains taken from fetuses and neonates up to 3 months of age revealed that the fetal selenium concentration decreases with age, but increases with age postnatally (Vahter et al. 1997).

9.3.2 Role of Selenium in the Brain

Selenium exists naturally in organic (e.g. selenomethionine, selenocysteine) and in inorganic forms (e.g. selenite, selenate, selenide) (Birringer et al. 2002); however, it is not known in which biochemical form selenium enters the brain. Research in animal models strongly suggests that selenium levels in the brain are dependent, at least partially, on the expression of the glycoprotein selenoprotein P (SelP), supporting a role for this enzyme in the transfer of selenium into the brain (Chen & Berry 2003; Schweizer et al. 2004). It is proposed that SelP binds to a specific apolipoprotein–SelP receptor complex at the blood–brain barrier. This complex is then endocytosed and selenium is released from selenoprotein P via the action of selenocysteine lyase, releasing the selenium into the brain interstitial space where it binds to other selenoproteins and transported for use within the brain tissue. Selenoproteins can be found in the human neurons and astrocytes and glial cells, and their roles include antioxidant, involvement in redox reactions, and activation of thyroid hormones. A comprehensive list of all the mammalian selenoproteins, their location in the brain, and their functions have been described in a comprehensive review (Schweizer et al. 2004) and includes roles within the neurons, astrocytes, and glial cells. Changes in the structure and function of selenoprotein P result in a fall in selenium concentrations in the brain, and studies in animal models indicate that selenium deficiency is associated with neurological damage and altered motor function (Torres-Vega et al. 2012).

9.3.3 Evidence from Human Studies

Evidence that selenium has a role in the human brain comes from the studies of mood. There have been a number of studies in the 1990s demonstrating a positive association between selenium supplementation and mood, particularly in those who had a low dietary intake (Benton & Cook 1991; Hawkes & Hornbostel 1996). In addition, in a study comparing the impact of consuming a high selenium diet (226.5 μg/day) or a low selenium diet (32.6 μg/day), Finley and Penland demonstrated that glutathione peroxidase activity was significantly associated with seven mood scales, with higher activity associated with a more positive mood (Finley & Penland 1998). The mechanism by which selenium deficiency depresses mood is not fully understood; however, evidence from studies in rats suggests that it may be related to its role in the conversion of thyroxine (T4) to 3,3′,5-triiodothyronine (T3) by iodothyronine deiodinases, a selenium-dependent family of enzymes (Beckett et al. 1989). Alternatively, it may be related to the turnover of neurotransmitters dopamine, serotonin, and noradrenaline which have been shown to respond to changes in selenium intake in the prefrontal cortex of rats (Castano et al. 1993, 1997). In contrast, a double-blind, placebo-controlled trial involving around 500 participants receiving either 100, 200, or 300 μg selenium/day for 6 months failed to demonstrate any positive impact on mood or quality of life (Rayman et al. 2006) despite a dose–responsive increase in plasma selenium concentration. This difference in findings could be partly explained by age-related changes in brain function because of the difference in participants' ages between the studies, with the mean age in this recent study being 67 years compared with the previous studies where the mean age was mid-30s. In addition, a recent study that examined the relationship between plasma selenium concentration, depressive symptoms, and mood in 978 young adults described a U-shaped relationship with optimal plasma selenium concentrations in the range of 82–85 μg/L. This range approximates to the values at which glutathione peroxidase is maximal, implicating a possible link between selenium antioxidant pathways and mood (Conner et al. 2015).

9.3.4 Role of Selenium in the Developing Brain: Evidence from Humans

There is a paucity of epidemiological studies examining the impact of chronic selenium deficiency on neonatal development; however, a large-scale mother–infant cohort study was conducted recently in Shanghai, China. One of the aims of the study was to examine the relationship between umbilical cord selenium and neurobehavioural development. The study included 927 healthy pregnant women, and neonatal Behavioural Neurological Assessment (NBNA) was administered when the infants were 3 days old. After adjusting for maternal age, gender, maternal and paternal education, maternal and paternal occupation, and family income, an inverted U-shaped relationship was observed between cord serum selenium and NBNA score. Thus, both low and high cord selenium levels had a deleterious impact on NBNA scores (Yang et al. 2013).

9.4 CONCLUSION

Copper and selenium both play essential roles, primarily as cofactors for enzymes involved in brain tissue function and it is not therefore surprising that sophisticated mechanisms are in place at the cellular level to ensure homeostasis to prevent the damaging impact of both deficiency and toxicity. Studying the impact of the consequences of a failure of this homeostatic response provides insights into the specific roles of these nutrients in the CNS; however, there is still much to be learned. Studies of genetic conditions where normal copper metabolism is disrupted reveal that a lack of catalytic activity of copper-dependent enzymes results in neuronal degeneration, impaired neurotransmitter metabolism, mitochondrial function, and brain energy metabolism. The neurological consequences are manifested in physical as well as functional symptoms (Tables 9.1 and 9.2). The prevalence of copper deficiency, in the absence of generalized malnutrition, is low; however, potential issues relating to copper deficiency are not easily defined due to a lack of specific and sensitive indicator of copper status. In contrast, suboptimal dietary selenium intake is prevalent in some parts of the world, and the correlation between maternal selenium status, transfer to the fetus, and breast milk concentration is therefore of concern.

An interesting feature of selenium is the relatively narrow range between deficiency, essentiality, and toxicity doses (Nogueira & Rocha 2011) which when coupled with the U-shaped relationship between cord selenium concentration and neonatal neurological development indicates that a cautious approach to optimizing dietary intakes is warranted.

REFERENCES

Aghini Lombardi, F. A., Pinchera, A., Antonangeli, L., Rago, T., Chiovato, L., Bargagna, S., Bertucelli, B. et al. 1995. Mild iodine deficiency during fetal/neonatal life and neuropsychological impairment in Tuscany. *J Endocrinol Invest*, 18, 57–62.

Ala, A., Walker, A. P., Ashkan, K., Dooley, J. S., & Schilsky, M. L. 2007. Wilson's disease. *Lancet*, 369, 397–408.

Arredondo, M., Munoz, P., Mura, C. V., & Nunez, M. T. 2003. DMT1, a physiologically relevant apical Cu^{1+} transporter of intestinal cells. *Am J Physiol Cell Physiol*, 284, C1525–C1530.

Arredondo, M. & Nunez, M. T. 2005. Iron and copper metabolism. *Mol Aspects Med*, 26, 313–327.

Beckett, G. J., Macdougall, D. A., Nicol, F., & Arthur, J. R. 1989. Inhibition of type-I and type-II iodothyronine deiodinase activity in rat-liver, kidney and brain produced by selenium deficiency. *Biochem J*, 259, 887–892.

Bekris, L. M., Yu, C. E., Bird, T. D., & Tsuang, D. W. 2010. Genetics of Alzheimer disease. *J Geriatr Psychiatry Neurol*, 23, 213–227.

Benton, D. & Cook, R. 1991. The impact of selenium supplementation on mood. *Biol Psychiatry*, 29, 1092–1098.

Birringer, M., Pilawa, S., & Flohe, L. 2002. Trends in selenium biochemistry. *Nat Prod Rep*, 19, 693–718.

Brtkova, A. & Brtko, J. 1996. Selenium: Metabolism and endocrines (mini review). *Endocr Regul*, 30, 117–128.

Burk, R. F., Brown, D. G., Seely, R. J., & Scaief, C. C., III. 1972. Influence of dietary and injected selenium on whole-body retention, route of excretion, and tissue retention of $^{75}SeO_3^{2-}$ in the rat. *J Nutr*, 102, 1049–1055.

Castano, A., Ayala, A., Rodriguezgomez, J. A., Herrera, A. J., Cano, J., & Machado, A. 1997. Low selenium diet increases the dopamine turnover in prefrontal cortex of the rat. *Neurochem Int*, 30, 549–555.

Castano, A., Cano, J., & Machado, A. 1993. Low selenium diet affects monoamine turnover differentially in substantia-nigra and striatum. *J Neurochem*, 61, 1302–1307.

Cengiz, B., Soylemez, F., Ozturk, E., & Cavdar, A. O. 2004. Serum zinc, selenium, copper, and lead levels in women with second-trimester induced abortion resulting from neural tube defects: A preliminary study. *Biol Trace Elem Res*, 97, 225–235.

Chen, J. 2012. An original discovery: Selenium deficiency and Keshan disease (an endemic heart disease). *Asia Pac J Clin Nutr*, 21, 320–326.

Chen, J. & Berry, M. J. 2003. Selenium and selenoproteins in the brain and brain diseases. *J Neurochem*, 86, 1–12.

Choi, B. S. & Zheng, W. 2009. Copper transport to the brain by the blood-brain barrier and blood-CSF barrier. *Brain Res*, 1248, 14–21.

Conner, T. S., Richardson, A. C., & Miller, J. C. 2015. Optimal serum selenium concentrations are associated with lower depressive symptoms and negative mood among young adults. *J Nutr*, 145, 59–65.

Desai, V. & Kaler, S. G. 2008. Role of copper in human neurological disorders. *Am J Clin Nutr*, 88, 855S–858S.

Dorea, J. G. 2002. Selenium and breast-feeding. *Br J Nutr*, 88, 443–461.

Dziezyc, K., Karlinski, M., Litwin, T., & Czlonkowska, A. 2014. Compliant treatment with anti-copper agents prevents clinically overt Wilson's disease in pre-symptomatic patients. *Eur J Neurol*, 21, 332–337.

EFSA Panel on Dietetic Products. 2014. Scientific opinion on Dietary Reference Values for selenium. *EFSA J*, 12, 67.

Fairweather-Tait, S. J., Bao, Y., Broadley, M. R., Collings, R., Ford, D., Hesketh, J. E., & Hurst, R. 2011. Selenium in human health and disease. *Antioxid Redox Signal*, 14, 1337–1383.

Finley, J. W. & Penland, J. G. 1998. Adequacy or deprivation of dietary selenium in healthy men: Clinical and psychological findings. *J Trace Elem Exp Med*, 11, 11–27.

Food and Nutrition Board; Institute of Medicine. 2001. Dietary Reference Intakes for vitamins and micronutrients. A report of the panel for micronutrients. In: Institute of Medicine (ed.). Washington, DC: National Academy Press.

Fu, X., Zhang, Y., Jiang, W., Monnot, A. D., Bates, C. A., & Zheng, W. 2014. Regulation of copper transport crossing brain barrier systems by Cu-ATPases: Effect of manganese exposure. *Toxicol Sci*, 139, 432–451.

Gupta, A. & Lutsenko, S. 2009. Human copper transporters: Mechanism, role in human diseases and therapeutic potential. *Future Med Chem*, 1, 1125–1142.

Gybina, A. A., Tkac, I., & Prohaska, J. R. 2009. Copper deficiency alters the neurochemical profile of developing rat brain. *Nutr Neurosci*, 12, 114–122.

Haug, A., Graham, R. D., Christophersen, O. A., & Lyons, G. H. 2007. How to use the world's scarce selenium resources efficiently to increase the selenium concentration in food. *Microb Ecol Health Dis*, 19, 209–228.

Hawkes, W. C. & Hornbostel, L. 1996. Effects of dietary selenium on mood in healthy men living in a metabolic research unit. *Biol Psychiatry*, 39, 121–128.

Henderson, L. I. K., Gregory, J., Bates, C., Prentice, A., Perks, J., Swan, G., & Farron, M. 2004. *Vitamin and Mineral Intake and Urinary Analytes. The National Diet & Nutrition Survey: Adults Aged 19 to 64 Years*. London, UK: HMSO.

Institute of Medicine. 2000. *Dietary Reference Intakes for Vitamin C, Vitamin E, Selenium, and Carotenoids*. Washington, DC: National Academy Press.

Institute of Medicine, Food and Nutrition Board. 2001. Dietary Reference Intakes for Vitamins and Micronutrients. A Report of the Panel for Micronutrients. Institute of Medicine. Washington, DC: National Academy Press.

Iwase, T., Nishimura, M., Sugimura, H., Igarashi, H., Ozawa, F., Shinmura, K., Suzuki, M., Tanaka, M., & Kino, I. 1996. Localization of Menkes gene expression in the mouse brain; its association with neurological manifestations in Menkes model mice. *Acta Neuropathol*, 91, 482–488.

Kantola, M. & Vartiainen, T. 1991. Selenium content of breast milk in Finland after fertilization of soil with selenium. *J Trace Elem Electrolytes Health Dis*, 5, 283–284.

Kuo, Y. M., Gybina, A. A., Pyatskowit, J. W., Gitschier, J., & Prohaska, J. R. 2006. Copper transport protein (Ctrl) levels in mice are tissue specific and dependent on copper status. *J Nutr*, 136, 21–26.

Linder, M. C., Wooten, L., Cerveza, P., Cotton, S., Shulze, R., & Lomeli, N. 1998. Copper transport. *Am J Clin Nutr*, 67, 965S–971S.

Mcardle, H. J., Andersen, H. S., Jones, H., & Gambling, L. 2008. Copper and iron transport across the placenta: Regulation and interactions. *J Neuroendocrinol*, 20, 427–431.

Mitchell, J. H., Nicol, F., Beckett, G. J., & Arthur, J. R. 1998. Selenoprotein expression and brain development in preweanling selenium- and iodine-deficient rats. *J Mol Endocrinol*, 20, 203–210.

Nandakumaran, M., Dashti, H. M., & Al-Zaid, N. S. 2002. Maternal-fetal transport kinetics of copper, selenium, magnesium and iron in perfused human placental lobule: In vitro study. *Mol Cell Biochem*, 231, 9–14.

Nogueira, C. W. & Rocha, J. B. 2011. Toxicology and pharmacology of selenium: Emphasis on synthetic organoselenium compounds. *Arch Toxicol*, 85, 1313–1359.

Olivares, M. & Uauy, R. 1996. Copper as an essential nutrient. *Am J Clin Nutr*, 63, 791S–796S.

Oster, O., Schmiedel, G., & Prellwitz, W. 1988. The organ distribution of selenium in German adults. *Biol Trace Elem Res*, 15, 23–45.

Petris, M. J., Mercer, J. F., Culvenor, J. G., Lockhart, P., Gleeson, P. A., & Camakaris, J. 1996. Ligand-regulated transport of the Menkes copper P-type ATPase efflux pump from the Golgi apparatus to the plasma membrane: A novel mechanism of regulated trafficking. *EMBO J*, 15, 6084–6095.

Pieczynska, J. & Grajeta, H. 2015. The role of selenium in human conception and pregnancy. *J Trace Elem Med Biol*, 29, 31–38.

Prohaska, J. R. 1986. Genetic diseases of copper metabolism. *Clin Physiol Biochem*, 4, 87–93.

Prohaska, J. R. 2008. Role of copper transporters in copper homeostasis. *Am J Clin Nutr*, 88, 826S–829S.

Qian, Y., Tiffany-Castiglioni, E., Welsh, J., & Harris, E. D. 1998. Copper efflux from murine microvascular cells requires expression of the menkes disease Cu-ATPase. *J Nutr*, 128, 1276–1282.

Rayman, M., Thompson, A., Warren-Perry, M., Galassini, R., Catterick, J., Hall, E., Lawrence, D., & Bliss, J. 2006. Impact of selenium on mood and quality of life: A randomized, controlled trial. *Biol Psychiatry*, 59, 147–154.

Rayman, M. P. 2004. The use of high-selenium yeast to raise selenium status: How does it measure up? *Br J Nutr*, 92, 557–573.

Rayman, M. P. 2008. Food-chain selenium and human health: Emphasis on intake. *Br J Nutr*, 100, 254–268.

Rayman, M. P. 2012. Selenium and human health. *Lancet*, 379, 1256–1268.

Rice, D. & Barone, S., Jr. 2000. Critical periods of vulnerability for the developing nervous system: Evidence from humans and animal models. *Environ Health Perspect*, 108(Suppl 3), 511–533.

Roberts, E. A. 2011. Wilson's disease. *Medicine*, 39, 602–604.

Schwarz, K. & Foltz, C. M. 1999. Selenium as an integral part of factor 3 against dietary necrotic liver degeneration. 1951. *Nutrition*, 15, 255.

Schweizer, U., Brauer, A. U., Kohrle, J., Nitsch, R., & Savaskan, N. E. 2004. Selenium and brain function: A poorly recognized liaison. *Brain Res Brain Res Rev*, 45, 164–178.

Torres-Vega, A., Pliego-Rivero, B. F., Otero-Ojeda, G. A., Gomez-Olivan, L. M., & Vieyra-Reyes, P. 2012. Limbic system pathologies associated with deficiencies and excesses of the trace elements iron, zinc, copper, and selenium. *Nutr Rev*, 70, 679–692.

Tumer, Z. & Moller, L. B. 2010. Menkes disease. *Eur J Hum Genet*, 18, 511–518.

Turnlund, J. R. 1998. Human whole-body copper metabolism. *Am J Clin Nutr*, 67, 960S–964S.

Uauy, R., Olivares, M., & Gonzalez, M. 1998. Essentiality of copper in humans. *Am J Clin Nutr*, 67, 952S–959S.

Uriu-Adams, J. Y., Scherr, R. E., Lanoue, L., & Keen, C. L. 2010. Influence of copper on early development: Prenatal and postnatal considerations. *Biofactors*, 36, 136–152.

Vahter, M., Lutz, E., Lind, B., Herin, P., Bui, T. H., & Krakau, I. 1997. Concentrations of copper, zinc and selenium in brain and kidney of second trimester fetuses and infants. *J Trace Elem Med Biol*, 11, 215–222.

Walsh, C. T., Sandstead, H. H., Prasad, A. S., Newberne, P. M., & Fraker, P. J. 1994. Zinc: Health effects and research priorities for the 1990s. *Environ Health Perspect*, 102(Suppl 2), 5–46.

Walshe, J. M. 1962. Wilson's disease. The presenting symptoms. *Arch Dis Child*, 37, 253–256.

White, T., Cullen, K., Rohrer, L. M., Karatekin, C., Luciana, M., Schmidt, M., Hongwanishkul, D., Kumra, S., Charles Schulz, S., & Lim, K. O. 2008. Limbic structures and networks in children and adolescents with schizophrenia. *Schizophr Bull*, 34, 18–29.

Wilson, S. A. K. 1912. Progressive lenticular degeneration: A familial nervous disease associated with cirrhosis of the liver. *Brain*, 34, 295–509.

Yang, X., Yu, X., Fu, H., Li, L., & Ren, T. 2013. Different levels of prenatal zinc and selenium had different effects on neonatal neurobehavioral development. *Neurotoxicology*, 37, 35–39.

Zachara, B. A., Pawluk, H., Bloch-Boguslawska, E., Sliwka, K. M., Korenkiewicz, J., Skok, Z., & Ryc, K. 2001. Tissue level, distribution, and total body selenium content in healthy and diseased humans in Poland. *Arch Environ Health*, 56, 461–466.

Zhang, Y., Zhou, Y., Schweizer, U., Savaskan, N. E., Hua, D., Kipnis, J., Hatfield, D. L., & Gladyshev, V. N. 2008. Comparative analysis of selenocysteine machinery and selenoproteome gene expression in mouse brain identifies neurons as key functional sites of selenium in mammals. *J Biol Chem*, 283, 2427–2438.

Zucconi, G. G., Cipriani, S., Scattoni, R., Balgkouranidou, I., Hawkins, D. P., & Ragnarsdottir, K. V. 2007. Copper deficiency elicits glial and neuronal response typical of neurodegenerative disorders. *Neuropathol Appl Neurobiol*, 33, 212–225.

10 Nutrient Interactions and Multiple Micronutrient Supplementation

Parul Christian and Laura E. Murray-Kolb

CONTENTS

10.1 INTRODUCTION

Brain growth and development are rapid in early life, especially in the first 1000 days – a critical period when nutritional insults can exert long-lasting effects on health and function into childhood and adulthood. Deficiencies of vitamins and minerals, referred to as micronutrients, during pregnancy, in infancy, and in preschool and even through the school years, may play a vital role singly or in interaction with the environment in influencing central nervous system (CNS) growth and development, cognitive and motor function, and socio-emotional and behavioural development. Numerous pathways of how early nutrition factors can lead to neurocognitive development have been postulated (Prado & Dewey 2014). Specifically, nutritionally driven processes during fetal and infancy periods may be linked to neuronal and synaptic maturation, neurochemistry and brain metabolism, and myelination. Most of the evidence for this from animal and human studies exists for iron, zinc, iodine, and B vitamins during pregnancy and infancy/early childhood, but other micronutrients may also play a role (Georgieff 2007; Levenson & Morris 2011; Morse 2012; Williams 2008). In the context of low- and middle-income countries (LMIC), where over a billion women and children are known to experience some form of micronutrient deficiency (Black et al. 2013) and children may not likely meet their full developmental potential (Walker et al. 2011), the relationship between the two requires urgent attention. Also highly prevalent in these settings are conditions of fetal growth restriction and preterm birth (Lee et al. 2013), which have been shown to increase the risk of poor cognitive development (Christian et al. 2014) and in turn are influenced by prenatal micronutrient interventions.

Multiple micronutrient deficiencies among women of reproductive age, especially during pregnancy when requirements increase, have led to a growing interest in antenatal supplementation as a strategy. A once-a-day antenatal supplement, as taken commonly in high-income settings, has been considered feasible and cost-effective for addressing, simultaneously, multiple deficiencies in LMIC contexts. An international micronutrient supplement called the UNIMMAP (United Nations Multiple Micronutrient Antenatal Preparation), containing 15 vitamins and minerals, each at an approximate RDA for pregnant women, was designed for this purpose. Over the past decade, close to 15 randomized controlled trials (RCTs) have been undertaken to test the effect of a multiple micronutrient supplement versus a placebo, or iron–folic acid as the current standard of care control, on outcomes of low birthweight and infant mortality. Meta-analyses reveal the impact of the intervention on these birth outcomes briefly summarized in the following texts (Haidar & Bhutta 2012; Ramakrishnan et al. 2012). The trials included in the meta-analyses tested multiple micronutrient supplementation from early to mid-pregnancy through the end of pregnancy on birth outcomes using a randomized design. Although supplements tested were not uniform, several of the trials used the UNIMMAP formulation. Ramakrishnan et al. (2012) reported that significant, albeit modest improvements in birthweight of 52.6 g (95% CI: 43.2–62.0 g) in a meta-analysis of multiple micronutrient vs. iron-folic acid supplementation, accompanied by reductions in low birthweight (relative risk, RR = 0.86, 95% CI: 0.81–0.91) and small-for-gestational age (RR = 0.83, 95% CI: 0.73–0.95), an indicator of fetal growth restriction. Haidar & Bhutta (2012) found similar effect sizes. Stunting in childhood, which is strongly associated with child cognition, has also been examined as an outcome in follow-up studies of prenatal multiple micronutrient supplementation, although a meta-analysis of four trials found no impact on height-for-age and weight-for-height Z-scores in children under 5 years of age whose mothers participated in these trials (Lu et al. 2014). Although a recommendation for the use of prenatal supplements for women in low-income countries does not exist, the evidence to support policy and programmatic action is clear and it is anticipated that such a recommendation is forthcoming. Although the main goal of these trials was to show improvements in birth outcomes and most did not examine cognitive development in infancy, medium- to long-term effects of these interventions are increasingly becoming of interest to examine.

Among infants and young children, single-micronutrient supplementation, such as with high-dose vitamin A, has long been done programmatically to improve child survival. Similarly, salt iodization for reducing iodine deficiency–related cognitive deficit has also been globally adopted. Increasingly, however, home-based fortification strategies with iron and multiple micronutrient powders are being tested, largely to assess their impact on child growth and improve nutrient status and reduce anaemia. Systematic reviews of numerous trials using both traditional food fortification and home-based fortification strategies exist. One such review identified 39 trials of food fortification with multiple micronutrients and reported overall benefits on the outcome of anaemia but not on linear or ponderal growth (Das et al. 2013). Similarly, a Cochrane review that included eight trials of home fortification of foods with multiple micronutrient powders conducted in low-income countries among children under 2 years of age found significant reduction in anaemia by 31% and in iron deficiency anaemia by 51% when compared with no intervention or placebo, but showed no impact on growth (De-Regil et al. 2013).

The field of work called the 'developmental origins of health and disease (DOHaD)' brings recognition to the idea that early life exposures, including nutritional and micronutrient deficiencies, will, through numerous biologic and metabolic pathways, result in impacting chronic disease risk (Christian and Stewart 2010). The DOHaD concept has been extended to cognitive development and function, linking early life nutritional insults to later outcomes. Critical are the early intrauterine and early postnatal periods when rapid brain growth and development is occurring and deficiencies of micronutrients such as iron and iodine have shown to have powerful negative influence on cognitive functions. These links are increasingly being examined in studies; for example, the NUTRIMENTHE project is a collaborative study among European researchers undertaken to investigate the effects of early life nutritional factors on later outcomes of cognitive performance and to elucidate mechanisms by which nutrients influence these outcomes (Anjos et al. 2013). Numerous large birth cohorts and interventions are included in this project that will generate the much needed information on early life nutrient influences on cognitive and behavioural outcomes, although the results are only likely to be applicable to other high-income settings, where prevalence of micronutrient deficiencies is unlikely to be high. In several instances, RCT birth cohorts from the multiple micronutrient studies in LMIC have been followed postnatally to examine the effects of both prenatal and in some instances supplementation in the first 2 years of life on childhood cognitive and behavioural outcomes. We review the studies which were undertaken to examine such effects.

For the purposes of this chapter, we define 'multiple' as two or more micronutrients. This allows us to examine important synergistic as well as antagonistic interactions between at least two nutrients. We use a life-stage framework in reviewing the evidence for a link between multiple micronutrient deficiencies and child development (Figure 10.1). Each life stage has its specific consideration and factors which influence both immediate and long-term outcomes of mental and psychomotor development and function. Both immediate supplementation effects and long-term outcomes are reviewed, although evidence is limited in some areas. We relied mostly on evidence from supplementation trials, but observational studies of micronutrient status during pregnancy or infancy and childhood linked with neurodevelopmental outcomes are also covered.

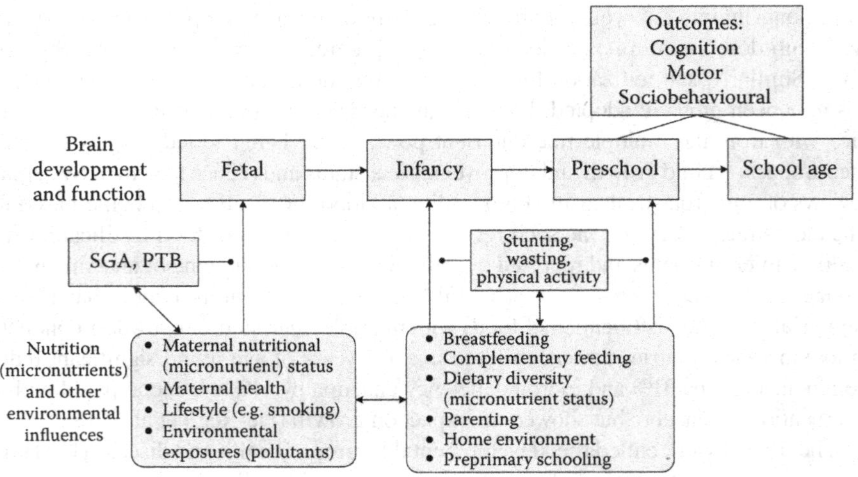

FIGURE 10.1 A life-cycle framework for examining nutritional and environmental influences on child development (SGA, small-for-gestational-age; PTB, preterm birth).

10.2 EFFECT OF MATERNAL (PRENATAL) MULTIPLE MICRONUTRIENT SUPPLEMENTATION ON CHILD DEVELOPMENT

Pregnancy is a period when the fetal brain develops rapidly, and maternal diet during this time can influence the structural and functional development of the brain with long-term consequences. The influence of individual nutrient deficiencies has been recorded in animal and human studies, which indicate that the adequacy of several nutrients, including both macronutrients and micronutrients, is important in promoting adequate fetal brain and CNS growth (Georgieff 2007; Levenson & Morris 2011; Morse 2012; Prado & Dewey 2014; Williams 2008). Cognitive development in the postnatal period is influenced by numerous environmental factors which can further influence cognitive development both independently and in interaction with fetal/intrauterine ones. We address the question of whether prenatal multiple micronutrients have a role in influencing child neurocognitive development.

Few studies have linked maternal diet and offspring cognitive development, although causal inferences are hard to make from such observational studies given the myriad of factors that influence child development (Figure 10.1). In Project Viva, a prospective birth cohort in Massachusetts, maternal intake of foods that provided nutrients that are methyl donors was associated with improved cognitive outcomes in 3-year-old children using the Peabody Picture Vocabulary Test III (PPVT-III) and the Wide Range Assessment of Visual Motor Abilities (Villamor et al. 2012). In a model in which several social, behavioural, and nutritional factors were adjusted, modest positive and linear increases in PPVT-III scores were observed with increasing intakes of folate during the first trimester. A weak association with PPVT scores was also shown with vitamin B_{12} intake in the second trimester (Villamor et al. 2012).

Similarly, one observational study examined maternal folate and vitamin B_{12} status and cognitive function in children (n = 536) at 9–10 years of age in the Mysore Parthenon birth cohort in India (Veena et al. 2010). They showed similar results in that maternal serum concentrations of folate but not vitamin B_{12}, at 30 weeks of gestation, were positively associated with children's cognitive function. Every 1 SD increase in serum folate resulted in a 0.1–0.2 SD increase in various test scores using the Kaufman Assessment Battery and additional tests of learning ability, attention and concentration, and visual-spatial and verbal abilities, among others, which were independent of a number of socio-economic, demographic, and birth-related factors. Levels of homocysteine were not associated with childhood cognitive ability (Veena et al. 2010). One study also examined antioxidant vitamin status (vitamins A, E, and C) during pregnancy and fetal transfer and intellectual development in 2-year-olds (Chen et al. 2009). Maternal serum and cord blood were examined for these vitamins and linked to child development outcomes. The study revealed both higher levels of vitamins A and E, but not C, in cord blood, and placental transfer rate of vitamin E was positively associated with cognitive and behavioural development domains at 2 years of age after adjusting for other confounders. Again, the observational nature of these data does not allow causal inferences.

We found five RCTs in the literature which have examined the effect of prenatal multiple micronutrient supplementation on development in the offspring across a range of ages in follow-up studies (Table 10.1). In one study, alternative combinations of micronutrients (3 or more versus 1) were examined (Christian et al. 2010), and the findings of each combination of nutrients are described in the following text separately. One trial in Tanzania among HIV-infected pregnant women, which tested a multivitamin preparation containing B-complex and C and E vitamins versus a placebo for its impact on vertical transmission and progression, followed children born in the study at 6, 12, and 18 months of age (n = 327) and tested their development using the Bayley Scales of Infant Development-II (BSID-II) (McGrath et al. 2006). Supplementation was beneficial as there were increases in the Psychomotor Development Index (PDI) score of 2.6 (95% CI: 0.1–5.1) and reduction in the risk of developmental delay on the motor scale of 60% (McGrath et al. 2006), although the clinical significance of these findings and generalizability to non-HIV populations is not clear and the multivitamin supplement was a formulation containing multiple RDAs of several B vitamins and lacked other essential nutrients. Iron–folic acid supplements in the study were provided through antenatal care to all women.

Similarly, Li et al. (2009) also tested, using BSID, children (n = 1305) of mothers who had participated in an RCT of prenatal multiple micronutrient supplementation versus folic acid–iron and folic acid alone in two rural communities in Western China. In contrast to the study from Tanzania, multiple micronutrient supplementation increased the mental development raw scores at age 1 year by 1.0 and 1.2 points compared with folic acid and folic acid–iron, respectively, but did not impact PDI scores. However, how meaningful these differences were in raw scores for predicting future intellectual performance remains unclear.

In a small study involving 184, 54-month-old children born to mothers who received daily iron–folic acid–zinc versus iron–folic acid during pregnancy in an RCT in Peru, no differences were found between groups across a range of domains

TABLE 10.1
Studies Examining the Effect of Prenatal Maternal Multiple Micronutrient Supplementation on Child Development

Location	Number Randomized	Age at Assessment	Control Group	Intervention Groups	Outcome/Domain	Main Findings
Tanzania (HIV-infected mothers) (McGrath et al. 2006)	327	6, 12, 18 months	No multivitamins	Multivitamins (multi-RDAs of B complex, vitamin C)	Mental, psychomotor	Increase in Psychomotor Development Index; reduced risk of developmental delay on the motor scale but no impact on overall score
China (Li et al. 2009)	1305	3, 6, 12 months	Folic acid	Multiple micronutrient supplement (15 nutrients plus folic acid)	Mental, psychomotor	Increase in mental development raw scores but not psychomotor development scores
Peru (Caulfield et al. 2010)	184	54 months	Iron–folic acid	Zinc, iron–folic acid	Intelligence, language and number skills, representational ability, behaviour, interpersonal	No differences in cognitive, social, or behavioural development
Nepal (Christian et al. 2010)	676	7–9 years	Vitamin A	Vitamin A, iron–folic acid	Intelligence, memory, executive function, motor (gross and fine)	Significant improvements in intellectual, motor, and executive functions

(Continued)

TABLE 10.1 (*Continued*)
Studies Examining the Effect of Prenatal Maternal Multiple Micronutrient Supplementation on Child Development

Location	Number Randomized	Age at Assessment	Control Group	Intervention Groups	Outcome/Domain	Main Findings
Nepal (Christian et al. 2010)	676	7–9 years	Vitamin A	Vitamin A, iron–folic acid, zinc	Intelligence, memory, executive function, motor (gross and fine)	No difference in outcomes
Nepal (Christian et al. 2010)	676	7–9 years	Vitamin A	Multiple micronutrient supplement (15 nutrients including vitamin A)	Intelligence, memory, executive function, motor (gross and fine)	No difference in outcomes
Indonesia (Prado et al. 2012)	487	42 months	Iron–folic acid	Iron–folic acid, 13 other micronutrients	Cognition, motor dexterity, and mood	No overall impact; increased motor ability among children with low MUAC and improved visual attention/spatial ability among children with low MUAC and of anaemic mothers

MUAC, mid-upper arm circumference.

of function tested including intelligence, language and math, and social and behavioural development (Caulfield et al. 2010). This trial included a three-nutrient supplement, but in fact, it was testing the effect of zinc when added to a standard of care and control group of iron–folic acid.

A follow-up study in Nepal tested neurocognitive outcomes in school-age children (7–9 years) related to prenatal supplementation with different combinations of micronutrients versus vitamin A alone in an RCT originally designed to look at the impact on birth outcomes, which improved (Christian et al. 2003). The three types of supplements were iron, folic acid, and vitamin A alone and with added zinc and a 15-nutrient micronutrient supplement containing all the aforementioned four nutrients. All these were compared with vitamin A alone as the standard of care in this population in which it had been shown to reduce maternal mortality (West et al. 2010) and risk of maternal night blindness (Christian et al. 1998). Tests of intelligence (using the Universal Nonverbal Intelligence Test, UNIT), executive function, and gross and fine motor control were administered to children by trained psychologists at the follow-up (Table 10.1) (Christian et al. 2010). Briefly, the combination of prenatal iron–folic acid–vitamin A compared with vitamin A alone showed significant increases in the meant UNIT T score of 2.4 (a one-quarter SD), reduced failure on a Stroop test, a higher score on the backward digit span, and improved fine motor control and speed using the finger tapping test. Neither the group with added zinc nor the multiple micronutrient supplement revealed the same benefits across these various domains of child development. We interpret these findings as suggestive of a potential inhibition of iron with zinc, especially in an environment in which maternal iron deficiency was high and perhaps more limiting for the early development of brain and neuronal development. Overall, maternal iron–folic acid supplementation during pregnancy improved general intellectual ability and aspects of executive and motor function in offspring at 7–9 years of age, although multiple micronutrient supplementation, which also included iron–folic acid, failed to show the same benefit (Christian et al. 2010).

Similar to these findings, an RCT in Indonesia also found no overall impact of prenatal multiple micronutrient supplementation compared with iron–folic acid as a standard of care on cognitive outcomes in 42-month-old preschool children (Prado et al. 2012). Small-sized effects were shown in motor ability and visual attention/spatial ability in a stratified analysis of mothers with low mid-upper arm circumference and anaemia, although these data should be interpreted with caution and considered exploratory.

10.3 EFFECTS OF MULTIPLE MICRONUTRIENT SUPPLEMENTATION IN CHILDHOOD ON CHILD DEVELOPMENT

Most studies evaluating the effects of postnatal micronutrient supplementation on child cognitive, motor, and socio-emotional development have tested a single micronutrient versus placebo. However, simultaneous micronutrient deficiencies typically occur, especially in children from LMIC. As such, more recent studies have aimed to understand the effects of supplementation with multiple micronutrients on child development. Here, we review those studies which included multiple micronutrient supplementation to children aged 0–18 years and evaluate the effect on development. These studies can be divided by age (supplementation occurring between birth and 5 years versus supplementation occurring between 6 and 18 years), type of intervention (supplement/powder versus fortified food), and primary outcome of interest (mental development, motor development, language development, socio-emotional development, executive functioning, and academic performance). We include trials that were conducted in apparently healthy children. Those that enrolled a select group of individuals specific for a chronic health condition were excluded. However, we include trials that selected children who had a low length-for-age Z-score and/or who were small for gestational age at birth, but we are careful to point this out when discussing the results.

Additionally, we review trials in which children were supplemented with ≥2 different micronutrients versus a placebo and studies in which children were provided with foods fortified with ≥2 different micronutrients versus non-fortified foods. Trials providing micronutrients to the control group are included as long as the intervention group received those same micronutrients plus at least two others. We also review studies that used interventions that were additional to the micronutrients (macronutrients, deworming, etc.) as long as the multiple micronutrients were the only difference between the intervention and control groups.

10.3.1 Multiple Micronutrient Supplementation during Early Postnatal Life and Child Development

Seventeen studies were identified in which children, at some point between birth and 5 years of age, were provided with multiple micronutrients and compared to a control group in which the outcomes of interest were assessed. In two of these studies (Black et al. 2004a; Colombo et al. 2014), the comparison group also received micronutrients and the intervention group was given one additional micronutrient, which does not allow for the assessment of the effects of multiple micronutrients. In one study (Manno et al. 2012), both groups received fortified foods with the only difference being the dose (which, once again, does not allow for the determination of the influence of multiple micronutrients on our outcomes of interest). These three studies are, therefore, not included in our review. The 14 studies which are included were conducted in North America (1 study) (Aburto et al. 2010), South America (1 study) (Lima et al. 2013), Africa (4 studies) (Adu-Afarwuah et al. 2007; Faber et al. 2005; Oelofse et al. 2003; Olney et al. 2006), and Asia (8 studies) (Aboud & Akhter 2011; Black et al. 2004b; Murray-Kolb et al. 2012; Pongcharoen et al. 2011; Sazawal et al. 2004; Siegel et al. 2011; Singla et al. 2014; Surkan et al. 2013) with most enrolling children between 1 and 36 months of age (with the exception of the study by Lima et al. [2013] in which children ranged from 3 months to 9 years of age at enrollment). The total number of subjects enrolled in these studies ranged from 60 to just over 700, and the intervention duration for most of the studies was 6 months to 1 year (one study had a treatment duration of 4 months [Aburto et al. 2010], one was 5 months [Singla et al. 2014], and one was up to 2 years, depending on the age of child at enrollment [Murray-Kolb et al. 2012]). Most of the studies assessed child development at the beginning of the study as well as immediately following the intervention period. However, three studies assessed the children several years after the intervention had ended: at 7–9 years of age (Murray-Kolb et al. 2012), at 9 years of age (Pongcharoen et al. 2011), and at up to 14 years of age (Lima et al. 2013). Of the 14 studies which used an appropriate control group for the present purposes, 11 used supplements or powders as the intervention, while 5 used food-based fortification (with 2 studies using both).

10.3.1.1 Supplement/Powder Interventions

Eleven studies used either supplements or powders as their vehicle for providing the children with multiple micronutrients. Table 10.2 summarizes the main outcome variables and findings from these studies. Multiple outcome domains were measured, including mental, motor, socio-emotional, language, executive functioning, and academic achievement. The mental and motor domains were assessed most often with mental outcomes being measured in six studies and motor outcomes in seven studies. The results of the studies which assessed mental outcomes are rather consistent, with only one study (Lima et al. 2013) reporting a significant improvement with multiple micronutrient supplementation, while five studies (Black et al. 2004; Murray-Kolb et al. 2012; Pongcharoen et al. 2011; Siegel et al. 2011; Singla et al. 2014) reported no improvements. Results from the studies which assessed motor outcomes are mixed with three (Abu-Afarwuah et al. 2007; Black et al. 2004b; Olney et al. 2006) of the seven studies (Adu-Afarwuah et al. 2007; Black et al. 2004b; Murray-Kolb et al. 2012; Olney et al. 2006; Pongcharoen et al. 2011; Singla et al. 2014; Surkan et al. 2013) reporting a significant improvement with multiple micronutrient supplementation. Language development was assessed in four of the studies (Aboud & Akhter 2011; Oelofse et al. 2003; Singla et al. 2014; Surkan et al. 2013), with two (Oelofse et al. 2003; Singla et al. 2014) reporting a benefit of multiple micronutrient supplementation. It should be noted that one of these studies enrolled only low birthweight infants (Singla et al. 2014). There are many possibilities for the mixed results such that the studies have been conducted in various settings throughout the world and have used various scales to measure the outcomes of interest as well as various assessors (investigator tested or observed, maternal report, etc.), used children of differing ages, and used different types and duration of micronutrient supplementation and that the nutritional status of participants in the studies likely varied. All of these differences make it very difficult to compare results across studies. Three studies assessed outcomes in the socio-emotional realm and the results are very consistent with all three reporting an improvement with multiple micronutrient supplementation (Aboud & Akhter 2011; Aburto et al. 2010; Black et al. 2004b). Interestingly, the length of intervention in these three studies was also similar. Two studies assessed executive functioning and neither reported improvements with multiple micronutrient supplementation (Murray-Kolb et al. 2012; Siegel et al. 2011). Only one study in this age group assessed the effects of multiple micronutrient supplementation on academic achievement, and they reported no significant improvement as a result of the supplementation (Pongcharoen et al. 2011).

TABLE 10.2
Studies Examining the Effect of Infancy and Preschool Multiple Micronutrient Supplementation Effects on Child Development

Location	n	Age at Enrollment (Months)	Intervention Duration (Months)	Age at Follow-Up (Months)	Control Group	Intervention Group(s)	Outcome Domain	Main Findings
Supplement/Powder Interventions								
Bangladesh (Black et al. 2004b)	221	6	6	12	B2	Fe, Zn, Fe + Zn, MM supplement	Mental and motor, socio-emotional	Motor development better in Fe + Zn and MM group, compared to control; orientation/engagement better in Fe, Zn, and Fe + Zn group, compared to control.
Zanzibar (Olney et al. 2006)	354	5–11	1–12	6–23	Placebo	Fe + FA, Zn, Fe + FA + Zn	Motor	Fe + FA with or without Zn reduced time it took for children to walk unassisted.
Bangladesh (Aboud & Akhter 2011)	302	8–20	6–7	16–28	Mothers received 12 information sessions on health	Mothers received six additional sessions and self-feeding and verbal responsiveness training; mothers received the same as other intervention group plus 6 months of MM-fortified food powder	Socio-emotional, language	All outcomes significantly higher in intervention versus control group; no difference between two intervention groups.

(Continued)

TABLE 10.2 (*Continued*)
Studies Examining the Effect of Infancy and Preschool Multiple Micronutrient Supplementation Effects on Child Development

Location	n	Age at Enrollment (Months)	Intervention Duration (Months)	Age at Follow-Up (Months)	Control Group	Intervention Group(s)	Outcome Domain	Main Findings
Thailand (Pongcharoen et al. 2011)	560	4–6	6	108	Placebo	Fe, Zn, Fe + Zn	Mental and motor, academic performance	No significant difference between groups on any of the outcomes; no interactions found as a result of combined Fe + Zn supplementation.
Nepal (Siegel et al. 2011)	367	12 or less	0–8.5	9 and 12	Placebo	Zn, Fe + FA, Fe + FA + Zn	Mental, executive functioning	Neither the individual nor combined MM supplements improved the performance on any outcomes.
Nepal (Murray-Kolb et al. 2012)	734	12–35	3–23	84–108	Placebo	Fe + FA, Zn, Fe + FA + Zn	Mental and motor, executive functioning	No significant differences found.

(*Continued*)

TABLE 10.2 (*Continued*)
Studies Examining the Effect of Infancy and Preschool Multiple Micronutrient Supplementation Effects on Child Development

Location	n	Age at Enrollment (Months)	Intervention Duration (Months)	Age at Follow-Up (Months)	Control Group	Intervention Group(s)	Outcome Domain	Main Findings
Brazil (Lima et al. 2013)	167	3–108	12	60 minimum; on avg. approx. 4 years after enrollment	Placebo	Glutamine, Zn, vit. A, glutamine + Zn, glutamine + vit. A, Zn + vit. A, glutamine + Zn + vit. A	Mental, language	Glutamine + Zn + vit. A group had higher verbal learning scores compared to placebo (true for girls but not for boys); glutamine + Zn + vit. A had higher verbal learning scores versus girls receiving Zn + vit. A alone (true for girls but not for boys).
Nepal (Surkan et al. 2013)	544	4–17	12	7–29	Placebo	Zn, Fe + FA, Zn + Fe + FA	Motor, language	Supplements did not improve attainment of motor or language milestones (no interaction seen for Zn + Fe + FA).

(*Continued*)

TABLE 10.2 (*Continued*)
Studies Examining the Effect of Infancy and Preschool Multiple Micronutrient Supplementation Effects on Child Development

Location	n	Age at Enrollment (Months)	Intervention Duration (Months)	Age at Follow-Up (Months)	Control Group	Intervention Group(s)	Outcome Domain	Main Findings
Bangladesh (Singla et al. 2014)	231	7–12	5	16–22	Mothers received nutrition, health, and hygiene education	Nutrition, health, and hygiene education plus MM-fortified powder	Mental and motor, language	Expressive language scores higher in MM fortified group.
Fortified Food Interventions								
S. Africa (Oelofse et al. 2003)	60	6	6	12	No intervention	MM-fortified complementary food	Motor	No benefit of MM complementary food.
India (Sazawal et al. 2004)	638	12–36	12	18–48	Unfortified milk	MM-fortified milk	Mental and motor	No significant differences between groups.
S. Africa (Faber et al. 2005)	361	6–12	6	12–18	Unfortified porridge	Fortified porridge	Motor	Higher motor scores (maternal report of milestones) in fortified group; improvement in Fe status; no change in Zn status; inconsistent results in retinol status.

(*Continued*)

TABLE 10.2 (*Continued*)
Studies Examining the Effect of Infancy and Preschool Multiple Micronutrient Supplementation Effects on Child Development

Location	n	Age at Enrollment (Months)	Intervention Duration (Months)	Age at Follow-Up (Months)	Control Group	Intervention Group(s)	Outcome Domain	Main Findings
Ghana (Adu-Afarwuah et al. 2007)[a]	313	6	6	12	No intervention	Sprinkles, nutritabs, nutributter	Motor	Lower % of control infants could walk independently compared to the three supplemented groups.
Mexico (Aburto et al. 2010)[a]	187	4–12	4	8–16	No intervention	MM-fortified milk-based food supplement, MM liquid syrup, MM powder	Socio-emotional	Liquid syrup and powder groups had increased odds of being in the high activity cluster.

[a] Studies with both a fortified food intervention and a supplement/powder intervention.

10.3.1.2 Fortified Food Interventions

Five studies used food-based fortification as the vehicle for providing the children with multiple micronutrients (Table 10.2). Multiple outcome domains were measured, including mental, motor, and socio-emotional development. The motor domain was assessed most often (four studies [Adu-Afarwuah et al. 2007; Faber et al. 2005; Oelofse et al. 2003; Sazawal et al. 2004]). Two (Adu-Afarwuah et al. 2007; Faber et al. 2005) of these four studies report an improvement in motor scores with multiple micronutrient supplementation. It should be noted that the control groups for two of these four studies (one of which reported an improvement on the motor outcome with supplementation (Adu-Afarwuah et al. 2007) were non-intervention groups and, as such, there is no true placebo group comparison). Only one of the food-based fortification studies assessed mental development (Sazawal et al. 2004) and one assessed socio-emotional development (Aburto et al. 2010). Neither report improvements in development as a result of the food-based multiple micronutrient supplementation.

10.3.1.3 Long-Term Follow-Up

Of the 14 studies providing multiple micronutrient supplementation between birth and 5 years of age, 3 studies (Lima et al. 2013; Murray-Kolb et al. 2012; Pongcharoen et al. 2011) examined child development outcomes in multiple years (4–8 years) after the intervention period. Outcomes assessed were intelligence (Lima et al. 2013; Murray-Kolb et al. 2012; Pongcharoen et al. 2011), motor functioning (Murray-Kolb et al. 2012; Pongcharoen et al. 2011), academic performance (Pongcharoen et al. 2011), and executive functioning (Murray-Kolb et al. 2012). The studies conducted in Thailand (Pongcharoen et al. 2011) and Nepal (Murray-Kolb et al. 2012) used similar supplementation schemes with the multiple micronutrient groups containing iron and zinc in the Thai study and iron, folic acid, and zinc in the Nepali study. Neither study reported an improvement in any of the outcome domains as a result of the multiple micronutrient supplementation. In contrast, the study conducted in Brazil (Lima et al. 2013) had several supplementation groups containing two or more micronutrients and one macronutrient (glutamine and zinc, glutamine and vitamin A, zinc and vitamin A, and glutamine, zinc, and vitamin A). The authors report higher verbal learning scores in the group that received glutamine, zinc, and vitamin A compared to the placebo group but only among the girls in the study. It should be noted that all of the participants in the Brazil study were below the median height-for-age Z-score and the sample sizes of each of the groups were quite small and below the necessary sample size calculated.

10.3.1.4 Summary of Early Life Supplementation

Of the 14 studies assessing the effects of multiple micronutrients given in early life, the domains of development that were most often tested were motor, mental, and language. Other outcomes assessed were socio-emotional development, executive functioning, and academic achievement. Overall, six of the studies (Murray-Kolb et al. 2012; Oelofse et al. 2003; Pongcharoen et al. 2011; Sazawal et al. 2004; Siegel et al. 2011; Surkan et al. 2013) reported no difference between the control group and the multiple micronutrient group on any of the outcomes tested, while eight studies (Aboud & Akhter 2011; Aburto et al. 2010; Adu-Afarwuah et al. 2007;

Black et al. 2004b; Faber et al. 2005; Lima et al. 2013; Olney et al. 2006; Singla et al. 2014) reported a significant improvement on at least one of the measured outcomes in the multiple micronutrient group compared with the control group. Only three studies (Lima et al. 2013; Murray-Kolb et al. 2012; Pongcharoen et al. 2011) have assessed the long-term effects of early life multiple micronutrient supplementation, with two (Murray-Kolb et al. 2012; Pongcharoen et al. 2011) reporting no differences between the supplemented groups and the placebo, and one (Lima et al. 2013) finding an improvement in verbal learning but only in a subset of the population (girls). The heterogeneity in the studies makes it difficult to directly compare the findings. The results appear equivocal but do provide some evidence that multiple micronutrient supplementation during early life may benefit child development, especially motor and socio-emotional development. There are still many unanswered questions, however, including the best combination of supplements, the best age at which to provide the supplements, the best length and dose of intervention, and the domains of development most likely to benefit. An additional question is whether or not the provision of multiple micronutrients has any differential benefit than that seen with the provision of a single micronutrient. Out of 14 studies, 7 studies (Black et al. 2004b; Lima et al. 2013; Murray-Kolb et al. 2012; Olney et al. 2006; Pongcharoen et al. 2011; Siegel et al. 2011; Surkan et al. 2013) tested both a single- and multiple micronutrient supplementation versus a control/placebo. Five of the studies (Murray-Kolb et al. 2012; Olney et al. 2006; Pongcharoen et al. 2011; Siegel et al. 2011; Surkan et al. 2013) do not report any improvements in the multiple micronutrient group that were not already seen in at least one of the single-micronutrient groups, with only two (Black et al. 2004b; Lima et al. 2013) reporting improvements in the multiple micronutrient group which were not experienced by the single-micronutrient groups.

10.3.2 Multiple Micronutrient Supplementation during School Years and Child Development

During some period between 5.5 and 16 years of age, 22 studies were identified in which children were provided with multiple micronutrients and compared to a control group and the outcomes of interest were assessed. In one study (Muthayya et al. 2009), all groups received fortified foods with the only difference being the dose (which does not allow for the determination of the influence of multiple micronutrients on the outcomes of interest). This study is, therefore, not included in our review. The 21 studies which are included were conducted in North America (3 studies) (Rico et al. 2006; Schoenthaler 1991; Schoenthaler et al. 2000), Europe (6 studies) (Benton & Buts 1990; Benton & Cook 1991; Benton & Roberts 1988; Crombie et al. 1990; Nelson et al. 1990; Snowden 1997), Africa (3 studies) (Gewa et al. 2009; Jinabhai et al. 2001; Taljaard et al. 2013), and Asia (8 studies) (Kumar & Rajagopalan 2007, 2008; Lien et al. 2009; Manger et al. 2008; Nga et al. 2011; Solon et al. 2003; Thankachan et al. 2012; Vazir et al. 2006), and 1 study was conducted in both Asia and Australia (Osendarp et al. 2007). The total number of subjects enrolled in these studies ranged from 30 to over 800, and the intervention duration for the studies ranged from 1 to 24 months. Most of the studies assessed child development at the beginning of the study as well as immediately following the intervention period. Of the 21 studies that used an appropriate control group for the present purposes, 12 used supplements or micronutrient powders added to foods such as salt as the vehicle, while nine used food-based multiple micronutrient fortification.

10.3.2.1 Supplement/Powder Interventions

Twelve studies used either supplements or powders to be added in foods for providing the children with multiple micronutrients. Table 10.3 summarizes the main outcome variables and findings from these studies. Multiple outcome domains were measured; the most frequently measured ones were intelligence, attention, and memory and those less frequently measured were processing speed, executive functioning, and academic achievement. The results of the studies that assessed intelligence are mixed, with six studies (Benton & Buts 1990; Benton & Cook 1991; Benton & Roberts 1988; Schoenthaler 1991; Schoenthaler et al. 2000; Snowden 1997) reporting a significant improvement with multiple micronutrient supplementation, while four studies (Crombie et al. 1990; Kumar & Rajagopalan 2007, 2008; Nelson et al. 1990) reported no improvements with the supplementation. Of the studies reporting an improvement with supplementation, an improvement in non-verbal intelligence as opposed to verbal intelligence was recorded for all. Results from the studies that assessed attention are also mixed, with three (Benton & Cook 1991; Kumar & Rajagopalan 2007, 2008) of the five studies (Benton & Cook 1991; Kumar & Rajagopalan 2007, 2008; Manger et al. 2008; Rico et al. 2006) reporting a significant improvement with multiple micronutrient supplementation. Memory was assessed in four of the studies and the results are more consistent, with three (Kumar & Rajagopalan 2007, 2008; Manger et al. 2008) reporting a benefit of multiple micronutrient supplementation and one (Rico et al. 2006) reporting no benefit. The mixed results which are seen for the intelligence and attention outcomes could be due to numerous possibilities including that the studies were conducted in various settings throughout the world, had differences in scales used to measure the outcomes of interest, had variable ages of the children between studies, tested several different combinations of micronutrient supplementation, had variable length of interventions, with likely varying levels of nutritional deficiencies among participants in the studies. All of these differences make it very difficult to compare the results across studies. The outcomes which were less studied were those of processing speed (Schoenthaler 1991), executive functioning (Benton & Cook 1991), and academic achievement with one study (Rico et al. 2006). None of these studies reported a significant improvement in these outcomes with multiple micronutrient supplementation.

10.3.2.2 Fortified Food Interventions

Nine studies used food-based fortification as the vehicle for providing the children with multiple micronutrients. Table 10.3 summarizes the main outcome variables and findings from these studies. Multiple outcome domains were measured, with memory, intelligence, attention, and executive functioning being assessed most often and academic achievement, learning, language abilities, and speed of processing being assessed less often. Of the studies assessing memory, three report an improvement in memory scores with multiple micronutrient supplementation

TABLE 10.3
Studies Examining the Effect of Multiple Micronutrient Supplementation during School Years and Child Development

Location	n	Age at Enrollment (Years)	Intervention Duration (Months)	Control Group	Intervention Groups	Outcome Domain	Main Findings
				Supplement/Powder Interventions			
Wales (Benton & Roberts 1988)	60	12–13	8	Placebo	No intervention Bioflavonoids, vit. A, B1, B2, B3, B6, B7, B_{12}, C, D, E, and K, choline, FA, inositol, pantothenic acid, PABA, Ca, Cr, Mg, Mn, Mo, I, Fe, Zn	Verbal and non-verbal intelligence	Significant increase in non-verbal intelligence in the MM group.
Scotland (Crombie et al. 1990)	94	11–13	7	Placebo	Bioflavonoids, vit. A, B1, B2, B3, B6, B7, B_{12}, C, D, E, and K, choline, FA, inositol, pantothenic acid, PABA, Ca, Cr, Mg, Mn, Mo, I, Fe, Zn	Verbal and non-verbal intelligence	No significant difference between groups on any of the tests.
Belgium (Benton & Buts 1990)	167	13	7	Placebo	Vit. A, B1, B2, B6, B_{12}, D2, C, and E, PP, FA, Ca, Cu, Fe, Mg, Mn, Zn	Verbal and non-verbal intelligence	Supplementation versus 'better diet' did not have a significant effect. Supplementation improved non-verbal scores in boys versus poorer diet. No difference for girls.

(Continued)

TABLE 10.3 (*Continued*)
Studies Examining the Effect of Multiple Micronutrient Supplementation during School Years and Child Development

Location	n	Age at Enrollment (Years)	Intervention Duration (Months)	Control Group	Intervention Groups	Outcome Domain	Main Findings
England (Nelson et al. 1990)	227	7–12	1	Placebo	Vit. B1, B2, B3, B5, B6, B7, B_{12}, D, E, and K, REs, FA, AA, Ca, Fe, Zn, Cr, Cu, I, Mg, Mn, Mo, Se	Verbal and non-verbal intelligence	No significant difference in performance between the groups.
Wales (Benton & Cook 1991)	47	6.5	1.5–2	Placebo	Bioflavonoids, vit. A, B1, B2, B3, B5, B6, B7, B_{12}, C, D, E, and K, choline, FA, inositol, para-aminobenzoic acid, Ca, Cr, Cu, Fe, Mg, Mn, Mo, I, Zn	Verbal and non-verbal intelligence, attention, frustration	Supplementation improved intelligence score, primarily non-verbal; supplementation improved attention.
United States (Schoenthaler 1991)	615	12–13/15–16	3	Placebo	Vit. A, B1, B2, B3, B5, B6, B7, B_{12}, D, E, C, and K, FA, Ca, Mg, Fe, Zn, I, Cu, Mn, Cr, Se, Mo At 50%, 100%, and 200% of RDA	Verbal and non-verbal intelligence; reaction time	Nonverbal scores improved (fluid intelligence) in those taking supplement providing 100% of RDA.

(*Continued*)

TABLE 10.3 (*Continued*)
Studies Examining the Effect of Multiple Micronutrient Supplementation during School Years and Child Development

Location	n	Age at Enrollment (Years)	Intervention Duration (Months)	Control Group	Intervention Groups	Outcome Domain	Main Findings
England (Snowden 1997)	30	9–10	2.5	Placebo	Bioflavonoids, vit. A, B1, B2, B3, B6, B7, B_{12}, C, D, E, and K, choline, FA, inositol, pantothenic acid, PABA, Ca, Cr, Mg, Mn, Mo, I, Fe, Zn	Verbal and non-verbal intelligence	Significant improvement in non-verbal IQ scores in supplemented group (not observed for verbal intelligence).
United States (Schoenthaler et al. 2000)	245	6–12	3	Placebo	Vit. A, D, E, C, B1, B2, B3, B5, B6, and B_{12}, FA, Fe, Zn, Cr, Mn, Mo, Se, Cu ~50% RDA	Non-verbal intelligence	Significantly higher IQ scores for those assigned to supplement.
Mexico (Rico et al. 2006)	602	6–8	6	Placebo	Fe, Zn, Fe + Zn	Receptive vocabulary, academic achievement, memory, attention, executive functioning	No significant difference between Fe + Zn group and placebo on any of the outcomes.
India (Kumar & Rajagopalan 2007)	129	7–11	12	Deworming	Deworming and fortified salt (vit. A, B1, B2, B3, B6, and B_{12}, FA, Ca, Fe, I)	Memory, attention, intelligence	Memory and attention improved significantly in experimental group, intelligence did not.

(*Continued*)

TABLE 10.3 (*Continued*)
Studies Examining the Effect of Multiple Micronutrient Supplementation during School Years and Child Development

Location	n	Age at Enrollment (Years)	Intervention Duration (Months)	Control Group	Intervention Groups	Outcome Domain	Main Findings
India (Kumar & Rajagopalan 2008)	123	7–11	12	No intervention	Fortified sprinkles (vit. A, B2, B3, B6, B_{12}, C, and E, FA, Fe, Ca, lysine)	Memory, attention, intelligence	Memory and attention improved significantly in experimental group, intelligence did not.
Thailand (Manger et al. 2008)	569	5.5–13.4	7	Unfortified powder	Fortified seasoning powder (vit. A, Fe, I, Zn)	Learning, memory, attention	Memory improved significantly in experimental group; no significant difference between groups for other outcomes.
Fortified Food Interventions							
S. Africa (Jinabhai et al. 2001)	579	8–10	4	Not dewormed unfortified biscuits	Dewormed, fortified biscuits (vit. A and B, Fe, Ca, Zn) Dewormed, biscuits with vit. A Dewormed, non-fortified biscuits Not dewormed, MM-fortified biscuits (vit. A and B, Fe, Ca, Zn) Not dewormed biscuits with vit. A	Intelligence; memory; attention; academic achievement	No significant differences between groups on any of the outcomes.

(*Continued*)

TABLE 10.3 (*Continued*)
Studies Examining the Effect of Multiple Micronutrient Supplementation during School Years and Child Development

Location	n	Age at Enrollment (Years)	Intervention Duration (Months)	Control Group	Intervention Groups	Outcome Domain	Main Findings
Philippines (Solon et al. 2003)	851	7–12	4	Non-fortified beverage and placebo antihelminthic therapy	Fortified beverage (vit. A, B2, B3, B6, B_{12}, C, and E, FA, Fe, I, Zn) and antihelminthic therapy Fortified beverage (vit. A, B2, B3, B6, B_{12}, C, and E, FA, Fe, I, Zn) and placebo antihelminthic therapy Non-fortified beverage and antihelminthic therapy	Verbal and non-verbal intelligence; quantitative	Consuming MM-fortified beverage did not result in any difference in cognitive changes overall; however, those who were anaemic and iodine deficient at baseline showed significant increases in total, non-verbal, and verbal abilities; changes in quantitative scores were inconsistent; antihelminthic treatment showed no or a negative effect.
India (Vazir et al. 2006)	608	6–15	14	Beverage with macronutrients (same profile as treatment group)	Fortified beverage (vit. A, B1, B2, B3, B6, B_{12}, C, and D, folate, Ca, Fe, Zn) and macronutrients	Intelligence, attention, memory, academic achievement	Supplementation improved attention scores, but none of the other outcomes were different between groups.

(Continued)

TABLE 10.3 (*Continued*)
Studies Examining the Effect of Multiple Micronutrient Supplementation during School Years and Child Development

Location	n	Age at Enrollment (Years)	Intervention Duration (Months)	Control Group	Intervention Groups	Outcome Domain	Main Findings
Australia/ Indonesia (Osendarp et al. 2007)	396 in Australia and 384 in Indonesia	6–10	12	Unfortified beverage	Fortified beverage (vit. A, B6, B_{12}, and C, FA, Fe, Zn) Fortified beverage with EPA, DHA MM-fortified beverage (vit. A, B6, B_{12}, and C, FA, Fe, Zn) plus EPA and DHA	Executive functioning, memory, attention, non-verbal reasoning, verbal learning/memory, academic achievement, language development	MM supplementation improved verbal learning and memory in Australia (also seen in girls in Indonesia). No effects of DHA/EPA on cognition were seen.
Kenya (Gewa et al. 2009)	554	6.3–8.9	24	No intervention	Vegetarian supplement based on maize, beans, and vegetables Milk supplement Meat supplement	Intelligence	Those who received meat supplement scored better than control, vegetarian, and milk.
Vietnam (Lien et al. 2009)	454	7–8	6	No intervention	Regular milk Fortified milk (vit. A, D, E, B1, and B2, inulin, taurine, Ca, Fe, Zn, I, Mn, Mg)	Memory	Those who drank milk had better memory scores than those who did not, fortified milk group had the best scores.

(*Continued*)

TABLE 10.3 (*Continued*)
Studies Examining the Effect of Multiple Micronutrient Supplementation during School Years and Child Development

Location	n	Age at Enrollment (Years)	Intervention Duration (Months)	Control Group	Intervention Groups	Outcome Domain	Main Findings
Vietnam (Nga et al. 2011)	510	6–8	4	Non-fortified biscuit	Fortified biscuit (vit. A, B1, B2, B3, B5, B6, B_{12}, C, D3, E, and K, biotin, FA, Ca, Mg, Se, K, P, Fe, I, Zn) Fortified biscuit (same as earlier) plus deworming	Intelligence, memory, attention, speed of processing, executive functioning	Groups consuming the fortified biscuits scored better on cognitive performance and attention tasks compared to other groups; deworming had no significant effect on scores.
India (Thankachan et al. 2012)	258	6–12	6	Unfortified rice	Fortified rice (low iron and vit. A, B1, B3, B6, and B_{12}, FA, Zn) Fortified rice (high iron and vit. A, B1, B3, B6, and B_{12}, FA, Zn)	Attention, memory, language, spatial abilities, executive functioning	None of the cognitive outcomes were different between groups at end line.
S. Africa (Taljaard et al. 2013)	414	6–11	8.5	Control beverage with non-nutritive sweetener	Control beverage with sugar Fortified beverage (vit. A, B2, B3, B6, B_{12}, C, and E, FA, Ca, Fe, I, Zn) and sugar-fortified beverage (vit. A, B2, B3, B6, B_{12}, C, and E, FA, Ca, Fe, I, Zn) and non-nutritive sweetener	Learning, memory, executive functioning	Groups with just sugar, just micronutrients, or both had higher cognitive scores than the control group; there was a sugar*micronutrients interaction that attenuated the findings.

(Lien et al. 2009; Osendarp et al. 2007; Taljaard et al. 2013); one of these studies reported an improvement in their Australian population, an improvement only seen in the girls in their counterpart Indonesian study (Osendarp et al. 2007). In contrast, four (Jinabhai et al. 2001; Nga et al. 2011; Thankachan et al. 2012; Vazir et al. 2006) indicated no improvement with multiple micronutrient supplementation. Five out of the nine food-based fortification studies assessed intelligence as an outcome. Two of these studies report an improvement with multiple micronutrient fortification (Gewa et al. 2009; Solon et al. 2003), while three (Jinabhai et al. 2001; Nga et al. 2011; Vazir et al. 2006) report no significant improvement (although, in one study reporting no significant improvement, stratification revealed a significant improvement in those who were anaemic at baseline and received the multiple micronutrients (Solon et al. 2003). It should be noted that one of the studies reporting an improvement used various food-based interventions (vegetarian based, milk based, meat based), so it is difficult to know what exactly is responsible for the differences between groups (Gewa et al. 2009). Five of the food-based fortification studies also assessed attention as an outcome and, once again, two report an improvement in attention with multiple micronutrients (Nga et al. 2011; Vazir et al. 2006), while three (Jinabhai et al. 2001; Osendarp et al. 2007; Thankachan et al. 2012) report no such findings. The four studies that assessed executive functioning as an outcome all report no improvement after multiple micronutrient treatment (Osendarp et al. 2007; Nga et al. 2011; Thankachan et al. 2012; Taljaard et al. 2013). Of the outcomes that were less measured, the studies reporting on academic achievement (Jinabhai et al. 2001; Osendarp et al. 2007; Vazir et al. 2006), language abilities (Osendarp et al. 2007; Thankachan et al. 2012), and speed of processing (Nga et al. 2011), all report no improvement with multiple micronutrients. However, the two studies that assessed learning both report an improvement as a result of the food-based multiple micronutrient supplementation (Osendarp et al. 2007; Taljaard et al. 2013).

10.3.2.3 Summary of School-Age Child Supplementation

Of the 21 studies assessing the effects of multiple micronutrients given during the school years, the cognitive domains which were most often tested were intelligence, memory, attention, and executive functioning. Other outcomes assessed were academic achievement, learning, language abilities, and speed of processing. Overall, 6 of the studies reported no difference between the control group and the multiple micronutrient group on any of the outcomes tested (Crombie et al. 1990; Jinabhai et al. 2001; Nelson et al. 1990; Rico et al. 2006; Solon et al. 2003; Thankachan et al. 2012), while 15 studies reported a significant improvement on at least one of the measured outcomes in the multiple micronutrient group compared to the control group (Benton & Buts 1990; Benton & Cook 1991; Benton & Roberts 1988; Gewa et al. 2009; Kumar & Rajagopalan 2007, 2008; Lien et al. 2009; Manger et al. 2008; Nga et al. 2011; Osendarp et al. 2007; Schoenthaler 1991; Schoenthaler et al. 2000; Snowden 1997; Taljaard et al. 2013; Vazir et al. 2006). It is difficult to directly compare most of the studies, given the heterogeneity that exists between studies. When analyzed as a whole, results from multiple micronutrient supplementation trials in children during the school years appear to provide some evidence that such supplementation during this period in life may benefit child cognitive abilities, with most evidence for the outcomes of intelligence and memory. However, more evidence is needed on the best combination of supplements, the best age at which to provide the supplements, the best length and dose of intervention, and the domains of cognition most likely to be impacted. As with supplementation in early life, an additional question is which micronutrient specifically had an impact and whether all micronutrients are equally essential. Of the 21 studies reviewed here, 20 did not contain one or more groups that received a single micronutrient, so this question could not be assessed in most of the studies. The one study that contained both single-micronutrient (an iron group and a zinc group) and multiple micronutrient groups (iron plus zinc) does not report any differential improvements in the multiple micronutrient group that were not seen in at least one of the single-micronutrient groups (Rico et al. 2006).

10.4 COMBINED EFFECTS OF MATERNAL AND PRESCHOOL MULTIPLE MICRONUTRIENT INTERVENTIONS

The majority of studies examining the effects of multiple micronutrient interventions on mental and motor development provided supplementation to the child during early life or the school years. There are some studies (reviewed in the previous text), which supplemented the mother, during pregnancy, and subsequently measured child cognitive development, after birth. Only one study, thus far, has reported on the combined effects of micronutrient supplementation during pregnancy and the preschool years on later cognitive abilities (Christian et al. 2011). In an examination of the effects of multiple micronutrient supplementation, the study team reported improvements in mental, motor, and executive functioning outcomes in school-aged children who had received iron–folic acid in utero (Christian et al. 2010). We also reported no long-term cognitive effect of micronutrient supplementation when the supplementation occurred during the preschool years (Murray-Kolb et al. 2012). To examine the combined effects of supplementation occurring in utero and during the preschool years, the authors designated the in utero iron–folic acid group as the control group (given the previous findings of better cognitive development in the children receiving this supplementation). We then compared children who received the iron–folic acid in utero (but no supplementation during the preschool years) to (1) those who received iron–folic acid in utero plus iron–folic acid during the preschool years as well as (2) those who received iron–folic acid in utero plus iron–folic acid–zinc during the preschool years. The combined supplementation (in utero and during the preschool years) did not impact scores on general intelligence nor executive functioning when compared to the *in utero* supplementation alone. For the domains of memory and motor functioning, the children who received in utero supplementation with iron–folic acid and preschool supplementation with iron–folic acid–zinc scored lower than those who received just the in utero supplementation. Also, on one of the fine motor outcomes, lower scores were reported in children who received iron–folic acid both in utero and during the preschool years compared to those who received the supplementation only *in utero*. The authors concluded that supplementation with multiple micronutrients (iron, folic acid, zinc) during the preschool years does not provide any additional cognitive benefit to children, when compared to in utero supplementation of iron–folic acid. They also indicate that the timing of the preschool supplementation (which did not start until 12 months of age), may have been a factor in the findings.

10.5 CONCLUSION

Micronutrient deficiencies in under-resourced contexts exist and affect in some cases large swathes of populations during the critical periods of early growth and development.

Strategies for improving micronutrient status are increasingly being applied in many programmatic contexts due to the evidence related to many functional benefits including improved pregnancy-related health, birth outcomes, and infant and child growth. Food fortification, supplementation, and dietary diversification, among others, are all approaches which are used singly or in complementary fashion to ameliorate the large burden of hidden hunger, globally. Among strategies, supplementation with multiple micronutrients during pregnancy and through the use of powders admixed with complementary foods in young children is simple, cost-effective, delivers up to an RDA of a range of essential vitamins and minerals, and has the potential for high coverage in many settings. Our chapter was undertaken to examine whether such micronutrient supplementation approaches benefit outcomes of child development. Our critical review of the literature revealed the following key findings:

- Prenatal supplementation with multiple micronutrients has not been examined extensively for its impact on childhood outcomes. Some evidence exists to show short-term benefits in early infancy/childhood, but long-term benefits are equivocal. Rather, smaller combinations which included iron–folic acid had wide-ranging benefits across multiple domains of outcomes, based on one rigorous trial.
- With regard to multiple micronutrient supplementation during early postnatal life, there may be some benefit on outcomes of motor and socio-emotional development although the heterogeneity of studies makes it hard to generalize the findings.
- Results from multiple micronutrient supplementation trials in children during the school years provide some evidence that supplementation during this period in life may benefit child cognitive abilities, with most evidence for the outcomes of intelligence and memory.
- Overall data are lacking or limited on the best timing and the right combination of micronutrients that will benefit specific domains of child developmental outcomes.

Despite the limited evidence for clear benefits, future research, policy, and programmatic efforts are likely to continue to examine multiple micronutrient supplementation strategies in settings where deficiencies are common. These will allow future studies to continue to examine the benefit of such strategies on child developmental outcomes. Also important is to seize the opportunity to conduct follow-up cognitive and developmental assessments in the numerous trials of prenatal multiple micronutrient interventions to further evaluate the long-term effects on child development, in addition to including assessments of child developmental outcomes in new micronutrient intervention studies being planned in the future.

REFERENCES

Aboud FE & Akhter S. (2011) A cluster-randomized evaluation of a responsive stimulation and feeding intervention in Bangladesh. *Pediatrics.* 127(5). 1191–1197.

Aburto NJ, Ramirez-Zea M, Neufeld LM, & Flores-Ayala R. (2010) The effect of nutritional supplementation on physical activity and exploratory behavior of Mexican infants aged 8–12 months. *Eur J Clin Nutr.* 64(6). 644–651.

Adu-Afarwuah S, Lartey A, Brown KH, Zlotkin S, Briend A, & Dewey KG. (2007) Randomized comparison of 3 types of micronutrient supplements for home fortification of complementary foods in Ghana: Effects on growth and motor development. *Am J Clin Nutr.* 86(2). 412–420.

Anjos T, Altmäe S, Emmett P, Tiemeier H, Closa-Monasterolo R, Luque V, Wiseman S et al. (2013) Nutrition and neurodevelopment in children: Focus on NUTRIMENTHE project. *Eur J Nutr.* 52(8). 1825–1842.

Benton D & Buts JP. (1990) Vitamin/mineral supplementation and intelligence. *Lancet.* 335(8698). 1158–1160.

Benton D & Cook R. (1991) Vitamin and mineral supplements improve the intelligence scores and concentration of six-year-old children. *Pers Individ Diff.* 12(11). 1151–1158.

Benton D & Roberts G. (1988) Effect of vitamin and mineral supplementation on intelligence of a sample of schoolchildren. *Lancet.* 1(8578). 140–143.

Black MM, Baqui AH, Zaman K, Ake Persson L, El Arifeen S, Le K, McNary SW, Parveen M, Hamadani JD, & Black RE. (2004a) Iron and zinc supplementation promote motor development and exploratory behavior among Bangladeshi infants. *Am J Clin Nutr.* 80(4). 903–910.

Black MM, Sazawal S, Black RE, Khosla S, Kumar J, & Menon V. (2004b) Cognitive and motor development among small-for-gestational-age infants: Impact of zinc supplementation, birth weight, and caregiving practices. *Pediatrics.* 113(5). 1297–1305.

Black RE, Victora CG, Walker SP, Bhutta A, Christian P, de Onis M, Ezzati M et al. (2013) Maternal and child undernutrition over overweight in low-income and middle-income countries. *Lancet.* 382(9890). 427–451.

Caulfield LE, Putnick DL, Zavaleta N, Lazarte F, Albornoz C, Chen P, Dipietro JA, & Bornstein MH. (2010) Maternal gestational zinc supplementation does not influence multiple aspects of child development at 54 mo of age in Peru. *Am J Clin Nutr.* 92(1). 130–136.

Chen K, Zhang X, Wei XP, Qu P, Liu YX, & Li TY. (2009) Antioxidant vitamin status during pregnancy in relation to cognitive development in the first two years of life. *Early Hum Dev.* 85(7). 421–427.

Christian P, Khatry SK, Katz J, Pradhan EK, LeClerq SC, Shrestha SR, Adhikari RK, Sommer A, & West KP Jr. (2003) Effects of alternative maternal micronutrient supplements on low birth weight in rural Nepal: Double blind randomised community trial. *BMJ.* 326(7389). 571.

Christian P, Morgan M, Murray-Kolb L, LeClerq SC, Khatry SK, Schaefer B, Cole PM, Katz J, & Tielsch JM. (2011) Preschool iron-folic acid and zinc supplementation in children exposed to iron-folic acid in utero confers no added cognitive benefit in early school-age. *J Nutr.* 141(11). 2042–2048.

Christian P, Murray-Kolb LE, Khatry SK, Katz J, Schaefer BA, Cole PM, Leclerq SC, & Tielsch JM. (2010) Prenatal micronutrient supplementation and intellectual and motor function in early school-aged children in Nepal. *JAMA*. 304(24). 2716–2723.

Christian P, Murray-Kolb LE, Tielsch JM, Katz J, LeClerq SC, & Khatry SK. (2014) Associations between preterm birth, small-for-gestational age, and neonatal morbidity and cognitive function among school-age children in Nepal. *BMC Pediatr.* 14. 58.

Christian P & Stewart CP. (2010) Maternal micronutrient deficiency, fetal development, and the risk of chronic disease. *J Nutr.* 140(3). 437–445.

Christian P, West KP Jr, Khatry SK, Katz J, LeClerq S, Pradhan EK, & Shrestha SR. (1998) Vitamin A or beta-carotene supplementation reduces but does not eliminate maternal night blindness in Nepal. *J Nutr.* 128(9). 1458–1463.

Colombo J, Zavaleta N, Kannass KN, Lazarte F, Albornoz C, Kapa LL, & Caulfield LE. (2014) Zinc supplementation sustained normative neurodevelopment in a randomized, controlled trial of Peruvian infants aged 6–18 months. *J Nutr.* 144(8). 1298–1305.

Crombie IK, Todman J, McNeill G, Florey CD, Menzies I, & Kennedy RA. (1990) Effect of vitamin and mineral supplementation on verbal and non-verbal reasoning of schoolchildren. *Lancet.* 335(8692). 744–747.

Das JK, Salam RA, Kumar R, & Bhutta ZA. (2013) Micronutrient fortification of food and its impact on women and child health: A systematic review. *Syst Rev.* 2. 67.

De-Regil LM, Suchdev PS, Vist GE, Walleser S, & Pena-Rosas JP. (2013) Home fortification of foods with multiple micronutrient powders for health and nutrition in children under two years of age (review). *Evid Based Child Health.* 8(1). 112–201.

Faber M, Kvalsvig JD, Lombard CJ, & Benadé AJS. (2005) Effect of a fortified maize-meal porridge on anemia, micronutrient status, and motor development of infants. *Am J Clin Nutr.* 82(5). 1032–1039.

Georgieff MK. (2007) Nutrition and the developing brain: Nutrient priorities and measurement. *Am J Clin Nutr.* 85(2). 614S–620S.

Gewa CA, Weiss RE, Bwibo NO, Whaley S, Sigman M, Murphy SP, Harrison G, & Neumann CG. (2009) Dietary micronutrients are associated with higher cognitive function gains among primary school children in rural Kenya. *Br J Nutr.* 101(9). 1378–1387.

Haidar BA & Bhutta ZA. (2012) Multiple-micronutrient supplementation for women during pregnancy. *Cochrane Database Syst Rev.* (11). CD004905.

Jinabhai CC, Taylor M, Coutsoudis A, Coovadia HM, Tomkins AM, & Sullivan KR. (2001) A health and nutritional profile of rural school children in KwaZulu-Natal, South Africa. *Ann Trop Paediatr.* 21(1). 50–58.

Kumar MV & Rajagopalan S. (2007) Multiple micronutrient fortification of salt and its effect on cognition in Chennai school children. *Asia Pac J Clin Nutr.* 16(3). 505–511.

Kumar MV & Rajagopalan S. (2008) Trial using multiple micronutrient food supplement and its effect on cognition. *Indian J Pediatr.* 75(7). 671–678.

Lee AC, Katz J, Blencowe H, Cousens S, Kozuki N, Vogel JP, Adair L et al. (2013) National and regional estimates of term and preterm babies born small for gestational age in 138 low-income and middle-income countries in 2010. *Lancet Glob Health.* 1(1). e26–e36.

Levenson CW & Morris D. (2011) Zinc and neurogenesis: Making new neurons from development to adulthood. *Adv Nutr.* 2(2). 96–100.

Li Q, Yan H, Zeng L, Cheng Y, Liang W, Dang S, Wang Q, & Tsuji I. (2009) Effects of maternal multimicronutrient supplementation on the mental development of infants in rural western China: Follow-up evaluation of a double-blind, randomized, controlled trial. *Pediatrics.* 123(4). e685–e692.

Lien DTK, Nhung BT, Khan NC, Hop le T, Nga NT, Hung NT, Kiers J, Shigeru Y, & te Biesebeke R. (2009) Impact of milk consumption on performance and health of primary school children in rural Vietnam. *Asia Pac J Clin Nutr.* 18(3). 326–334.

Lima AAM, Kvalsund MP, de Souza PPE, Figueiredo ÍL, Soares AM, Mota RM, Lima NL et al. (2013) Zinc, vitamin A, and glutamine supplementation in Brazilian shantytown children at risk for diarrhea results in sex-specific improvements in verbal learning. *Clinics (Sao Paulo).* 68(3). 351–358.

Lu WP, Lu MS, Li ZH, & Zhang CX. (2014) Effects of multimicronutrient supplementation during pregnancy on postnatal growth of children under 5 years of age: A meta-analysis of randomized controlled trials. *PLoS One.* 9(2). e88496.

Manger MS, McKenzie JE, Winichagoon P, Gray A, Chavasit V, Pongcharoen T, Gowachirapant S, Ryan B, Wasantwisut E, & Gibson RS. (2008) A micronutrient-fortified seasoning powder reduces morbidity and improves short-term cognitive function, but has no effect on anthropometric measures in primary school children in northeast Thailand: A randomized controlled trial. *Am J Clin Nutr.* 87(6). 1715–1722.

Manno D, Kowa PK, Bwalya HK, Siame J, Grantham-McGregor S, Baisley K, De Stavola BL, Jaffar S, & Filteau S. (2012) Rich micronutrient fortification of locally produced infant food does not improve mental and motor development of Zambian infants: A randomised controlled trial. *Br J Nutr.* 107(4). 556–566.

McGrath N, Bellinger D, Robins J, Msamanga GI, Tronick E, & Fawzi WW. (2006) Effect of maternal multivitamin supplementation on the mental and psychomotor development of children who are born to HIV-1-infected mothers in Tanzania. *Pediatrics.* 117(2). e216–e225.

Morse NL. (2012) Benefits of docosahexaenoic acid, folic acid, vitamin D and iodine on foetal and infant brain development and function following maternal supplementation during pregnancy and lactation. *Nutrients.* 4(7). 799–840.

Murray-Kolb LE, Khatry SK, Katz J, Schaefer BA, Cole PM, LeClerq SC, Morgan ME, Tielsch JM, & Christian P. (2012) Preschool micronutrient supplementation effects on intellectual and motor function in school-aged Nepalese children. *Arch Pediatr Adolesc Med.* 166(5). 404–410.

Muthayya S, Eilander A, Transler C, Thomas T, van der Knaap HC, Srinivasan K, van Klinken BJ, Osendarp SJ, & Kurpad AV. (2009) Effect of fortification with multiple micronutrients and n-3 fatty acids on growth and cognitive performance in Indian schoolchildren: The CHAMPION (Children's Health and Mental Performance Influenced by Optimal Nutrition) study. *Am J Clin Nutr.* 89(6). 1766–1775.

Nelson M, Naismith DJ, Burley V, Gatenby S, & Geddes N. (1990) Nutrient intakes, vitamin-mineral supplementation, and intelligence in British schoolchildren. *Br J Nutr.* 64(1). 13–22.

Nga TT, Winichagoon P, Dijkhuizen MA, Khan NC, Wasantwisut E, & Wieringa FT. (2011) Decreased parasite load and improved cognitive outcomes caused by deworming and consumption of multi-micronutrient fortified biscuits in rural Vietnamese schoolchildren. *Am J Trop Med Hyg.* 85(2). 333–340.

Oelofse A, Van Raaij JM, Benade AJ, Dhansay MA, Tolboom JJ, & Hautvast JG. (2003) The effect of a micronutrient-fortified complementary food on micronutrient status, growth and development of 6- to 12-month-old disadvantaged urban South African infants. *Int J Food Sci Nutr.* 54(5). 399–407.

Olney DK, Pollitt E, Kariger PK, Khalfan SS, Ali NS, Tielsch JM, Sazawal S, Black R, Allen LH, & Stoltzfus RJ. (2006) Combined iron and folic acid supplementation with or without zinc reduces time to walking unassisted among Zanzibari infants 5- to 11-mo old. *J Nutr.* 136(9). 2427–2434.

Osendarp SJ, Baghurst KI, Bryan J, Calvaresi E, Hughes D, Hussaini M, Karyadi SJ et al. (2007) Effect of a 12-mo micronutrient intervention on learning and memory in well-nourished and marginally nourished school-aged children: 2 parallel, randomized, placebo-controlled studies in Australia and Indonesia. *Am J Clin Nutr.* 86(4). 1082–1093.

Pongcharoen T, DiGirolamo AM, Ramakrishnan U, Winichagoon P, Flores R, & Martorell R. (2011) Long-term effects of iron and zinc supplementation during infancy on cognitive function at 9 y of age in northeast Thai children: a follow-up study. *Am J Clin Nutr.* 93(3). 636–643.

Prado EL, Alock KJ, Muadz H, Ullman MT, & Shankar AH. (2012) Maternal multiple micronutrient supplements and child cognition: A randomized trial in Indonesia. *Pediatrics.* 130(3). e536–e546.

Prado EL & Dewey KG. (2014) Nutrition and brain development in early life. *Nutr Rev.* 72(4). 267–287.

Ramakrishnan U, Grant FK, Goldenberg T, Bui V, Imdad A, & Bhutta ZA. (2012) Effect of multiple micronutrient supplementation on pregnancy and infant outcomes: A systematic review. *Paediatr Perinat Epidemiol.* 26(Suppl 1). 153–167.

Rico JA, Kordas K, López P, Rosado JL, Vargas GG, Ronquillo D, & Stoltzfus RJ. (2006) Efficacy of iron and/or zinc supplementation on cognitive performance of lead-exposed mexican schoolchildren: A randomized, placebo-controlled trial. *Pediatrics.* 117(3). e518–e527.

Sazawal S, Dhingra P, Menon VP, Vernma P, Sood M, Juyal R, Sarkar A, Black M, Kumar J, & Black RE. (2004) P1169 Effect of zinc and iron fortification of milk along with vitamin C, E and A on development, activity and growth of children over one year follow up – A community based double masked randomized controlled trial. *J Pediatr Gastroenterol Nutr.* 39(Suppl 1). ps501.

Schoenthaler S. (1991) Brains and vitamins. *Lancet.* 337(8743). 728–729.

Schoenthaler SJ, Bier ID, Young K, Nichols D, & Jansenns S. (2000) The effect of vitamin-mineral supplementation on the intelligence of American schoolchildren: A randomized, double-blind placebo-controlled trial. *J Altern Complement Med.* 6(1). 19–29.

Siegel EH, Kordas K, Stoltzfus RJ, Katz J, Khatry SK, LeClerq SC, & Tielsch JM. (2011) Inconsistent effects of iron-folic acid and/or zinc supplementation on the cognitive development of infants. *J Health Popul Nutr.* 29(6). 593–604.

Singla DR, Shafique S, Zlotkin SH, & Aboud FE. (2014) A 22-element micronutrient powder benefits language but not cognition in Bangladeshi full-term low-birth-weight children. *J Nutr.* 144(11). 1803–1810.

Snowden W. (1997) Evidence from an analysis of 2000 errors and omissions made in IQ tests by a small sample of schoolchildren, undergoing vitamin and mineral supplementation, that speed of processing is an important factor in IQ performance. *Pers Individ Diff.* 22(1). 131–134.

Solon FS, Sarol JN, Bernardo ABI, Solon JA, Mehansho H, Sanchez-Fermin LE, Wambangco LS, & Juhlin KD. (2003) Effect of a multiple-micronutrient-fortified fruit powder beverage on the nutrition status, physical fitness, and cognitive performance of schoolchildren in the Philippines. *Food Nutr Bull.* 24(Suppl 4). 129–140.

Surkan PJ, Siegel EH, Patel SA, Katz K, Khatry SK, Stoltzfus RJ, LeClerq SC, & Tielsch JM. (2013) Effects of zinc and iron supplementation fail to improve motor and language milestone scores of infants and toddlers. *Nutrition.* 29(3). 542–548.

Taljaard C, Covic NM, van Graan AE, Kruger HS, Smuts CM, Baumgartner J, Kvalsvig JD, Wright HH, van Stuijvenberg ME, & Jerling JC. (2013) Effects of a multi-micronutrient-fortified beverage, with and without sugar, on growth and cognition in South African schoolchildren: A randomised, double-blind, controlled intervention. *Br J Nutr.* 110(12). 2271–2284.

Thankachan P, Rah JK, Thomas T, Selvam S, Amalrajan V, Srinivasan K, Steiger G, & Kurpad AV. (2012) Multiple micronutrient-fortified rice affects physical performances and plasma vitamin B-12 and homocysteine concentrations of Indian school children. *J Nutr.* 142(5). 846–852.

Vazir S, Nagalla B, Thangiah V, Kamasamudram V, & Bhattiprolu S. (2006) Effect of micronutrient supplement on health and nutritional status of schoolchildren: Mental function. *Nutrition.* 22(Suppl 1). s26–s32.

Veena SR, Krishnaveni GV, Srinivasan K, Srinivasan K, Wills AK, Muthaya S, Kurpad A Yajnik C, & Fall CHD. (2010) Higher maternal plasma folate but not vitamin B-12 concentrations during pregnancy are associated with better cognitive function scores in 9–10 year old children in South-India. *J Nutr.* 140(5). 1014–1022.

Villamor E, Rifas-Shiman SL, Gillman MW, & Oken E. (2012) Maternal intake of methyl-donor nutrients and child cognition at 3 years of age. *Paediatr Perinat Epidemiol.* 26(4). 328–335.

Walker SP, Wachs TD, Grantham-McGregor S, Black MM, Nelson CA, Huffman SL, Baker-Henningham H et al. (2011) Inequality in early childhood: Risk and protective factors for early child development. *Lancet.* 378(9799). 1325–1338.

West KP Jr, Christian P, Katz J, Labrique A, Klemm R, & Sommer A. (2010) Effect of vitamin A supplementation on maternal survival. *Lancet.* 376(9744). 873–874.

Williams, G.R. (2008) Neurodevelopmental and neurophysiological actions of thyroid hormone. *J Neuroendocrinol.* 20(6). 784–794.

11 Early Brain Development

Influence of Integrated Nutrition, Child Development, and Environmental Factors

Maureen M. Black and Jennifer M. Reid

CONTENTS

11.1 INTRODUCTION

The origins of adult health and well-being stem from genetic–environmental interactions that begin in the first 1000 days (conception through 24 months) (Pongcharoen et al. 2012; Shonkoff & Garner 2012). Children with adequate nutrition and opportunities for early learning and responsive caregiving have the best chances of thriving. In contrast, children raised in adverse conditions, characterized by poverty, nutritional deprivation, and limited access to opportunities for early learning and responsive caregiving, are at risk for negative health and social outcomes throughout their life course, including chronic diseases, mental illness, and lack of economic productivity. Estimates have found that over one-third of children under the age of 5 years in low- and middle-income countries (LMIC) are disadvantaged (not reaching their developmental potential) due to poverty, stunting, nutritional deficiencies, and lack of opportunities for early learning and responsive caregiving (Grantham-McGregor et al. 2007).

The global community is becoming increasingly aware of the threat that poverty, nutritional deprivation, and lack of opportunities for learning and responsive caregiving are having on children and ultimately on societies. This chapter focuses on associations among nutrition, environment, and brain development in LMIC, where the deficiencies and threats are the greatest. Section 11.2 examines relations among child development, poverty, and nutritional deprivation (stunting). Section 11.3 examines how prenatal maternal nutrition relates to children's brain development and functioning. Section 11.4 examines associations among specific nutritional deficiencies in early life and children's early brain development. Section 11.5 examines the evidence on early interventions designed to overcome the nutritional and environmental threats and to promote early child development.

11.2 BRAIN DEVELOPMENT, CHILD DEVELOPMENT, POVERTY, AND STUNTING

11.2.1 Brain Development

Brain development begins shortly after conception with the formation and closure of the neural tube by the 28th day (Cavalli 2008), a process that is dependent on adequate nutrition, particularly folic acid, and occurs before many women have recognized that they are pregnant. Cell division occurs during gestation and, through migration, cells become specialized. Synapses, or connections, are formed between cells. Through the process of synaptogenesis and pruning, neural pathways are formed and eliminated. This process extends through childhood and is influenced by experience in an activation-dependent 'use it or lose it' process (Johnson 2001). Early brain development occurs rapidly and is characterized by both vulnerability and plasticity. Nutrients have specific effects on specific areas of the developing brain and are influenced by the timing of development, the dose of the nutrient available, and the duration of availability (Georgieff 2007). Table 11.1 illustrates the role of key nutrients that have been associated with neurodevelopment during fetal and neonatal brain development.

TABLE 11.1
Important Nutrients during Late Fetal and Neonatal Brain Development

Nutrient	Brain Requirement for the Nutrient	Predominant Brain Circuitry or Process Affected by Deficiency
Protein energy	Cell proliferation, cell differentiation	Global
	Synaptogenesis	Cortex
	Growth factor synthesis	Hippocampus
Iron	Myelin	White matter
	Monoamine synthesis	Striatal–frontal
	Neuronal and glial energy metabolism	Hippocampal–frontal
Zinc	DNA synthesis	Autonomic nervous system
	Neurotransmitter release	Hippocampus, cerebellum
Copper	Neurotransmitter synthesis, neuronal and glial energy metabolism, antioxidant activity	Cerebellum
LC-PUFAs	Synaptogenesis	Eye
	Myelin	Cortex
Choline	Neurotransmitter synthesis	Global
	DNA methylation	Hippocampus
	Myelin synthesis	White matter

Source: Georgieff, M.K., *Am. J. Clin. Nutr.*, 85(2), 614S, 2007.

11.2.2 Child Development

Child development is a maturational and interactive process whereby children acquire an orderly progression of motor, cognitive, language, and socio-emotional skills. The order of the skills is similar across cultures, but the timing of skill acquisition may vary. In addition, children acquire culture-specific attitudes, approaches, and behaviours that guide interpersonal relationships and personality development.

The recognition that the link between nutritional deprivation and child development depends on non-nutritional factors and can be influenced by environmental opportunities has had an important impact on research involving nutritionally deprived children. Caregiving variables, such as the quality of parent–child interaction, have been incorporated into models of child development, moving away from models that merely control for socio-economic differences (Sameroff 2009).

Interactions between children and parents are conceptualized through a transactional system that emphasizes the active contributions of children. Parents' reactions to their children are influenced by perceptions, such as their children's size, health status, and temperament. Likewise, parents serve as a buffer and mediator between environmental factors and children's development (Sameroff 2009). Applied to nutrition, the transactional system provides the conceptual grounding for responsive feeding (Black & Aboud 2011). Responsive feeding refers to the interactive nature of feeding, whereby caregivers establish mealtime patterns and rules and react to their child's signals promptly, and in a developmentally appropriate and respectful manner (Black & Hurley 2007). Unresponsive feeding interactions are characterized either by negative, coercive strategies to promote eating or by permissive, overindulgent strategies. These strategies are likely to undermine children's appetite, increasing mealtime stress as children hold out for snacks.

11.2.3 Poverty

Multiple studies have reported negative associations between poverty and children's cognitive and brain functioning (Duncan & Magnuson 2012; Luby et al. 2013). Until recently, a principal explanation for the association was thought to be limited access to resources. For example, stunting and poor weight gain throughout childhood among children in LMIC has been associated with poverty, food insecurity, low dietary diversity, infections, and poor hygiene (Prentice et al. 2013). Children's development is also likely to be compromised by the same factors. In addition, child development may be further hindered by the lack of enriching resources, such as books (Bradley & Corwyn 2002).

11.2.4 Poverty and Neuroscience

Evidence from neuroscience has shown that poverty early in life is associated with disruptions to neural structures and functions, including smaller white and cortical grey matter and hippocampal and amygdala volumes, areas of the brain that are associated with cognitive performance (Hackman et al. 2015; Luby et al. 2013). These findings suggest that poverty impacts specific aspects of brain development and functioning, raising major concerns about the mechanisms and longitudinal effects of poverty on children's growth and development.

11.2.5 Poverty and the Stress Response

Poverty is often associated with parenting stress and other co-morbidities that could undermine responsive parenting, leading to dysregulation. Stress reactivity refers to an increase in cortisol production following a stress-inducing task. Reactions to early life stress, such as maternal deprivation, vary, with both hyper-responsivity of the hypothalamic–pituitary–adrenal (HPA) axis and blunted or hypo-responsivity reported. Dysregulation of the stress response system is an important mechanism that may explain how early life adversity is associated with children's developmental and behavioural problems (Gunnar & Donzella 2002). In response to stressors, the adrenal cortex releases glucocorticoid hormones (cortisol), which mobilize glucose and increase cardiovascular tone in preparation for a response. Under optimal conditions, when the stress ends, the organism returns to homeostatic balance. However, if the glucocorticoid receptors restrain the HPA axis from returning to baseline, the organism remains in a hyper-vigilant state that is associated with hypo-responsivity to subsequent stressors. This blunted process results in 'weathering', which has negative consequences on the inflammatory system and other immune functions, increasing the risk for subsequent health and behavioural problems.

The Bucharest Early Intervention Project is a randomized controlled trial in which institution-raised children in Bucharest were randomly assigned either to foster care or to prolonged institutional care and were compared with similar-aged children who had never been institutionalized (Zeanah et al. 2003). At mean age 12.9 years, the children's stress response was evaluated (McLaughlin et al. 2015). The children randomized to remain in institutional care had significantly blunted responses to psychosocial stress compared to the children randomized to foster care and to the comparison group. There were no significant differences in stress response in the latter two groups, suggesting that the foster care experience may have attenuated the dysregulated HPA system experienced by the institutionalized group prior to their randomization to foster care.

11.2.6 Stunting

Stunting, a general indicator of children's chronic nutritional status, is a gradual process that occurs in response to chronic biological insults, including undernutrition and infectious diseases, during periods of linear bone growth. It often begins in utero and extends through the first 2 years (Victora et al. 2010). Childhood stunting is closely associated with poverty and is often used as a population-based indicator to compare nutritional adequacy across countries. Stunting represents significant inequities and remains a major threat to children's health and development.

A recent meta-analysis on the association between linear growth and children's cognitive, motor, and socio-emotional development included 68 reports from 29 LMIC (Sudfeld et al. 2015). Findings were strongest for children <2 years, with each unit increase in height-for-age z-score associated with a +0.24 SD increase in concurrent cognition and a +0.22 SD increase in cognition at ages 5–12 years. Thus, early growth restriction is associated with lower cognitive scores through childhood. There were similar findings related to motor development, often indexed by onset of walking. Findings related to socio-emotional development were less clear, primarily due to the small number of studies and differences in measurement of socio-emotional development across differing ages.

The long-term consequences of stunting extend into adulthood, including lower height, less schooling, and reduced economic productivity (Hoddinott et al. 2013; Victora et al. 2008). Studies into the next generation have shown associations between first-generation stunting and offspring birth size (Victora et al. 2008). A recent study from Jamaica found that children born to parents who had been stunted prior to aged 2 years were shorter than children of non-stunted parents and had low scores on measures of cognitive assessments between 12 and 72 months (Walker et al. 2015).

There are several mechanisms that may link stunting to children's development. The biological insults that compromise early linear growth may also disrupt early brain development. Another possibility is that delayed motor skills associated with poor growth may disrupt the exploration associated with cognitive development. Finally, in response to children's short stature, expectations from parents and peers may be reduced, thereby limiting the acquisition of developmental skills. Associations between early stunting and children's long-term performance are relatively strong, and stunting has been used as an indicator to estimate the number of children worldwide who do not reach their developmental potential (UNICEF 2014).

However, interventions to promote child development are likely to be strongest if they extend beyond the factors that led to stunting and include the responsive parenting and educational factors associated with child development.

11.3 PRENATAL MATERNAL NUTRITION

Many nutritional deficiencies begin prenatally, or perhaps prior to conception, setting children onto negative trajectories prior to birth (Bhutta et al. 2013; Victora et al. 2010). Recent attention has turned to ensure adequate maternal nutrition during pregnancy. Prenatal vitamins, including folic acid and iron, have been widely recommended. However, compliance has been variable, especially in LMICs (Bhutta et al. 2013). Multiple micronutrient (MMN) supplements have also been recommended (Leung et al. 2011).

11.3.1 Iron and Folic Acid

Current evidence supports a strong association between prenatal iron and folate status and healthy brain development (Anjos et al. 2013). Iron deficiency during pregnancy can have consequences for the offspring's development due to iron's role in neuron myelination and neurotransmitter production, including serotonin and dopamine. It is hypothesized that iron deficiency during critical periods of brain development could result in neurotransmitter metabolism abnormalities, decreased myelination, and impaired energy metabolism in the brain (Andersson et al. 2015; Szajewska et al. 2010).

Trials examining iron deficiency and nutritional interventions have met with limited success in illuminating this relationship. Although the last trimester of gestation is indicated as a peak developmental period requiring adequate iron status for myelination, striatum, and hippocampus development, a recent systematic review showed prenatal maternal iron supplementation to have no effect on child IQ or behavioural status (Szajewska et al. 2010).

Folic acid plays a critical role in brain development due to its functions in DNA synthesis and methylation (Skorka et al. 2012). While the importance of maternal folate status during pregnancy on prevention of neural tube defects is well established, the effect of maternal folic acid status on child mental development is less certain (Anjos et al. 2013). A recent systematic review showed no benefit to child mental performance with prenatal multivitamin supplementation containing folic acid (Skorka et al. 2012). However, these results should be interpreted with caution due to the limited number of studies examined. Children born to folate-deficient mothers have been shown to exhibit increased risk of internalizing and externalizing behaviours, and cohort studies have shown that children born to folate supplemented mothers have fewer behavioural problems at 18 months (Anjos et al. 2013).

11.3.2 Multiple Micronutrients

Reviews suggest a positive impact of prenatal MMN supplementation on fetal growth (e.g. reductions in low birthweight [LBW] and small for gestational age [SGA]), particularly in areas where deficiencies are common. However, the impact on children's development has been mixed (Fall et al. 2009; Haider et al. 2013; Leung et al. 2011; Ramakrishnan et al. 2012) and largely limited to beneficial effects on motor development. Three studies provide examples of the emerging information on the nature of relations between prenatal nutrition and infants' cognitive and motor performances. The first, a study in Benin, found an inverted U-shaped relation between maternal prenatal haemoglobin concentration and infants' motor performance at 1 year of age, with optimal prenatal haemoglobin concentrations between 90 and 110 g/L (Mireku et al. 2015). There were no associations with cognitive performance and no clear explanations for the curvilinear relation with motor performance in which optimal maternal concentrations were in the range of anaemia. The second was a randomized controlled trial of delayed cord clamping (≥180 seconds versus ≤10 seconds) among women in Sweden (Andersson et al. 2015). At the age of 4 years, children in the delayed cord clamping group had better scores in fine motor and social tasks compared to control children, especially boys. The third was a trial in Nepal which found better scores on multiple measures of executive functioning in school-age children whose mothers received iron, folic acid, and vitamin A during pregnancy (as compared to a single nutrient) (Christian et al. 2010). In addition, three pregnancy trials conducted in Bangladesh, Tanzania, and China measured development between 6 and 18 months. Two found beneficial effects on motor development and one on cognition. In the randomized controlled trial in China, the offspring of pregnant women supplemented with multiple micronutrients had increased mental development raw scores at 1 year of age compared to the offspring of mothers receiving folic acid and iron or folic acid alone (Li et al. 2009).

A systematic review of 18 prenatal nutrition trials found substantial variation in methods and measures and concluded that there was no convincing evidence that enhancing the prenatal environment through micronutrient supplementation was associated with better cognitive or mental performance among children (Leung et al. 2011).

The mixed findings are often attributed to variations in timing, duration, and formulation of nutritional supplements (Bhutta et al. 2013). To date, most trials have begun after conception, often well into the second trimester of pregnancy, leading to the possibility that preconceptual nutritional status may be necessary to ensure an adequate environment for fetal development. Interventions which do not begin until the pregnancy is established may expose the young fetus to an inadequate nutritional environment, increasing the risk for intrauterine growth restriction (IUGR), LBW, and low birth length (LBL) (Mook-Kanamori et al. 2010; Smith 2010). Evidence from Bangladesh comparing prenatal interventions initiated at 9 and 20 weeks gestation showed benefits in birthweight and mother–infant interactions associated with the 9-week intervention, emphasizing the importance of early intervention (Frith et al. 2012; Persson et al. 2012).

When examining maternal outcomes, a trial in Indonesia among undernourished women found that receipt of MMN during pregnancy was associated with better scores on measures of cognition and reading efficiency, than receipt of iron and folic acid (Prado et al. 2012). At 42 months, children of MMN-supplemented mothers achieved higher scores on measures of motor and visual attention/spatial ability than children of iron-/folic acid–supplemented mothers, with no difference in scores from children of well-nourished mothers (Prado et al. 2012). These studies raise the possibility that improving women's nutritional status prenatally leads to enhancement of the offspring's nutritional status and developmental capabilities and enhancement of the mother's nutritional status and caregiving skills.

In summary, beyond ensuring iodine repletion to avoid cretinism and folate repletion to avoid neural tube disorders prior to conception, there have been few nutrient-specific findings from prenatal supplementation. Iron–folic acid has been adopted as a prenatal vitamin by many countries and recommendations often include MMN supplementation. Additional long-term follow-up is warranted to examine the impact of MMN supplementation.

11.3.3 Maternal Stress

Since important fetal brain systems developing during the last trimester rely on adequate nutrient supply, a low-stress, healthy pregnancy is vital to ensure optimal nutrient delivery to the developing fetal brain (Wachs et al. 2014). A recent review found prenatal maternal psychological stress (stress, anxiety, depression, psychiatric diagnosis) adversely impacts offspring cognitive, behavioural, and psychomotor development (Kingston et al. 2012). Prenatal stress is also known to increase anxiety behaviour in the offspring and alter brain structure and function, particularly the hippocampus (Wachs et al. 2014).

High stress during pregnancy is a risk factor for maternal depression, which is negatively associated with early child development. As both maternal stress and depression are independent risk factors for poor child development, the two may interact for multilevel, cumulative consequences for offspring development (Walker et al. 2011). Until recently, limited attention has been directed to preparing women for pregnancy. However, recognition that maternal nutritional status impacts the health of both the mother and the infant and that rates of maternal anaemia are high in LMIC has led to increased attention to preconception maternal health (Black et al. 2013; Dean et al. 2014).

11.4 NUTRITIONAL DEFICIENCIES AND BRAIN DEVELOPMENT

11.4.1 Micronutrients

Essential micronutrients are small quantities of vitamins and minerals required for specific physiological functions and not made by the body. Several micronutrients have been linked to brain development (iron, zinc, iodine, vitamin B_{12}, choline) (Prado & Dewey 2014). Some of these key micronutrients will be discussed briefly in the following, but for a more detailed description, please refer to other chapters in this book.

11.4.2 Iron

Iron deficiency is a global health concern associated with impaired cognitive, motor, and behavioural development. The first year of life (particularly 6–12 months) is a high-risk period for iron deficiency due to high growth velocity yet limited capacity to absorb iron (Andersson et al. 2015; Bhutta et al. 2013). Since iron is necessary for haemoglobin synthesis, adequate iron is essential for oxygen delivery to all tissues, especially the brain. From 6 months to 3 years of age, iron is in peak demand for developmental processes such as myelination, frontal cortex, and basal ganglia development (Wachs et al. 2014). In infancy, iron deficiency has been associated with slower neural transmission in auditory and visual responses, potentially indicating hypomyelination (Lozoff et al. 2006). In toddlerhood, iron deficiency has been associated with impaired social-emotional behaviour, including shyness, wariness, and low responsivity (Lozoff et al. 2006). Should iron deficiency occur during these peak developmental periods, the adverse effects are potentially irreversible, even with subsequent iron supplementation (Wachs et al. 2014).

Although the associations between iron deficiency and infant and child development are strong, nutritional interventions early in life, when children's rate of growth is rapid and nutritional demands are high, have met with limited success either in alleviating nutritional deficiencies or in promoting early development (Bhutta et al. 2013). A recent meta-analysis of iron supplementation trials among children 4–23 months found reductions in anaemia, but no effects on mental or motor development (Pasricha et al. 2013). One possibility is that the origins of nutritional deficiency occur prenatally or prior to conception, and interventions targeting infancy and early childhood are too late. In addition, iron deficiency often occurs in the context of other micronutrient deficiencies, leading to recommendations to focus on multiple micronutrient deficiencies (Allen 2005).

Another recent review of iron supplementation to infants in LMIC found positive outcomes in all five studies reviewed, including improved motor development (n = 5), improved cognitive/language development (n = 2), and improved socio-emotional development (n = 3) (Ramakrishnan et al. 2012). One possible explanation for the variability in findings is that the studies took place in LMIC where iron deficiency is usually high, suggesting that iron supplementation may be more effective when targeted to at-risk populations. Iron deficiency anaemia in early infancy is a strong risk factor for impaired mental and motor development (Prado & Dewey 2014) and has been associated with long-term negative functional consequences, including non-completion of secondary school, negative emotions, and lack of a marital partner (Lozoff et al. 2013). Additional research is necessary to determine the optimal timing, dose, and combination of micronutrients necessary to prevent iron deficiency.

11.4.3 Zinc

Zinc is a trace mineral critical for central nervous system development due to its roles in enzymes required for brain growth, proteins involved in neurotransmission, and neurotransmitters involved in memory (Black 2011). Zinc is the fourth most abundant ion in the brain and can be found in high concentrations in the hippocampus, cerebellum, prefrontal cortex, cortex, and limbic system (Colombo et al. 2014; Prado & Dewey 2014). Late gestation and older infancy (beginning at 6 months) are important stages of development when zinc is in high demand and accordingly, there is a high risk for zinc deficiency (Colombo et al. 2014; Wachs et al. 2014).

The impact of zinc status during infancy on child cognitive development remains unclear. Current research supports zinc's contribution to neuron formation, migration, and synapse generation (Anjos et al. 2013). Although animal studies have corroborated zinc's important role in neurodevelopment, recent reviews found no evidence from human randomized trials for a positive association between prenatal or infant zinc supplementation and child cognitive development, although some positive effects on motor development following zinc supplementation in infants were more commonly found (Black 2011; Prado & Dewey 2014). However, studies examining zinc's effect on neurodevelopment and cognition in infancy are relatively limited.

From a recent study in Peru, infants aged 6 months were randomized into a control (iron and copper supplementation) or experimental (zinc, iron, and copper supplementation) group to examine zinc's impact on cognitive and sensorimotor development during infancy. The zinc-supplemented group showed normal developmental trajectories in habituation and multiple object free play tasks during the first 18 months of life. However, there were no group differences related to any of the psychophysiological variables of attention, the *Bayley Scales of Infant Development* (2nd edition), or the A-not-B error task. These results suggest that zinc may play a more substantial role in processing speed and motor aspects of attention and thus motor development (Colombo et al. 2014).

11.4.4 Iodine

Iodine deficiency disrupts normal production and levels of thyroid hormones, thyroxine (T4) and triiodothyronine (T3), which play integral roles in central nervous system development, such as neurogenesis, neuronal migration, synaptogenesis, and myelination (Bougma et al. 2013; Prado & Dewey 2014). While severe iodine deficiency early in life is known to cause neurological damage, studies show that even mild to moderate deficiency is associated with delayed mental development (Bougma et al. 2013).

A recent review of iodine supplementation trials and prospective cohort studies among pregnant women and infants examined the effects of iodine on mental development of children under 5 years old. Regardless of study design, this review showed iodine deficiency to have a biologically important impact on mental development. Among observational cohort prospective studies examined in which mental development was stratified by newborn iodine status, a mean effect size of 0.54 translating to 8.1 IQ points was observed (Bougma et al. 2013).

11.4.5 Vitamin B_{12}

The developing fetus is supplied with vitamin B_{12} by the placenta with the amount dependent upon maternal vitamin B_{12} status (Bhate et al. 2008). Vitamin B_{12} deficiency in infants can arise from a variety of sources including low dietary intake from animal sources (including vegetarianism and veganism), maternal bariatric surgery, Crohn's disease, celiac disease, and pernicious anaemia (Pepper & Black 2011). Vitamin B_{12} participates in a series of biological processes important for fetal development. Vitamin B_{12} functions in haemoglobin synthesis and fat and protein metabolism via its catalytic role in succinyl-CoA production. Vitamin B_{12} also participates in DNA methylation and epinephrine synthesis by serving as a cofactor for methionine synthesis (Pepper & Black 2011).

An association between prenatal vitamin B_{12} deficiency and cognitive effects has been shown by longitudinal studies, but more research is needed to elucidate vitamin B_{12}'s role in neurodevelopment. In a 2008 follow-up study, cognitive function at 9 years of age was compared between children born to mothers with high (>224 pM B_{12}) and low (<77 pM B_{12}) vitamin B_{12} status at 28 weeks gestation. This study showed negative association between low maternal B_{12} status and frontal lobe (exhibited by perceptual tracking and simple sequencing tasks) and temporal lobe (short-term memory) function at age 9 (Bhate et al. 2008). This association was significant after adjusting for possible confounders, including age, sex, head size, socio-economic status, education, and B_{12} status at 6 years (Bhate et al. 2008).

The association between vitamin B_{12} deficiency and abnormal behaviour and development can potentially be explained through two mechanisms: demyelination and inflammation. Vitamin B_{12} deficiency in infants has been associated with demyelination, which alters the speed of neuronal conduction and can ultimately result in delayed cognitive development. Additionally, vitamin B_{12} deficiency has been associated with gastric inflammatory states, possibly indicating an inflammation-induced autoimmune process blocking intrinsic factor and thus preventing vitamin B_{12} absorption (Black et al. 2007).

11.4.6 Essential Fatty Acids

Essential fatty acids (EFAs) play an important role in membrane function, synapse function, and myelination (Prado & Dewey 2014). Essential fatty acids are supplied to the fetus by the placenta prenatally and by breast milk after birth (Anjos et al. 2013). Placental EFA transfer to the brain is heightened during the third trimester, placing preterm infants at greater risk of EFA deficiency (Prado & Dewey 2014).

The European Food Safety Authority has confirmed a causal relationship between adequate docosahexaenoic acid (DHA) status and improved visual function at 1 year. However, the relationship between essential fatty acids and neurodevelopment is less clear (Anjos et al. 2013). In a recent meta-analysis of n-3 polyunsaturated fatty acids (PUFAs) that included 7 infant trials, the n-3 PUFAS were administered through formula or capsules (Jiao et al. 2014). The n-3 PUFA supplementation was associated with improved scores on the Mental Developmental Index and Psychomotor Developmental Index of the Bayley Scales of Infant Development (effect sizes of 0.33 and 0.27, respectively). In addition, the supplemented groups had better scores on measures of language, motor, and cognitive abilities. These effects were specific to infants, with no effects in trials involving children, adults, or the elderly.

11.4.7 Multiple Micronutrients

Micronutrient deficiencies often cluster, and as such, interventions supplementing multiple micronutrients may prove to be more beneficial than single micronutrient trials for child development. If children are deficient in multiple micronutrients, single micronutrient supplementation may not have a positive impact on their brain development or functioning. A recent review identified three randomized trials from Ghana, China, and South Africa, reporting benefit of multiple micronutrient supplementation during infancy on motor development in children between 12 and 18 months (Prado & Dewey 2014).

11.4.8 Summary

Many of the intervention trials suffer from low quality, including small sample size, lack of clarity on design or methods, and use of non-standardized measurement strategies. Many investigators relied on global measures of child development. However, micronutrients may impact specific brain areas or regions, leading to specific aspects of development. Executive function tasks, including attention, inhibitory control, working memory, problem-solving, and decision-making, may be more sensitive to micronutrient deficiencies and repletion than are global assessments. As Colombo and colleagues showed in the zinc supplementation trial in Peru, micronutrient supplementation may be associated with subtle findings that underlie the skills used in global assessments (Colombo et al. 2014).

A recent meta-analysis examined the effects of 18 nutritional interventions delivered during the first 24 months of life on mental development, measured as cognitive or language development (Aboud & Yousafzai 2015). The effects were very small ($d = 0.086$), indicating limited impact on mental development. In contrast, there was a much larger effect on mental development among the 21 trials of stimulation interventions identified ($d = 0.420$). In addition to the differing content between the nutrition and stimulation interventions, they differed in site, contact time, and labour intensity. The nutrition trials were more likely to be conducted in low-income countries, whereas the stimulation trials were in low- and middle-income countries. The nutrition trials required minimal contact, usually just delivery of the supplement or fortificant, whereas the stimulation trial often required 30–40 minute contact with the caregiver. Finally, the nutrition trials had much lower labour demands than the stimulation trials, which generally included a specific behaviour change component.

11.5 INTERVENTIONS

This section examines postnatal interventions which have been associated with early child development: breastfeeding, responsive feeding, and stimulation/early learning.

11.5.1 Breastfeeding

The first postnatal nutrition is received from breast milk. Exclusive breast milk is recommended by the World Health Organization (WHO) for the first 6 months, with continued breastfeeding for at least the first year (WHO 2001). The health and nutritional benefits of breast milk and breastfeeding for children and mothers are widely recognized (Gartner et al. 2005) and support for breastfeeding initiation, exclusivity, and duration are major goals in many nutrition interventions (Lassi et al. 2014).

In spite of the nutritional benefits of breastfeeding, the effects of breast milk on children's cognition are controversial. Most studies of breastfeeding are unable to eliminate the likelihood of bias and confounding. A recent commentary (Smithers et al. 2015) reviews the methodological challenges related to the study of breastfeeding. The longitudinal cohort, the most frequently used design to study breastfeeding, is often biased, because it may be influenced by maternal factors associated with the decision to breastfeed, including intelligence, motivation, socio-economic status, and education. These factors may also influence cognition, raising concerns about confounding. In a notable exception, a recent population-based study conducted in Brazil, where rates of breastfeeding are high, had limited confounding (Victora et al. 2015). Breastfeeding for 12 months was associated with higher cognition scores, more schooling, and high income, compared to breastfeeding for less than 1 month (Victora et al. 2015). In sibling-pair designs, where siblings who differed in consumption of breast milk are compared, there may also be important decisions in the reasons to provide breast milk that could influence children's cognition. Cross-population studies examine comparability of findings across different populations where decisions regarding breastfeeding may differ. Randomized trials remove bias through random assignment. However, there are ethical concerns related to random assignment of breastfeeding.

A recent trial in Belarus involving over 13,000 infants overcame the ethical dilemma by randomizing breastfeeding promotion at the hospital level (Kramer et al. 2008). Infants in the experimental condition were exclusively breastfed longer and at school age had higher standardized cognitive test scores and higher teacher-reported academic performance than children in the control condition. Additional research is necessary to examine the mechanisms linking breast milk/breastfeeding to cognition and brain development.

11.5.2 Responsive Caregiving

In addition to nutritional deficiencies, a lack of appropriate caregiver–child interactions can contribute to the loss of developmental potential. Appropriate interactions include positive emotionality, sensitivity, and responsiveness from the caregiver towards the child (Walker et al. 2011). Responsive caregiving is a central component of several theories related to early child health and development, including attachment theory and social cognitive theory, and has been promoted as a critical component of early childhood prevention programs (Black & Dewey 2014). Caregivers and young children co-regulate their interactions through mutual communication, leading to child stress regulation (Tronick & Beeghly 2011). Caregivers are influenced by their child's behaviour and by perceptions of their child's temperament. Based on attachment theory, responsive caregiving is initiated by child's behaviour, followed by prompt and sensitive caregiver behaviour. The child experiences a positive interaction and the interaction continues. From a social cognitive perspective, responsive caregiving reinforces the child's behaviour and provides scaffolding opportunities. Children acquire skills through modelling from their caregivers, thereby promoting more advanced developmental skills.

Emerging evidence suggests that the absence of responsive caregiving (e.g. children raised in institutional or foster care) increases the risk for alterations in stress-responsive neurobiological systems (Bruce et al. 2013). Hostinar and colleagues (Hostinar et al. 2014) employ a developmental framework to examine the social buffering phenomenon and conclude that not only is the HPA axis regulated by social relationships early in life, but that responsive caregiving interventions can be protective against stress. For example, evidence from high-income countries has shown that foster children who receive Multidimensional Treatment Foster Care for Preschoolers, a preventive intervention that emphasizes responsive caregiving, are more likely to demonstrate typical diurnal cortisol slopes, compared to children who receive services as usual and demonstrate increasingly blunted diurnal cortisol slopes (Fisher et al. 2007) and their mothers experience less caregiver stress in response to child behaviour problems (Fisher & Stoolmiller 2008). Findings have linked disrupted mother–infant communication (during the still face procedure) and dysregulation in maternal and infant stress reactivity as early as 4 months of age (Crockett et al. 2013). These findings highlight the potential role of responsive caregiving as a prevention strategy in promoting early stress regulation. Evidence from LMIC has shown that parenting programmes are effective in altering parenting behaviour to include responsive caregiving (Engle et al. 2007, 2011).

11.5.3 Early Learning/Stimulation

Early learning/stimulation interventions have been well demonstrated in LMIC. For infants and toddlers, they are often delivered through home-visiting or group sessions and include methods to promote interactive play and communication. Through the use of home-made toys geared to the developmental level of the child, caregivers are shown developmentally appropriate toys and methods of play and interaction. For preschoolers, early learning opportunities often occur in preschools. Evaluations of programmes for both infants and preschoolers have been shown to be effective in promoting child development skills (Engle et al. 2007, 2011).

11.5.4 Integrated Interventions

Nutrient deficiencies and lack of opportunities for early learning and responsive caregiving can have detrimental effects on a child's developing brain. Several studies have shown that interventions addressing both have proven more effective than either alone in improving child development. In addition to an additive effect, integrated interventions may be more beneficial for child development if the success of one intervention depends on the presence of the other. For example, in a study in Jamaica, that exposed infants to psychosocial stimulation and/or zinc supplementation showed that only those infants receiving zinc supplementation benefitted from psychosocial stimulation (Gardner et al. 2005; Prado & Dewey 2014).

11.6 CONCLUSION

Brain development begins shortly after conception, guided by maturation and dynamic gene by environment interactions. Early in the process when plasticity is high, the foundations of adult health and well-being are established. Nutrition plays an important role throughout early brain development, and in the face of undernutrition, children may experience lasting deficits to their growth and development. The process is influenced by poverty and by opportunities for early learning and responsive caregiving. Through associations with adversity, poverty undermines brain development, potentially interfering with regulatory process and higher-order functioning. However, the nurturance associated with responsive caregiving can mitigate some of the neuropsychological effects of adversity, emphasizing the importance of interventions to children's health and well-being. In spite of the positive evaluations on the impact of early learning and responsive caregiving interventions, there are far fewer intervention options available for children and families. Future recommendations include strategies to effectively integrate, monitor, and sustain effective interventions for infants and preschoolers.

ACKNOWLEDGEMENT

Research reported in this chapter was supported by The Summer Program in Obesity, Diabetes and Nutrition Research Training (SPORT) under NIH Award Number T35DK095737.

REFERENCES

Aboud, F. A. & Yousafzai, A. K. (2015). Global health and development in early childhood. *Annual Review of Psychology*, 66, 433–457.

Allen, L. H. (2005). Multiple micronutrients in pregnancy and lactation: An overview. *American Journal of Clinical Nutrition*, 81(5), 1206S–1212S.

Andersson, O., Lindquist, B., Lindgren, M., Stjernqvist, K., Domellof, M., & Hellstrom-Westas, L. (2015). Effect of delayed cord clamping on neurodevelopment at 4 years of age: A randomized clinical trial. *JAMA Pediatrics*, 169(7), 631–638. doi: 10.1001/jamapediatrics.2015.0358.

Anjos, T., Altmae, S., Emmett, P., Tiemeier, H., Closa-Monasterolo, R., Luque, V. et al. (2013). Nutrition and neurodevelopment in children: Focus on NUTRIMENTHE project. *European Journal of Nutrition*, 52(8), 1825–1842. doi: 10.1007/s00394-013-0560-4.

Bhate, V., Deshpande, S., Bhat, D., Joshi, N., Ladkat, R., Watve, S. et al. (2008). Vitamin B12 status of pregnant Indian women and cognitive function in their 9-year-old children. *Food Nutrition Bulletin*, 29(4), 249–254.

Bhutta, Z. A., Das, J. K., Rizvi, A., Gaffey, M. F., Walker, N., Horton, S. et al. (2013). Evidence-based interventions for improvement of maternal and child nutrition: What can be done and at what cost? *Lancet*, 382(9890), 452–477. doi: 10.1016/s0140-6736(13)60996-4.

Black, M. & Aboud, F. (2011). Theoretical basis of responsive feeding among infants and young children in high and low income countries. *Journal of Nutrition*, 141(3), 490–494.

Black, M. M. (2011). Zinc deficiency and cognitive development. In Benton D. (ed.), *Lifetime Nutritional Influences on Cognition, Behaviour and Psychiatric Illness* (pp. 79–93). Cambridge, UK: Woodhead Publishing.

Black, M. M., Baqui, A. H., Zaman, K., McNary, S. W., Le, K., Arifeen, S. E. et al. (2007). Depressive symptoms among rural Bangladeshi mothers: Implications for infant development. *Journal of Child Psychology and Psychiatry*, 48(8), 764–772. doi: 10.1111/j.1469-7610.2007.01752.x.

Black, M. M. & Dewey, K. G. (2014). Promoting equity through integrated early child development and nutrition interventions. *Annals of the New York Academy of Sciences*, 1308(1), 1–10. doi: 10.1111/nyas.12351.

Black, M. M. & Hurley, K. M. (2007). Helping children develop health eating habits. In Tremblay, R. E., Barr, R. G., Peters, R., De V., & Boivin, M. (eds.), *Encyclopedia on Early Childhood Development* [online] (pp. 1–10). Montreal, Quebec, Canada: Canadian Centre of Excellence for Early Childhood Development. http://www.child-encyclopedia.com/pages/PDF/BlackANGxp_rev-Eating.pdf.

Black, R. E., Victora, C. G., Walker, S. P., Bhutta, Z. A., Christian, P., de Onis, M. et al. (2013). Maternal and child undernutrition and overweight in low-income and middle-income countries. *Lancet*, 382(9890), 427–451.

Bougma, K., Aboud, F. E., Harding, K. B., & Marquis, G. S. (2013). Iodine and mental development of children 5 years old and under: A systematic review and meta-analysis. *Nutrients*, 5(4), 1384–1416. doi: 10.3390/nu5041384.

Bradley, R. H. & Corwyn, R. F. (2002). Socioeconomic status and child development. *Annual Review of Psychology*, 53, 371–399. doi: 10.1146/annurev.psych.53.100901.135233.

Bruce, J., Gunnar, M. R., Pears, K. C., & Fisher, P. A. (2013). Early adverse care, stress neurobiology, and prevention science: Lessons learned. *Prevention Science*, 14(3), 247–256. doi: 10.1007/s11121-012-0354-6.

Cavalli, P. (2008). Prevention of neural tube defects and proper folate periconceptional supplementation. *Journal of Prenatal Medicine*, 2(4), 40–41.

Christian, P., Murray-Kolb, L. E., Khatry, S. K., Katz, J., Schaefer, B. A., Cole, P. M. et al. (2010). Prenatal micronutrient supplementation and intellectual and motor function in early school-aged children in Nepal. *Journal of the American Medical Association*, 304(24), 2716–2723. doi: 10.1001/jama.2010.1861.

Colombo, J., Zavaleta, N., Kannass, K. N., Lazarte, F., Albornoz, C., Kapa, L. L., & Caulfield, L. E. (2014). Zinc supplementation sustained normative neurodevelopment in a randomized, controlled trial of Peruvian infants aged 6–18 months. *Journal of Nutrition*, 144(8), 1298–1305. doi: 10.3945/jn.113.189365.

Crockett, E. E., Holmes, B. M., Granger, D. A., & Lyons-Ruth, K. (2013). Maternal disrupted communication during face-to-face interaction at 4 months: Relation to maternal and infant cortisol among at-risk families. *Infancy*, 18(6), 1111–1134. doi: 10.1111/infa.12015.

Dean, S. V., Lassi, Z. S., Imam, A. M., & Bhutta, Z. A. (2014). Preconception care: Closing the gap in the continuum of care to accelerate improvements in maternal, newborn and child health. *Reproductive Health*, 11(Suppl 3), S1. doi: 10.1186/1742-4755-11-s3-s1.

Duncan, G. J. & Magnuson, K. (2012). Socioeconomic status and cognitive functioning: Moving from correlation to causation. *Wiley Interdisciplinary Reviews: Cognitive Science*, 3(3), 377–386. doi: 10.1002/wcs.1176.

Engle, P. L., Black, M. M., Behrman, J. R., Cabral de Mello, M., Gertler, P. J., Kapiriri, L. et al. (2007). Strategies to avoid the loss of developmental potential in more than 200 million children in the developing world. *Lancet*, 369(9557), 229–242.

Engle, P. L., Fernald, L. C., Alderman, H., Behrman, J., O'Gara, C., Yousafzai, A. et al. (2011). Strategies for reducing inequalities and improving developmental outcomes for young children in low-income and middle-income countries. *Lancet*, 378(9799), 1339–1353. doi: 10.1016/S0140-6736(11)60889-1.

Fall, C. H., Fisher, D. J., Osmond, C., & Margetts, B. M. (2009). Multiple micronutrient supplementation during pregnancy in low-income countries: A meta-analysis of effects on birth size and length of gestation. *Food Nutrition Bulletin*, 30(4 Suppl), S533–S546.

Fisher, P. A. & Stoolmiller, M. (2008). Intervention effects on foster parent stress: Associations with child cortisol levels. *Development and Psychopathology*, 20(3), 1003–1021. doi: 10.1017/s0954579408000473.

Fisher, P. A., Stoolmiller, M., Gunnar, M. R., & Burraston, B. O. (2007). Effects of a therapeutic intervention for foster preschoolers on diurnal cortisol activity. *Psychoneuroendocrinology*, 32(8–10), 892–905. doi: 10.1016/j.psyneuen.2007.06.008.

Frith, A. L., Naved, R. T., Persson, L. A., Rasmussen, K. M., & Frongillo, E. A. (2012). Early participation in a prenatal food supplementation program ameliorates the negative association of food insecurity with quality of maternal-infant interaction. *Journal of Nutrition*, 142(6), 1095–1101. doi: 10.3945/jn.111.155358.

Gardner, J. M., Powell, C. A., Baker-Henningham, H., Walker, S. P., Cole, T. J., & Grantham-McGregor, S. M. (2005). Zinc supplementation and psychosocial stimulation: Effects on the development of undernourished Jamaican children. *American Journal of Clinical Nutrition*, 82(2), 399–405.

Gartner, L. M., Morton, J., Lawrence, R. A., Naylor, A. J., O'Hare, D., Schanler, R. J. et al. (2005). Breastfeeding and the use of human milk. *Pediatrics*, 115(2), 496–506. doi: 10.1542/peds.2004-2491.

Georgieff, M. K. (2007). Nutrition and the developing brain: Nutrient priorities and measurement. *American Journal of Clinical Nutrition*, 85(2), 614S–620S.

Grantham-McGregor, S., Cheung, Y., Cueto, S., Glewwe, P., Richter, L., & Strupp, B. (2007). Over two hundred million children fail to reach their developmental potential in the first five years in developing countries. *Lancet*, 369, 60–70.

Gunnar, M. R. & Donzella, B. (2002). Social regulation of the cortisol levels in early human development. *Psychoneuroendocrinology*, 27(1–2), 199–220.

Hackman, D. A., Gallop, R., Evans, G. W., & Farah, M. J. (2015). Socioeconomic status and executive function: Developmental trajectories and mediation. *Developmental Science*, 18(5), 686–702.

Haider, B. A., Olofin, I., Wang, M., Spiegelman, D., Ezzati, M., & Fawzi, W. W. (2013). Anaemia, prenatal iron use, and risk of adverse pregnancy outcomes: Systematic review and meta-analysis. *British Medical Journal*, 346, f3443.

Hoddinott, J., Behrman, J. R., Maluccio, J. A., Melgar, P., Quisumbing, A. R., Ramirez-Zea, M. et al. (2013). Adult consequences of growth failure in early childhood. *American Journal of Clinical Nutrition*, 98(5), 1170–1178.

Hostinar, C. E., Sullivan, R. M., & Gunnar, M. R. (2014). Psychobiological mechanisms underlying the social buffering of the hypothalamic-pituitary-adrenocortical axis: A review of animal models and human studies across development. *Psychological Bulletin*, 140(1), 256–282. doi: 10.1037/a0032671.

Jiao, J., Li, Q., Chu, J., Zeng, W., Yang, M., & Zhu, S. (2014). Effect of n-3 PUFA supplementation on cognitive function throughout the life span from infancy to old age: A systematic review and meta-analysis of randomized controlled trials. *American Journal of Clinical Nutrition*, 100(6), 1422–1436.

Johnson, M. H. (2001). Functional brain development in humans. *Nature Reviews Neuroscience*, 2(7), 475–483. doi: 10.1038/35081509.

Kingston, D., Tough, S., & Whitfield, H. (2012). Prenatal and postpartum maternal psychological distress and infant development: A systematic review. *Child Psychiatry and Human Development*, 43(5), 683–714. doi: 10.1007/s10578-012-0291-4.

Kramer, M. S., Aboud, F., Mironova, E., Vanilovich, I., Platt, R. W., Matush, L. et al. (2008). Breastfeeding and child cognitive development: New evidence from a large randomized trial. *Archives of General Psychiatry*, 65(5), 578–584. doi: 10.1001/archpsyc.65.5.578.

Lassi, Z. S., Mallick, D., Das, J. K., Mal, L., Salam, R. A., & Bhutta, Z. A. (2014). Essential interventions for child health. *Reproductive Health*, 11(Suppl 1), S4. doi: 10.1186/1742-4755-11-s1-s4.

Leung, B. M., Wiens, K. P., & Kaplan, B. J. (2011). Does prenatal micronutrient supplementation improve children's mental development? A systematic review. *BMC Pregnancy Childbirth*, 11, 12. doi: 10.1186/1471-2393-11-12.

Li, Q., Yan, H., Zeng, L., Cheng, Y., Liang, W., Dang, S. et al. (2009). Effects of maternal multimicronutrient supplementation on the mental development of infants in rural western China: Follow-up evaluation of a double-blind, randomized, controlled trial. *Pediatrics*, 123(4), e685–e692. doi: 10.1542/peds.2008-3007.

Lozoff, B., Kaciroti, N., & Walter, T. (2006). Iron deficiency in infancy: Applying a physiologic framework for prediction. *American Journal of Clinical Nutrition*, 84(6):1412–1421.

Lozoff, B., Smith, J. B., Kaciroti, N., Clark, K. M., Guevara, S., & Jimenez, E. (2013). Functional significance of early-life iron deficiency: Outcomes at 25 years. *Journal of Pediatrics*, 163(5), 1260–1266.

Luby, J., Belden, A., Botteron, K., Marrus, N., Harms, M. P., Babb, C. et al. (2013). The effects of poverty on childhood brain development: The mediating effect of caregiving and stressful life events. *JAMA Pediatrics*, 167(12), 1135–1142. doi: 10.1001/jamapediatrics.2013.3139.

McLaughlin, K. A., Sheridan, M. A., Tibu, F., Fox, N. A., Zeanah, C. H., & Nelson, C. A. (2015). Causal effects of the early caregiving environment on development of stress response systems in children. *Proceedings of the National Academy of Sciences*, 112(18), 5637–5642. doi: 10.1073/pnas.1423363112.

Mireku, M. O., Davidson, L. L., Koura, G. K., Ouédraogo, S., Boivin, M. J., Xiong, X. et al. (2015). Prenatal hemoglobin levels and early cognitive and motor functions of one-year-old children. *Pediatrics*. doi: 10.1542/peds.2015-0491.

Mook-Kanamori, D. O., Steegers, E. A., Eilers, P. H., Raat, H., Hofman, A., & Jaddoe, V. W. (2010). Risk factors and outcomes associated with first-trimester fetal growth restriction. *Journal of the American Medical Association*, 303(6), 527–534. doi: 10.1001/jama.2010.78.

Pasricha, S. R., Hayes, E., Kalumba, K., & Biggs, B. A. (2013). Effect of daily iron supplementation on health in children aged 4–23 months: A systematic review and meta-analysis of randomised controlled trials. *Lancet Global Health*, 1(2), e77–e86. doi: 10.1016/s2214-109x(13)70046-9.

Pepper, M. R. & Black, M. M. (2011). B12 in fetal development. *Seminars in Cell and Developmental Biology*, 22(6), 619–623. doi: 10.1016/j.semcdb.2011.05.005.

Persson, L. A., Arifeen, S., Ekstrom, E. C., Rasmussen, K. M., Frongillo, E. A., & Yunus, M. (2012). Effects of prenatal micronutrient and early food supplementation on maternal hemoglobin, birth weight, and infant mortality among children in Bangladesh: The MINIMat randomized trial. *Journal of the American Medical Association*, 307(19), 2050–2059. doi: 10.1001/jama.2012.4061.

Pongcharoen, T., Ramakrishnan, U., DiGirolamo, A. M., Winichagoon, P., Flores, R., Singkhornard, J., & Martorell, R. (2012). Influence of prenatal and postnatal growth on intellectual functioning in school-aged children. *Archives of Pediatrics and Adolescent Medicine*, 166(5), 411–416. doi: 10.1001/archpediatrics.2011.1413.

Prado, E. L., Alcock, K. J., Muadz, H., Ullman, M. T., & Shankar, A. H. (2012). Maternal multiple micronutrient supplements and child cognition: A randomized trial in Indonesia. *Pediatrics*, 130(3), e536–e546. doi: 10.1542/peds.2012-0412.

Prado, E. L. & Dewey, K. G. (2014). Nutrition and brain development in early life. *Nutrition Reviews*, 72(4), 267–284. doi: 10.1111/nure.12102.

Prado, E. L., Ullman, M. T., Muadz, H., Alcock, K. J., & Shankar, A. H. (2012). The effect of maternal multiple micronutrient supplementation on cognition and mood during pregnancy and postpartum in Indonesia: A randomized trial. *PLoS One*, 7(3), e32519. doi: 10.1371/journal.pone.0032519.

Prentice, A. M., Moore, S. E., & Fulford, A. J. (2013). Growth faltering in low-income countries. *World Review of Nutrition and Dietetics*, 106, 90–99. doi: 10.1159/000342563.

Ramakrishnan, U., Grant, F. K., Goldenberg, T., Bui, V., Imdad, A., & Bhutta, Z. A. (2012). Effect of multiple micronutrient supplementation on pregnancy and infant outcomes: A systematic review. *Paediatric and Perinatal Epidemiology*, 26(Suppl 1), 153–167. doi: 10.1111/j.1365-3016.2012.01276.x.

Sameroff, A. (ed.). (2009). *The Transactional Model of Development: How Children and Contexts Shape Each Other*. New York: Wiley.

Shonkoff, J. P. & Garner, A. S. (2012). The lifelong effects of early childhood adversity and toxic stress. *Pediatrics*, 129(1), e232–e246. doi: 10.1542/peds.2011-2663.

Skorka, A., Gieruszczak-Bialek, D., Piescik, M., & Szajewska, H. (2012). Effects of prenatal and/or postnatal (maternal and/or child) folic acid supplementation on the mental performance of children. *Critical Reviews in Food Science and Nutrition*, 52(11), 959–964. doi: 10.1080/10408398.2010.515042.

Smith, G. C. (2010). First-trimester determination of complications of late pregnancy. *Journal of the American Medical Association*, 303(6), 561–562. doi: 10.1001/jama.2010.102.

Smithers, L. G., Kramer, M. S., & Lynch, J. W. (2015). Effects of breastfeeding on obesity and intelligence: Causal insights from different study designs. *JAMA Pediatrics*, 169(8), 707–708. doi: 10.1001/jamapediatrics.2015.0175.

Sudfeld, C. R., Charles McCoy, D., Danaei, G., Fink, G., Ezzati, M., Andrews, K. G., & Fawzi, W. W. (2015). Linear growth and child development in low- and middle-income countries: A meta-analysis. *Pediatrics*, 135(5), e1266–e1275. doi: 10.1542/peds.2014-3111.

Szajewska, H., Ruszczynski, M., & Chmielewska, A. (2010). Effects of iron supplementation in nonanemic pregnant women, infants, and young children on the mental performance and psychomotor development of children: A systematic review of randomized controlled trials. *American Journal of Clinical Nutrition*, 91(6), 1684–1690. doi: 10.3945/ajcn.2010.29191.

Tronick, E. & Beeghly, M. (2011). Infants' meaning-making and the development of mental health problems. *American Psychologist*, 66(2), 107–119. doi: 10.1037/a0021631.

UNICEF. (2014). The state of the world's children 2014. http://www.unicef.org/sowc2014/numbers/. Accessed on April 10, 2016.

Victora, C. G., Adair, L., Fall, C., Hallal, P. C., Martorell, R., Richter, L., & Sachdev, H. S. (2008). Maternal and child undernutrition: Consequences for adult health and human capital. *Lancet*, 371, 340–357.

Victora, C. G., de Onis, M., Hallal, P. C., Blossner, M., & Shrimpton, R. (2010). Worldwide timing of growth faltering: Revisiting implications for interventions. *Pediatrics*, 125(3), e473–e480. doi: 10.1542/peds.2009-1519.

Victora, C. G., Horta, B. L., de Mola, C. L., Quevedo, L., Pinheiro, R. T., Gigante, D. P. et al. (2015). Association between breastfeeding and intelligence, educational attainment, and income at 30 years of age: A prospective birth cohort study from Brazil. *Lancet Global Health, 3*(4), e199–e205. doi: 10.1016/s2214-109x(15)70002-1.

Wachs, T. D., Georgieff, M., Cusick, S., & McEwen, B. S. (2014). Issues in the timing of integrated early interventions: Contributions from nutrition, neuroscience, and psychological research. *Annals of the New York Academy of Sciences*, 1308, 89–106. doi: 10.1111/nyas.12314.

Walker, S. P., Chang, S. M., Wright, A., Osmond, C., & Grantham-McGregor, S. M. (2015). Early childhood stunting is associated with lower developmental levels in the subsequent generation of children. *Journal of Nutrition*, 145(4), 823–828. doi: 10.3945/jn.114.200261.

Walker, S. P., Wachs, T. D., Grantham-McGregor, S., Black, M. M., Nelson, C. A., Huffman, S. L. et al. (2011). Inequality in early childhood: Risk and protective factors for early child development. *Lancet*, 378(9799), 1325–1338. doi: http://dx.doi.org/10.1016/S0140-6736(11)60555-2.

WHO. (2001). Report of the expert consultation of the optimal duration of exclusive breastfeeding. Geneva, Switzerland: World Health Organization.

Zeanah, C. H., Nelson, C. A., Fox, N. A., Smyke, A. T., Marshall, P., Parker, S. W., & Koga, S. (2003). Designing research to study the effects of institutionalization on brain and behavioral development: The Bucharest Early Intervention Project. *Development and Psychopathology*, 15(4), 885–907.

Index

D

Printed in the United States
by Baker & Taylor Publisher Services